Soft Robotics for Medical and Healthcare Applications

Soft robotics is an emerging field that involves the development and application of robots and robotic systems made from soft and flexible materials. *Soft Robotics for Medical and Healthcare Applications* discusses the use of soft robotics in minimally invasive vascular surgery, for clubfoot, and filariasis leg.

The title:

- Discusses soft robot design which is helpful for researchers and students to design the mechanisms for problems like filariasis leg, and personalized rehabilitation devices.
- Covers metal additive manufacturing processes used for soft robot parts printing.
- Explains design, actuation, manufacturing, and analysis of soft robots for healthcare applications.
- Explores 3D and 4D printing for soft robotics, data-driven soft robotics, and the use of soft robotics in drug delivery.
- Presents case studies including the creation of custom filariasis limbs and the application of soft robots in minimally invasive vascular surgery.

The text is primarily written for senior undergraduates, graduate students, and academic researchers in fields including electrical engineering, electronics and communications engineering, computer engineering, and biomedical engineering.

Computational and Intelligent Systems

Series Editor: Ramesh Chandra Poonia

CHRIST (Deemed to be University), Bangalore 560029, Karnataka, India

About the Series:

In today's world, the systems that integrate intelligence into machine-based applications are known as intelligent systems. In order to simplify the man–machine interaction, intelligent systems play an important role. The books under the proposed series will explain the fundamentals of intelligent systems, review the computational techniques, and also offer step-by-step solutions to the practical problems. Aimed at senior undergraduate students, graduate students, academic researchers, and professionals, the proposed series will focus on broad topics including artificial intelligence, deep learning, image processing, cyber physical systems, wireless security, mechatronics, cognitive computing, and industry 4.0.

Application of Soft Computing Techniques in Mechanical Engineering
Amar Patnaik, Vikas Kukshal, Pankaj Agarwal, Ankush Sharma and Mahavir Choudhary

Computational Intelligence based Optimization of Manufacturing Process for Sustainable Materials
Deepak Sinwar, Kamalakanta Muduli, Vijaypal Singh Dhaka and Vijander Singh

Advanced Mathematical Techniques in Computational and Intelligent Systems
Sandeep Singh, Aliakbar Montazer Haghighi and Sandeep Dalal

Natural Language Processing and Information Retrieval
Principles and Applications
Edited By Muskan Garg, Sandeep Kumar, and Abdul Khader Jilani Saudagar

Soft Robotics for Medical and Healthcare Applications
Edited by Shaik Himam Saheb, Tharakeshwar Appala, and Mohammad S Khan

For more information on this series page, please visit our website link: https://www.routledge.com/Computational-and-Intelligent-Systems/book-series/CRCCIS

Soft Robotics for Medical and Healthcare Applications

Edited by
Shaik Himam Saheb
Tharakeshwar Appala
Mohammad S Khan

CRC Press
Taylor & Francis Group
Boca Raton New York London

CRC Press is an imprint of the
Taylor & Francis Group, an **informa** business

Designed cover image: image credited to the editors.

First edition published 2025
by CRC Press

2385 NW Executive Center Drive, Suite 320, Boca Raton FL 33431
and by CRC Press
4 Park Square, Milton Park, Abingdon, Oxon, OX14 4RN

CRC Press is an imprint of Taylor & Francis Group, LLC

ISBN: 978-1-032-88767-8 (hbk)
ISBN: 978-1-032-88768-5 (pbk)
ISBN: 978-1-003-53961-2 (ebk)

DOI: 10.1201/9781003539612

Typeset in Sabon
by SPi Technologies India Pvt Ltd (Straive)

This book is dedicated to the parents of the editors, and to the Almighty God

Contents

Preface xvi
Acknowledgments xviii
Editors xix
Contributors xx

1 Introduction to soft robotics: Opportunities and challenges 1

1.1 Introduction 1
1.2 Digital twin and soft robotics 3
1.3 Applications of the soft robotics 4
1.3.1 Medical and healthcare 4
1.3.2 Agriculture and food industry 5
1.4 Soft robotics and 3D printing 5
1.5 Fabrication of soft robots 6
1.6 Conclusions 9
References 10

2 Recent developments and emerging trends in soft robotics 12

2.1 Introduction 12
2.1.1 Literature review 12
2.2 What is a soft robot 16
2.3 Actuation of a soft robot 16
2.3.1 Photosensitive actuators 19
2.3.2 Dielectric elastomer actuators 20
2.3.3 Combustion-driven actuators 20
2.4 Advances in smart robotic material technologies 21
2.5 Advanced manufacturing techniques 22
2.6 Trends in design and analysis of soft robots 23

2.7 *Future directions and challenges* 24
2.8 *Conclusions* 25
References 26

3 Soft Robotic Treatment for Club Foot 29

3.1 *Introduction* 29
3.2 *Clubfoot* 30
3.2.1 *Reasons for clubfoot* 31
3.2.2 *Symptoms of clubfoot* 32
3.3 *There are two main types of clubfoot* 33
3.3.1 *Idiopathic clubfoot* 33
3.3.2 *Nonidiopathic clubfoot* 34
3.4 *Soft robots in clubfoot treatment* 36
3.5 *Soft robotic materials used in clubfoot treatment* 37
3.5.1 *Chemical structure and resistance* 40
3.5.2 *Fungus resistance* 40
3.6 *Proposed treatment methods* 40
3.7 *Conclusions* 42
References 43

4 Medical applications of bio-inspired soft robotics 47

4.1 *Introduction* 47
4.2 *Design and mechanisms of bio-inspired soft robots* 47
4.2.1 *Actuation mechanisms* 48
4.3 *Sensing and control* 49
4.4 *Minimally invasive surgery* 50
4.4.1 *Endoscopic soft robots* 50
4.5 *Surgical instruments* 50
4.6 *Rehabilitation and prosthetics* 51
4.6.1 *Wearable soft exoskeletons* 51
4.6.2 *Soft prosthetic limbs* 52
4.7 *Drug delivery systems* 52
4.7.1 *Microscale soft robots* 52
4.7.2 *Implantable drug delivery devices* 53
4.8 *Diagnostic tools* 53
4.8.1 *Soft robotic biopsy devices* 53
4.8.2 *Flexible endoscopic tools* 54
4.9 *Case studies* 54
4.10 *Challenges and future prospects* 56
4.11 *Conclusions* 56
References 57

5 Motion control of soft robotic arm through servo motors 60

5.1 Introduction 60
5.2 Literature survey 62
5.3 Stepper motors 66
5.3.1 Operation 66
5.3.2 Advantages of stepper motors 67
5.3.3 Applications of stepper motors 68
5.3.4 Limitations of stepper motors 69
5.4 Servo motors 69
5.4.1 Advantages of servo motors over stepper motors 72
5.5 Motion control in soft robotics 72
5.5.1 Actuation mechanisms 73
5.5.2 Control strategies 73
5.6 Hardware configurations 74
5.7 Dynamic model of high-speed precision positional servo system 74
5.7.1 Motion control 75
5.8 Conclusion 75
References 76

6 Soft robotic applications to care elderly people 78

6.1 Introduction 78
6.2 Literature review 81
6.2.1 Soft robotics: Definition and characteristics 81
6.2.2 Mobility assistance for elderly individuals 81
6.3 Soft robotic exoskeletons 82
6.3.1 Lower-limb exoskeletons for walking assistance 82
6.3.2 Challenges in lower-limb exoskeletons 82
6.4 Soft wearable devices 83
6.4.1 Soft robotic belts for balance and postural control 83
6.4.2 Challenges in wearable devices 83
6.4.3 Fall prevention and stability support 83
6.4.4 Smart footwear and balance sensors 84
6.4.5 Wearable sensors for real-time monitoring 84
6.4.6 Challenges in fall prevention systems 84
6.5 Human–robot interaction and user acceptance 85
6.5.1 User-centered design 85
6.5.2 Perceived trust and safety 85

6.6 *Rehabilitation and therapy 85*
6.6.1 *Soft robotic exoskeletons for physical rehabilitation 86*
6.6.2 *Gait training and mobility improvement 86*
6.6.3 *Poststroke rehabilitation 86*
6.6.4 *Therapeutic robotics for joint mobility 87*
6.6.5 *Cognitive and physical rehabilitation integration 87*
6.6.6 *Challenges and future prospects 87*
6.7 *Activities of daily living (ADLs) support 88*
6.7.1 *Dressing assistance 88*
6.7.2 *Feeding assistance 88*
6.7.3 *Hygiene and bathing 89*
6.7.4 *Grooming and personal care 89*
6.7.5 *Challenges and future directions 89*
6.8 *Emotional support and companionship 90*
6.8.1 *Therapeutic robotic companions 90*
6.8.2 *Socially assistive robots (SARs) 90*
6.8.3 *Combating loneliness and social isolation 91*
6.8.4 *Ethical considerations: Authenticity of relationships 91*
6.9 *Challenges and limitations 92*
6.10 *Future directions 92*
6.10.1 *Ethical considerations and challenges 92*
6.10.2 *Autonomy and dependency 93*
6.10.3 *Privacy and data security 93*
6.10.4 *Informed consent and decision-making 93*
6.10.5 *Human–robot relationships and social isolation 93*
6.10.6 *Cost and accessibility 94*
6.10.7 *Dignity and emotional well-being 94*
6.11 *Conclusion 94*
References 95

7 Innovative soft robotics: Transforming care and quality of life for elderly persons 98

7.1 *Introduction 98*
7.2 *Soft robotics 98*
7.3 *Elderly person problems 99*
7.4 *Healthcare access and management 101*
7.5 *Case studies 106*

7.6 Conclusions 113
References 113

8 Comprehensive study on materials used in soft robotics for medical and healthcare industries 116

8.1 Introduction 116
8.2 Types of soft robotic materials 116
8.2.1 Elastomers 117
8.2.2 Hydrogels 120
8.3 TRA 122
8.3.1 Optically responsive actuators 123
8.3.2 Magnetically responsive hydrogel 123
8.3.3 Hydraulically responsive hydrogel 123
8.4 Shape-memory polymers (SMPs) 124
8.4.1 PLA 125
8.5 Conclusions 125
References 126

9 Data-driven soft robotics 128

9.1 Introduction to soft robotics 128
9.2 Fundamentals of soft robotics 130
9.2.1 Materials used in soft robotics 130
9.2.2 Design and fabrication techniques 131
9.2.3 3D printing 133
9.3 The role of data in soft robotics 135
9.3.1 Data collection and sensors 135
9.3.2 Data-driven modeling and simulation 136
9.4 Soft robotics control systems 137
9.4.1 Traditional control methods 138
9.4.2 Data-based control techniques 139
9.5 Architectures representing data-driven soft robotics 141
9.5.1 Sensor-actuator architecture 141
9.5.2 Control architecture 142
9.5.3 Simulation and modeling architecture 142
9.5.4 Adaptation and learning architecture 142
9.5.5 Integration and deployment architecture 143

9.6 *Applications of data-driven soft robotics 143*
9.6.1 *Medical applications 143*
9.6.2 *Industrial applications 144*
9.6.3 *Environmental and exploration applications 145*
9.7 *Challenges and future directions 146*
9.7.1 *Technical challenges 146*
9.7.2 *Ethical and societal implications 148*
9.7.3 *Future research directions 148*
9.8 *Conclusion 150*
References 150

10 Machine learning in soft robotics: Techniques and applications 153

10.1 *Introduction 153*
10.2 *Machine learning 155*
10.3 *Necessity of machine learning 156*
10.3.1 *Unsupervised method 157*
10.3.2 *Supervised method 157*
10.3.3 *Semi-supervised method 157*
10.3.4 *Reinforcement method 157*
10.4 *Soft robotics 158*
10.5 *Collaboration of soft robotics with machine learning 161*
10.6 *Notable examples of soft robotics 162*
10.7 *Conclusions 165*
References 166

11 3D and 4D printing: Revolutionizing soft robotics 170

11.1 *Introduction 170*
11.2 *Historical development 171*
11.2.1 *Principles and techniques 172*
11.3 *3D printing in soft robotics 172*
11.4 *Advancements expanding capabilities 173*
11.5 *4D printing in soft robotics 173*
11.5.1 *Multimaterial printing: A blend of functions 174*
11.5.2 *Microstructures: Nanoscale engineering 174*
11.6 *Challenges and constraints 176*

11.7 Recent progress and future prospects 178
11.8 Fabrication improvements 178
11.9 Conclusions 180
References 181

12 Designing bio-inspired soft robotics for medical applications 183

12.1 Introduction 183
12.2 Soft robotics 184
12.3 Classification of soft robots 185
12.4 Manufacturing (3D printing) technology for robotic soft actuator 185
12.4.1 Material selection 185
12.4.2 Design and modeling 186
12.4.3 Manufacturing techniques 186
12.4.4 Postprocessing 187
12.4.5 Integration and testing 189
12.4.6 Applications and customization 190
12.4.7 Fundamentals of bio-inspired soft robotics design 190
12.4.8 Material selection 190
12.4.9 Actuation mechanisms 190
12.5 Major applications of soft robotics 195
12.5.1 Medical applications 195
12.5.2 Drug delivery systems 195
12.5.3 Types of soft robotic drug delivery systems 196
12.5.4 Rehabilitation and assistive devices 196
12.5.5 Tissue engineering 196
12.6 Challenges and future directions 197
12.6.1 Bioinspired soft robotics: Challenges 197
12.6.2 Future directions of bio-inspired soft robotics 198
12.7 Future studies ought to concentrate on 199
12.8 Outlook 200
References 200

13 Advances in design and manufacturing of soft robotic applications **203**

13.1 Introduction 203
13.2 Importance of soft robotics design 203
13.2.1 Enhanced design accuracy 204
13.2.2 Complex geometries and topologies 206
13.2.3 Simulation and testing 207
13.2.4 Material optimization 207
13.2.5 Collaboration and prototyping 207
13.3 Manufacturing of soft robots 208
13.3.1 Manufacturing intelligence 212
13.4 Mechanisms used in soft robotics 213
13.5 Conclusions 214
References 214

14 Soft robotics: Current opportunities and challenges **217**

14.1 Introduction 217
14.2 Literature review 218
14.3 Current opportunities 220
14.3.1 Soft robotics compatible technology development 220
14.3.2 Complete conversion from hard robots to soft robots 220
14.3.3 Soft actuator development 220
14.3.4 Soft robots' control 221
14.3.5 μ-Organism-like soft robots' development 221
14.3.6 Wearable soft robots' development 221
14.3.7 Untethered soft robots' development 221
14.4 Encountered challenges 222
14.4.1 Wearable soft robots' challenges 222
14.4.2 M-Organism-like soft robots' development challenges 222
14.4.3 Soft actuator development challenges 222
14.4.4 Soft materials development challenges 222
14.4.5 Untethered soft robots' challenges 223
14.4.6 Soft robots control challenges 223
14.5 Softness characteristics 223
14.6 Conclusion 224
References 224

15 Current and future market trends in soft robotics: A management perspective **226**

15.1 Introduction 226
15.2 Current market overview 227
15.3 Economic implications and value creation 228
15.3.1 Case studies of economic impact 229
15.4 Competitive landscape and market entry challenges 229
15.5 Anticipated market growth and opportunities 230
15.6 Strategic management approaches 232
15.7 Conclusions 234
References 235

Index 237

Preface

In recent years, the field of soft robotics has emerged as a transformative force in various sectors, particularly within the medical and healthcare industries. As our understanding of human physiology and the intricacies of patient care deepens, the need for adaptable, safe, and effective technologies becomes increasingly apparent. This book, *Soft Robotics for Medical and Healthcare Applications*, aims to elucidate the innovative ways in which soft robotics is redefining patient interaction, surgical procedures, rehabilitation, control of soft robotics, smart materials, and advanced manufacturing processes.

Soft robotics stands apart from traditional robotics through its use of compliant materials and structures that mimic the flexibility and adaptability of biological organisms. This unique characteristic allows soft robots to perform surgeries, making them particularly well suited for medical applications. From soft grippers used in minimally invasive surgeries to wearable devices that assist in personalized rehabilitation, the potential for these technologies is vast and exciting. The clubfoot and paralysis problems are effectively solved by soft robotic applications.

This book is intended for a diverse audience, including researchers, clinicians, engineers, and students interested in the convergence of robotics and healthcare. Each chapter provides insights from leading experts in the field, offering a comprehensive overview of current advancements, challenges, and future directions. The ultimate goal of soft robotics in healthcare is to enhance the quality of life for patients and streamline processes for healthcare providers.

The opening chapter, "Introduction to soft robotics: Opportunities and challenges," lays the groundwork by outlining the unique advantages of soft robotics, such as its adaptability, history of soft robots, and effectiveness, and addressing the technical and ethical challenges that accompany these advancements. This sets the stage for understanding the landscape of soft robotics today.

Chapter 2, "Recent developments and emerging trends in soft robotics," highlighted the cutting-edge research and breakthroughs that are pushing the boundaries of what is possible in this field. Chapter 3, "Soft robotic treatment for clubfoot," more focused on applications, showcases how soft robotics can improve therapeutic outcomes for specific medical conditions.

Chapter 4, "Medical applications of bio-inspired soft robotics," demonstrates the rich interplay between nature-inspired design and advanced engineering, illustrating how these elements combine to create effective medical tools. Chapter 5, "Motion control of soft robotic arm through servo motors," explains the control strategies in soft robotics. Further, Chapter 6 and 7, emphasizes the importance of creating compassionate technologies that support aging populations These chapters also discussed the different robots available for elderly person care.

Chapter 8, "Comprehensive study on materials used in soft robotics for medical and healthcare industries" discusses the importance of the soft materials.

The advancement of machine learning is completely transforming the predictions and developments of robotics and its applications; for any machine learning algorithm, the complete data are a crucial step. Chapter 9, "Data-driven soft robotics," and Chapter 10, "Machine learning in soft robotics: Techniques and applications," discuss the integration of artificial intelligence and data analytics in optimizing soft robotic systems. These chapters illustrate how machine learning is not only enhancing robotic capabilities but also personalizing healthcare solutions.

The rapid manufacturing and additive manufacturing applications of soft robotics are addressed in Chapter 11, "3D and 4D printing: Revolutionizing soft robotics," describing how these technologies are enabling rapid prototyping and customization of soft robotic devices. This leads to a variety of designs and customizable products. Chapter 12, "Designing bio-inspired soft robotics for medical applications," describes the principles that guide the design process, ensuring that these innovations are effective and user-friendly. The identification of proper problem and steps to solve the problem and associated software are discussed in this chapter. Chapter 13 "Advances in design and manufacturing of soft robotic applications" explains the advanced manufacturing methods such as 4D printing, cloud printing, This chapter also discusses the Augmented Reality and Virtual Reality based designs.

Chapter 14 discusses the future challenges and opportunities of soft robotics. Chapter 15 demonstrates the present and future growth of soft robotics from a management perspective. The possible growth penetration of the soft robotics industry in medical and healthcare industries worldwide is discussed in this chapter. We are grateful to the contributing authors, whose expertise and dedication have shaped this work. The readers will explore the promising future of soft robotics in medicine and healthcare.

Shaik Himam Saheb
Department of Mechanical Engineering
Vignan's Foundation for Science, Technology and Research
Hyderabad

Acknowledgments

We would like to extend my heartfelt gratitude to several individuals whose support and guidance have been instrumental in the completion of this book. We thank Dr. Lavu Rathaiah Garu, Chairman of Vignan group of institutions, for his commitment to encourage a culture of innovation at Vignan's Foundation for Science, Technology and Research. We are deeply grateful to Vice-Chancellor Dr. P. Nagabhushan Garu, for his encouragement and support in pursuing research initiatives that bridge engineering and healthcare.

Our sincere thanks to Dr. M. Ramakrishna, Professor, Mechanical Engineering and Dean-IQAC, for his valuable insights and guidance. His guidance has greatly influenced our work.

We would like to thank staff members of VFSTR Hyderabad campus for their support throughout this journey. We thank Dr. K.L. Narayana, Director of ICFAI Tech, IFHE, for his support and encouragement. We thank Management and Principal of Sri Venkateswara College of Engineering, Tirupati. We thank your family members for their continuous support and encouragement. We extend our thanks to the Straive team, particularly Devaa, for their unwavering support throughout the publication process.

Special Thanks to all chapter contributors, for being an integral part of this journey.

Editors

Dr. Shaik Himam Saheb is a senior assistant professor in the Department of Mechanical and Robotics Engineering, Vignan's Foundation for Science, Technology and Research (Deemed to be University), Hyderabad, Telangana, India. His research interests are mechanisms, robotics, parallel manipulators, data science, and machine learning. He has published 52 research papers in national and international journals and international conferences. He has published four books. The team guided by him has received a national-level Go-Kart Championship with a rupees 100,000 cash prize in an event organized by the Indian Society of New Era Engineers. His professional affiliations are MISTE, LMIAENG, and MSMAE.

Dr Tharakeshwar Appala is a professor in the Department of Mechanical Engineering and the Vice Principal at Sri Venkateswara College of Engineering, Tirupati. His research interests are robotics, mechanisms, and multibody dynamics. He earned his doctorate degree from the Indian Institute of Science (IISc) in Bangalore and has over 20 years of teaching and research experience. He has published 10 national and international journals and conferences.

Dr. Mohammad S Khan (SM' 19) is an associate professor of Computing at East Tennessee State University and the Director of Network Science and Analysis Lab (NSAL). He earned his MSc and PhD degrees in computer science and computer engineering from the University of Louisville, Kentucky, USA, in 2011 and 2013, respectively. His primary areas of research are in ad-hoc networks, wireless sensor networks, network tomography, connected vehicles, and vehicular social networks. He currently serves as an associate editor of *IEEE Access*, *IET ITS*, *IET WSS*, and Springer's *Telecommunication Systems* and *Neural Computing and Applications*. He has been on the technical program committees of various international conferences and technical reviewer of various international journals in his field. He is a senior member of IEEE.

Contributors

A. Chandrashekhar
Department of Mechanical Engineering, FST
The ICFAI Foundation for Higher Education
Hyderabad, Telangana, India

E Devaraj
Department of Mechanical Engineering
CMR University
Bangalore, Karnataka, India

S Gopinath
Department of Mechanical Engineering
Sri Venkateswara College of Engineering
Tamil Nadu, India

Harpal Singh Kalra
Department of Mechanical Engineering
Asia Pacific Institute of Information Technology SD INDIA
Panipat, Haryana India

Shaik Mahaboob Syed
Vignan's Foundation for Science, Technology and Research
Hyderabad, Telangana, India

M. Sreedhar
Department of Mechanical Engineering
Guru Nanak University
Ibrahimpatnam, Hyderabad, Telangana, India

M. Avinash
Department of Mechanical Engineering, FST
The ICFAI Foundation for Higher Education
Hyderabad, Telangana, India

M.L. Pavan Kishore
Department of Mechanical Engineering, FST
The ICFAI Foundation for Higher Education
Hyderabad, Telangana, India

M Prasanna Kumar
Department of Mechanical Engineering
Centre for Post Graduate Studies
Visvesvaraya Technological University, Mysuru

P Sree Lakshmi
Department of Computer Science and Engineering

Koneru Lakshmaiah Education Foundation
Hyderabad, Telangana, India

P Rohini
Department of Computer Science and Engineering
Faculty of Science and Technology, ICFAI Foundation for Higher Education
Hyderabad, Telangana, India

Perabathula Satish
Department of Mechanical Engineering
Vignan's Foundation for Science Research and Technology
Guntur, India

Prateek Mishra
Department of Computer Science & Engineering
Asia Pacific Institute of Information Technology SD INDIA
Panipat, Haryana, India

A Ranjith Raj
Department of Mechanical Engineering
Sri Venkateswara College of Engineering
Chennai, Tamil Nadu, India

Shaik Himam Saheb
Department of Mechanical Engineering
Vignan's Foundation for Science Research and Technology
Hyderabad, Telangana, India

S Supreeth
Mechanical Department
Mysore College of Engineering and Management
Mysuru, Karnataka, India

Suresh Chandra Ch
Vignan's Foundation for Science, Technology and Research
Hyderabad, Telangana, India

Syed Quadir Moinuddin
Department of Mechanical Engineering
College of Engineering, King Faisal University
Al-Ahsa, Kingdom of Saudi Arabia

Tharakeshwar Appala
Department of Mechanical Engineering
Sri Venkateswara College of Engineering
Tirupati, Andhra Pradesh, India

Vinay K M
Department of Industrial & Production Engineering
University BDT College of Engineering
Davanagere, Karnataka, India

Chapter 1

Introduction to soft robotics

Opportunities and challenges

Shaik Himam Saheb and Tharakeshwar Appala

1.1 INTRODUCTION

Soft robotics, a rapidly evolving field in the realm of robotics, presents a paradigm shift in the way we approach the design and development of robotic systems. This innovative approach leverages flexible materials and adaptive systems, allowing robots to interact safely and effectively with their environments, ultimately enhancing capabilities in areas such as medical devices, rehabilitation, and search and rescue operations [1], which emphasize the importance of safety and adaptability in human–robot interactions [2, 3].

The field of soft robotics has gained significant attention in recent years, driven by its potential to revolutionize various applications, particularly in the medical and rehabilitation sectors. Soft robotic devices, characterized by their lightweight, compliant, and adaptable nature, offer unique advantages over traditional rigid robotic systems [4]. Stroke survivors often face significant challenges in hand rehabilitation, and soft robotic gloves have emerged as a promising solution [5]. These devices can provide cyclic stretching of the fingers, active-assisted exercise, and task-oriented training, helping to reduce hyperexcitability of the flexor muscles and improve hand function [6].

One study conducted a pilot investigation on the use of a soft robotic glove in chronic stroke survivors, where four participants underwent 300 repetitions of hand opening and closing over six training sessions. The results demonstrated the viability of this approach, suggesting that soft robotic devices can be a valuable tool in home-based hand rehabilitation for stroke survivors [7]. Soft robotic devices have also shown promise in other medical applications, such as prosthetics and assistive devices. These flexible, adaptable systems can better conform to the unique anatomy and movements of the human body, enhancing comfort and functionality for users [8]. The development of soft robotic devices for hand rehabilitation and assistance has seen a rapid increase in recent years, as evidenced by the growing body of research in this field. Soft robotics is a fascinating branch of robotics that emphasizes creating robots from highly flexible materials, in contrast to traditional robots which are often made of rigid materials [9, 10].

DOI: 10.1201/9781003539612-1

Materials like silicone rubber and polyurethane are commonly used because of their flexibility and durability called elastomers [11]. Hydrogels can absorb large amounts of water, allowing for significant changes in volume and shape [12]. Shape-memory materials are the materials that can return to a predefined shape when exposed to specific stimuli, such as heat. The actuation of the robot plays a major role in the soft robot design. The traditional soft materials are used as soft robotic materials with the addition of controller as shown in Figure 1.1. The pneumatic actuation often uses air pressure to create movement. Pneumatic actuators can create complex and flexible motions by inflating and deflating chambers within the robot. Whereas hydraulic actuation is similar to pneumatic actuators but uses fluids, hydraulic systems can provide precise and powerful movements. The soft actuators include materials that change shape or stiffness in response to external stimuli, such as temperature or electric fields.

Soft robotics is an exciting and rapidly growing field within robotics that focuses on creating robots from highly flexible and adaptable materials. Unlike traditional rigid robots, which are made from hard materials like metals and plastics, soft robots are constructed from materials that can deform, stretch, and compress. This allows them to handle delicate objects, navigate through tight or complex spaces, and interact with their environment in a more adaptable way. Their soft nature makes them safer for interactions with humans and fragile objects. Soft robotics can adapt their shape and movement to navigate complex environments. Their flexible materials can absorb impacts and recover from deformations, which can be useful in unpredictable or harsh conditions.

Soft robots can be difficult to control soft robots precisely due to their flexible nature and the complexity of their movements. The materials used

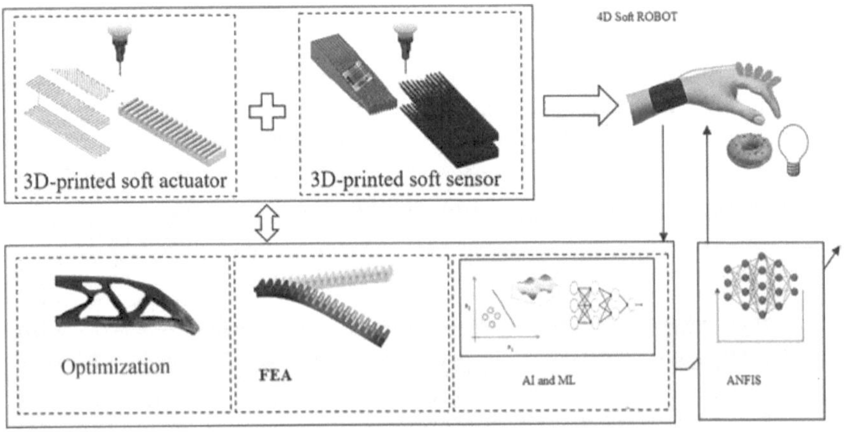

Figure 1.1 Integration of normal soft sensors with controller to get a variety of soft robots [13].

in soft robots may wear out or degrade over time, which can impact their performance and longevity. Soft robotics represents a shift toward more adaptable, flexible, and gentle robots, expanding the potential applications and capabilities of robotic technology.

1.2 DIGITAL TWIN AND SOFT ROBOTICS

A digital twin is a virtual replica of a physical object, system, or process. It uses real-time data and simulations to mirror the state and behavior of its physical counterpart. This concept is used to monitor, analyze, and optimize the physical object or process by allowing for predictions and scenario testing in a virtual environment. Digital twins are used across various industries, including manufacturing, healthcare, and urban planning. The intersection of digital twins and soft robotics represents an exciting frontier in robotics and automation. By integrating these two technologies, you can enhance the design, operation, and maintenance of soft robotic systems.

- **Enhanced Design and Development:** Digital twins allow engineers to create detailed virtual models of soft robots. These models can simulate how the robot will behave under various conditions, enabling the design of more effective and optimized soft robots. Engineers can test different materials, configurations, and control strategies in the virtual world before physical prototypes are built. Digital twins facilitate rapid prototyping and iterative design processes. By continuously updating the digital twin with data from physical tests, engineers can quickly identify design flaws and make necessary adjustments.
- **Real-Time Monitoring and Adaptation:** A digital twin can provide real-time insights into the performance of a soft robot. By analyzing data from sensors on the physical robot and comparing it with the digital twin, operators can monitor the robot's condition and performance, identifying issues such as wear and tear or deviations from expected behavior. The digital twin can be used to adjust control algorithms in real time. If the physical soft robot encounters unexpected conditions, the digital twin can simulate responses and guide adjustments to the robot's control system to adapt to the new conditions.
- **Predictive Maintenance:** Failure prediction is possible by continuously analyzing data from the digital twin; it is possible to predict when components of the soft robot might fail or require maintenance. This predictive capability can reduce downtime and extend the lifespan of the robot by addressing issues before they lead to failure. The digital twin can help schedule maintenance activities based on the predicted wear and tear of the robot, optimizing maintenance resources and minimizing disruptions to operations.

- **Training and Simulation:** Digital twins can be used for training operators and technicians in a virtual environment. By interacting with a digital twin, they can practice operating and troubleshooting the soft robot without risking damage to the actual hardware. New control algorithms or adjustments can be tested in the digital twin before being applied to the physical robot. This allows for thorough testing and optimization without the risks associated with direct experimentation on the physical robot.
- **Improved Interaction and Collaboration:** Digital twins can help refine how soft robots interact with their human counterparts. By simulating various human–robot interaction scenarios, designers can ensure that the soft robot operates safely and effectively alongside humans. In environments where multiple soft robots work together, digital twins can simulate and coordinate their activities, optimizing their collective performance and ensuring smooth cooperation. The digital twin and soft robotics integration leads to major implicational changes in the various disciplines.
- In medical applications, digital twins of soft surgical robots can be used to simulate complex procedures, refine robotic movements, and predict outcomes. This improves the precision of minimally invasive surgeries and enhances patient safety. Digital twins of soft robotic systems used for harvesting crops can simulate various harvesting conditions and optimize the robot's performance for different types of crops and environments. Soft robots used in search and rescue missions, digital twins can model different scenarios, helping to plan and execute rescue operations more effectively and adapt to dynamic and unpredictable environments. The integration of digital twins with soft robotics enhances the capabilities of both technologies, leading to more adaptable, efficient, and reliable robotic systems. As these technologies continue to evolve, their combined potential will likely drive innovation across various fields and applications.

1.3 APPLICATIONS OF THE SOFT ROBOTICS

Soft robotics presents numerous opportunities across various fields due to its unique characteristics and capabilities.

1.3.1 Medical and healthcare

- **Minimally Invasive Surgery:** Soft robots can navigate through the human body with minimal disruption, making them ideal for delicate procedures. Minimally invasive surgery (MIS) is a technique that allows surgeons to perform operations through small incisions, often with the aid of specialized instruments and imaging technologies. This approach typically results in less pain, reduced risk of infection, shorter recovery times, and minimal scarring compared to traditional open surgery. The operations such as Laparoscopic Surgery, Appendectomy, Cholecystectomy, Hernia Repair, Colorectal Surgery, Gastroscopy, Colonoscopy, Bronchoscopy, Prostatectomy, Gynecological Procedures like Hysterectomy, Myomectomy, and other procedures related to the female reproductive system. Kidney surgery, Endogenous Laser Therapy (EVLT), and all such operations need MIS, where the soft robotics gives better solutions than the existing processes.

- **Prosthetics and Orthotics:** Soft robotic devices can provide more natural movement and comfort in prosthetic limbs and orthotic devices, enhancing the quality of life for individuals with mobility impairments.
- **Rehabilitation:** Soft robots can be used in physical therapy to create adaptive and customizable rehabilitation devices that can gently assist in the recovery process.

1.3.2 Agriculture and food industry

- **Harvesting and Handling:** Soft robots can pick and handle delicate fruits and vegetables without causing damage, which is crucial for maintaining quality and reducing waste. Soft robots are revolutionizing the way we handle harvesting and handling tasks in agriculture by offering gentle, adaptable solutions for delicate operations. Their flexible, conformable materials allow them to pick fruits and vegetables with minimal damage, manage tender plants with care, and sort or pack produce efficiently. This technology reduces bruising and maintains high quality while improving safety for both the produce and operators. Although challenges such as durability, integration with existing systems, and cost need addressing, the benefits of soft robots in enhancing precision and efficiency make them a promising tool in modern agricultural practices.
- **Precision Agriculture:** Soft robot–based precision agriculture is transforming farming by offering adaptable and gentle solutions for a variety of tasks. These robots use flexible materials and advanced sensors to perform precise operations such as targeted planting, weeding, and harvesting. Their ability to conform to different plant shapes and sizes allows for delicate handling, reducing crop damage and optimizing yield. By integrating real-time data and adaptive control, soft robots enhance efficiency and accuracy in managing crops, leading to more sustainable and productive farming practices.

1.4 SOFT ROBOTICS AND 3D PRINTING

The integration of soft robotics with 3D printing represents an emerging advancement in manufacturing and design flexibility. By combining the adaptive and flexible characteristics of soft robotics with the precision and customization capabilities of 3D printing, this integration allows for the creation of highly specialized and complex robotic components with greater flexibility. 3D printing enables the fabrication of soft robots with intricate geometries and tailored properties, such as varying stiffness and elasticity, which are essential for handling delicate tasks and adapting to diverse environments. This synergy not only accelerates the development process but also reduces costs and enhances the performance and functionality of soft robots, paving the way for more innovative applications in fields like agriculture, healthcare, and manufacturing. This technology allows for the creation of intricate structures that can mimic natural movements and adapt to different tasks with high precision.

3D printing allows for the production of soft robots with tailored designs that match specific application requirements. This includes creating components with complex internal structures and varying material properties that would be difficult or impossible to achieve with traditional manufacturing methods. Advanced 3D-printing techniques use a range of soft, flexible materials, such as silicones and elastomers. These materials are essential for building soft robots that can perform delicate tasks, such as handling fragile objects or navigating tight spaces. The combination of 3D printing and soft robotics accelerates the prototyping and iteration process. Designers can quickly modify and test new concepts, reducing development time and costs.

3D printing can incorporate various functions into a single component, such as sensors and actuators, within the soft robotic structure. This integration enhances the robot's capabilities and performance by allowing it to perform complex tasks with fewer separate parts. The ability to produce custom soft robotic parts on demand reduces the need for expensive molds and tooling, making it more economical to manufacture low-volume or highly specialized robots. The collaboration between soft robotics and 3D printing opens up new possibilities for creating advanced, adaptable robots that can tackle a wide range of applications, from precision agriculture to medical procedures and beyond. There are many challenges with 3D printing of soft robotics; the major challenges are studied by Sachyani et al. [14], as shown in Figure 1.2.

1.5 FABRICATION OF SOFT ROBOTS

The manufacturing of soft robots is an intricate process that involves several stages, from initial design through to production and quality control. This chapter delves into the methodologies, materials, and techniques used to create soft robots, which are characterized by their flexibility and adaptability compared to traditional rigid robots.

The process begins with the design phase, which is crucial for defining the robot's intended functionality, size, and movement capabilities. Designers must consider the robot's tasks, whether it is for gripping, crawling, or

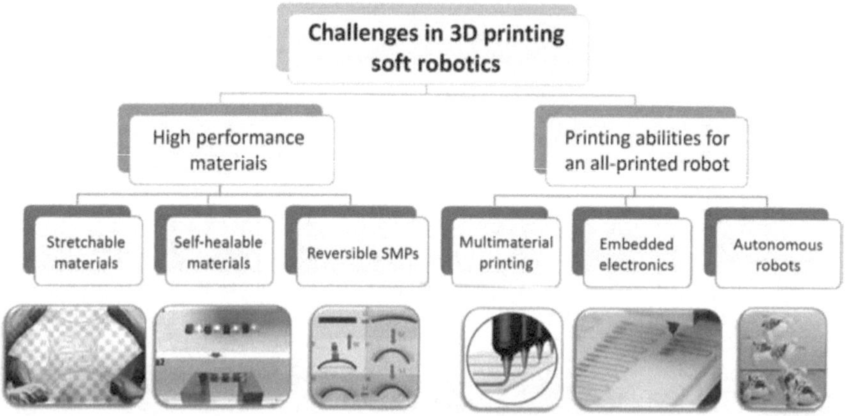

Figure 1.2 Challenges in 3D printing of soft robots [14].

expanding. The design must also account for the range of motion and flexibility required, as well as the material properties that will best achieve these goals. Prototyping plays a significant role in this stage, allowing for rapid testing and refinement of designs. Techniques such as 3D printing and soft lithography are employed to create preliminary models quickly. This iterative process helps identify potential design flaws and improvements before finalizing the model.

Material selection is a critical aspect of manufacturing soft robots. The choice of materials affects the robot's performance, durability, and responsiveness. Common materials used in soft robotics include silicone elastomers, hydrogels, and shape-memory polymers. Silicone elastomers are favored for their flexibility, durability, and ease of molding, making them suitable for a variety of applications. Hydrogels, which absorb water and change shape in response to environmental stimuli, are ideal for applications requiring significant deformation. Shape-memory polymers can revert to a predetermined shape when exposed to specific stimuli, such as heat, offering unique capabilities in soft robotic designs. The various processes for the fabrication of soft robots are shown in Figure 1.3. The selection of manufacturing process depends on various factors such as type of materials, melting point of the materials, and biocompatibility of the materials. Once materials are chosen, they must be prepared for fabrication. This preparation can involve mixing components to achieve the desired properties, curing materials through heat or chemical reactions, and conditioning materials for specific uses, such as adjusting the water content in hydrogels. The fabrication of soft robots employs several techniques to shape and assemble components. Molding is a prevalent method, where materials are poured or injected into molds to create various parts. Silicone molding and injection molding are typical approaches used to produce flexible, detailed components [15–17].

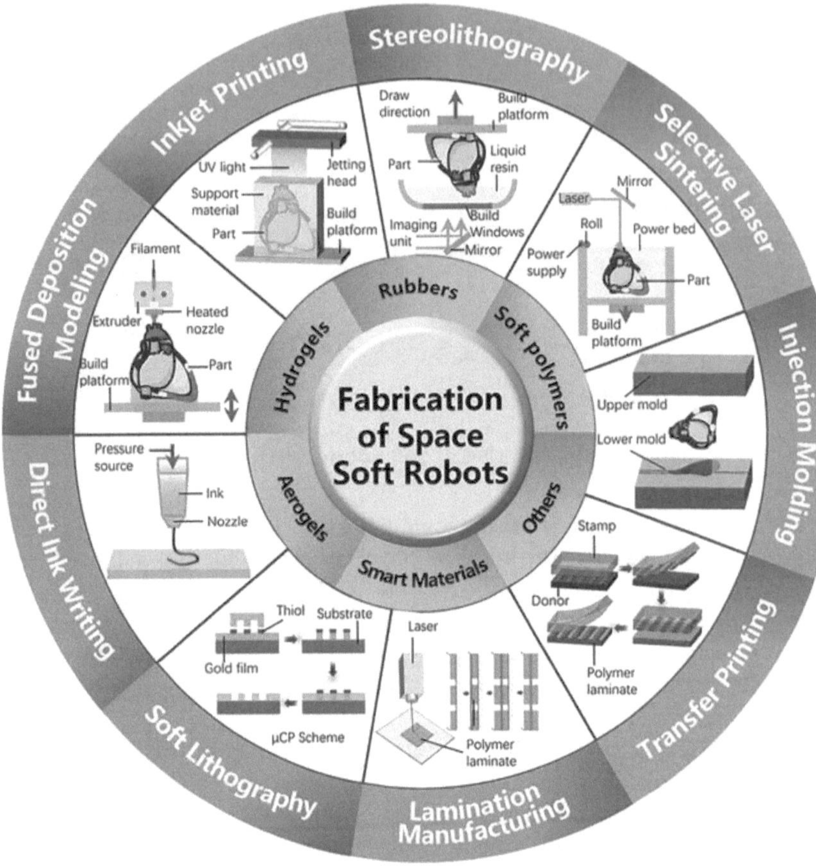

Figure 1.3 Various fabrication processes of soft robots based on the material [20].

3D printing has revolutionized the fabrication of soft robots, allowing for precise, layer-by-layer construction of parts. Technologies like fused deposition modeling (FDM) [18] and inkjet printing [19] enable the creation of complex geometries and integration of embedded features. Casting is another technique where liquid material is poured into molds and allowed to set, often used with silicone elastomers. Electrospinning, which involves spinning fine fibers from a polymer solution, can produce mesh structures or coatings that contribute to the robot's functionality.

The integration of components is a pivotal stage in manufacturing soft robots. This involves assembling different parts, such as soft actuators, sensors, and control systems, ensuring they fit together accurately and function as intended. Precision handling is crucial to maintain alignment and attachment of components. Additionally, embedding electronic components, sensors, or actuators within the soft materials is necessary for the robot's operation. Techniques such as encapsulation protect electronic components, while integration involves designing pathways or channels for fluidic or electrical systems.

Testing and validation are essential to ensure that the soft robot performs according to its design specifications. Functional testing assesses the robot's movement, flexibility, and responsiveness to stimuli and control inputs. Durability testing examines the robot's performance under various conditions, including stress and wear over time. Iterative improvement based on test results helps refine the design and manufacturing process, enhancing performance and reliability. Quality control ensures that the final product meets established standards and specifications. This involves inspecting the robot for defects or inconsistencies, both visually and through dimensional measurement. Functional testing is repeated to confirm that the robot operates as intended. Standardization of processes and documentation is vital to maintain consistency and reliability in manufacturing.

As production scales, manufacturers move from small-batch production to mass production. Small-batch production allows for initial testing and refinement, while mass production requires efficient processes and supply chains. Automation and supply chain management become crucial to meet the demands of larger-scale production. Deployment of soft robots involves integrating them into their intended applications, ensuring they function effectively in real-world environments. Ongoing support and maintenance are necessary to address any issues and ensure continued operation. Technical support, troubleshooting, and upgrades based on user feedback are integral to maintaining the robot's performance and relevance.

The manufacturing of soft robots encompasses a comprehensive approach, integrating material science, advanced fabrication techniques, and rigorous testing. By carefully managing each stage from design through production, manufacturers can create innovative soft robots that offer enhanced flexibility and adaptability for various applications.

1.6 CONCLUSIONS

The chapter provides an insightful overview of the burgeoning field of soft robotics, highlighting both its transformative potential and the obstacles that must be overcome. Soft robotics, characterized by its use of flexible, adaptive materials, offers significant advantages in a range of applications, from medical devices and manufacturing to exploration and environmental monitoring.

Soft robots excel in environments where adaptability and gentle interaction are crucial. Their ability to conform to various shapes and handle delicate objects with care makes them ideal for tasks in sensitive and unstructured settings. In healthcare, soft robots enhance minimally invasive procedures and patient rehabilitation, while in industrial contexts, they improve safety and efficiency. The potential for soft robots to explore challenging environments, such as deep-sea or extraterrestrial terrains, further underscores their versatility.

Despite their promise, the development of soft robots is fraught with challenges. Key issues include the need for advanced materials that combine flexibility with durability, scalable fabrication techniques, and sophisticated control systems capable of managing the unique dynamics of soft robots. Integrating sensors and actuators within soft materials without compromising performance is also a significant hurdle. Moreover, ensuring safety and reliability in real-world applications remains a critical concern.

These challenges require continued innovation in material science, robotics, and computational methods. The integration of machine learning and advanced control algorithms can enhance the autonomy and functionality of soft robots. Collaboration across disciplines and sectors will be essential for advancing the technology and expanding its applications. While soft robotics presents exciting opportunities for revolutionizing various fields, it also necessitates ongoing research and development to overcome its inherent challenges. By pushing the boundaries of current technology and fostering interdisciplinary collaboration, the full potential of soft robotics can be realized, leading to new possibilities and improvements in both industrial and everyday applications.

REFERENCES

[1] Ramadurai, K. W., & Bhatia, S. K. (2018). *Reimagining Innovation in Humanitarian Medicine: Engineering Care to Improve Health and Welfare.* USA: Springer.

[2] Zacharaki, A., Kostavelis, I., Gasteratos, A., & Dokas, I. (2020). Safety bounds in human robot interaction: A survey. *Safety Science*, 127, 104667.

[3] Casper, J., & Murphy, R. R. (2003). Human-robot interactions during the robot-assisted urban search and rescue response at the world trade center. *IEEE Transactions on Systems, Man, and Cybernetics, Part B (Cybernetics)*, 33(3), 367–385.

[4] Polygerinos, P., Correll, N., Morin, S. A., Mosadegh, B., Onal, C. D., Petersen, K., ... & Shepherd, R. F. (2017). Soft robotics: Review of fluid-driven intrinsically soft devices; manufacturing, sensing, control, and applications in human-robot interaction. *Advanced Engineering Materials*, 19(12), 1700016.

[5] Chandrashekhar, A., Saheb, S., & Pavan Kishore, M. L. (2021). Investigation of the static and dynamic path planning of mobile and aerial robots. *Computer Networks and Inventive Communication Technologies: Proceedings of Third ICCNCT 2020*, 1033–1044.

[6] Xiloyannis, M., Alicea, R., Georgarakis, A. M., Haufe, F. L., Wolf, P., Masia, L., & Riener, R. (2021). Soft robotic suits: State of the art, core technologies, and open challenges. *IEEE Transactions on Robotics*, 38(3), 1343–1362.

[7] Jumet, B., Bell, M. D., Sanchez, V., & Preston, D. J. (2022). A data-driven review of soft robotics. *Advanced Intelligent Systems*, 4(4), 2100163.
[8] Jyothish, K. J., & Mishra, S. (2024). A Survey on Robotic Prosthetics: Neuroprosthetics, Soft Actuators, and Control Strategies. *ACM Computing Surveys*, 56(8), 1–44.
[9] Schmitt, F., Piccin, O., Barbé, L., & Bayle, B. (2018). Soft robots manufacturing: A review. *Frontiers in Robotics and AI*, 5, 84.
[10] Kwok, K. W., Wurdemann, H., Arezzo, A., Menciassi, A., & Althoefer, K. (2022). Soft robot-assisted minimally invasive surgery and interventions: Advances and outlook. *Proceedings of the IEEE*, 110(7), 871–892.
[11] Rahimi, A., & Mashak, A. (2013). Review on rubbers in medicine: Natural, silicone and polyurethane rubbers. *Plastics, rubber and composites*, 42(6), 223–230.
[12] Khandan, A., Jazayeri, H., Fahmy, M. D., & Razavi, M. (2017). Hydrogels: Types, structure, properties, and applications. *BiomatTiss Eng*, 4(27), 143–169.
[13] Polygerinos, P., Correll, N., Morin, S. A., Mosadegh, B., Onal, C. D., Petersen, K., ... & Shepherd, R. F. (2017). Soft robotics: Review of fluid-driven intrinsically soft devices; manufacturing, sensing, control, and applications in human-robot interaction. *Advanced engineering materials*, 19(12), 1700016.
[14] Sachyani, Ela, Kamyshny, Alexander, Totaro, Massimo, Beccai, Lucia, & Magdassi, Shlomo. (2020). 3D Printing Materials for Soft Robotics. *Advanced Materials*. 33. 2003387. doi:10.1002/adma.202003387
[15] Bell, M. A., Becker, K. P., & Wood, R. J. (2022). Injection molding of soft robots. *Advanced Materials Technologies*, 7(1), 2100605.
[16] Kalami, H., & Urbanic, R. J. (2019). Design and fabrication of a low-volume, high-temperature injection mould leveraging a 'rapid tooling' approach. *The International Journal of Advanced Manufacturing Technology*, 105, 3797–3813.
[17] Rosato, D. V., Rosato, D. V., & Rosato, M. G. (2000). Molding materials. In *Injection Molding Handbook* (pp. 479–622). Boston, MA: Springer US.
[18] Yap, H. K., Ng, H. Y., & Yeow, C. H. (2016). High-force soft printable pneumatics for soft robotic applications. *Soft Robotics*, 3(3), 144–158.
[19] Calvert, P. (2001). Inkjet printing for materials and devices. *Chemistry of materials*, 13(10), 3299–3305.
[20] Zhang, Yongchang, Li, Pengchun, Quan, Jiale, Li, Longqiu, Zhang, Guangyu, & Zhou, Dekai. (2022). Progress, challenges, and prospects of soft robotics for space applications. *Advanced Intelligent Systems*. 5. doi:10.1002/aisy.202200071

Chapter 2

Recent developments and emerging trends in soft robotics

M. L. Pavan Kishore and Shaik Himam Saheb

2.1 INTRODUCTION

Soft robotics is a rapidly expanding field that combines the principles of robotics and soft materials to create flexible, adaptable, and safe robots. These robots are designed to interact with humans and their environment in a more natural and gentle manner, making them particularly suitable for applications where traditional rigid robots may not be effective. The field has seen significant growth in recent years, with a substantial increase in both the quantity and quality of scientific publications [1, 2]. Soft robotics is a subfield of robotics that focuses on the design and fabrication of robots using soft and compliant materials. These robots are designed to mimic the properties of living tissues, such as flexibility, adaptability, and gentleness, which enable them to interact with humans and their environment in a more natural and safe manner [3]. Soft robots are particularly useful in applications where traditional rigid robots may not be effective, such as in medical procedures, search and rescue operations, and industrial tasks that require precision and delicacy [4].

The key components of soft robots include actuators, sensors, and control systems, which work together to provide the necessary dexterity and adaptability for a wide range of tasks. The design and fabrication of soft robots involve the use of various materials and techniques, including the processing and engineering of soft materials, the development of novel actuation and sensing mechanisms, and the integration of control systems that can accommodate imprecise feedback data and unpredictable reaction times. Soft robotics has seen significant growth in recent years, driven by advancements in materials science, biomechanics, and robotics engineering. The field is characterized by its interdisciplinary nature, drawing from biology, physics, and engineering to create innovative solutions for various applications.

2.1.1 Literature review

Over the past years, the field of soft robotics has witnessed a significant surge in interest, driven largely by advancements in additive manufacturing

 DOI: 10.1201/9781003539612-2

technologies such as 3D and 4D printing. In this chapter, we delve into key research contributions and milestones in the realm of 3D and 4D printing of soft robotics, spanning from 1975 to 2024.

2.1.1.1 1970s to 1980s: Early foundations

Toepperwein and Greenwood [5, 6]—"The Use of Flexible Materials in Robotic Systems": Explored the early concept of using flexible materials in robotic systems. This paper laid the groundwork for future research by discussing the advantages of compliance and adaptability in robotic design for safer interaction with humans.

Hagerty [7]—"Development of Flexible Pneumatic Actuators for Use in Soft Robots": Introduced the concept of flexible pneumatic actuators, marking an early step toward the development of soft actuation mechanisms. This paper discussed the design and potential applications of these actuators in creating more adaptable robotic systems.

2.1.1.2 1990s: Advancements in soft materials

Hirose [8]—"Biologically Inspired Robots Snake-like Locomotors and Manipulators": Detailed the design of snake-like robots using flexible materials, inspired by biological organisms. This work emphasized the importance of flexibility for achieving complex locomotion and manipulation tasks in robotics.

Arnold et al. [9]—"Artificial Muscles Based on Electroactive Polymers": Investigated the potential of electroactive polymers (EAPs) as artificial muscles. This study was crucial in highlighting the benefits of EAPs for creating soft, life-like robotic movements.

2.1.1.3 2000s: Emergence of soft robotics

Lauer et al. [10]—"Soft Robotics for Human Interaction": Discussed the need for soft robotics to enhance safety and compliance in human–robot interactions. This paper provided a comprehensive overview of the potential benefits of incorporating softness into robotic systems.

Dario et al. [11]—"Microsystems in Biomedical Applications": Explored the application of soft materials in medical robotics, particularly focusing on minimally invasive surgery. This work highlighted the significance of soft robotics in enhancing the precision and safety of medical procedures.

Choi et al. [12]—"Development of Soft Actuators using Dielectric Elastomers": Focused on the use of dielectric elastomers for soft actuation. This paper presented key advancements in actuator technology, which are essential for the development of soft robotic systems.

Amiet et al. [13]—"Design and Control of a Bio-inspired Soft Robotic Arm": Presented the design and control methodologies for a bio-inspired soft robotic arm. This study showcased the advantages of soft robotics in achieving adaptable and flexible movements.

2.1.1.4 2010s: Growth and diversification

Sitti et al. [14]—"Miniature Soft Robots with Bio-inspired Locomotion": Described the development of small-scale soft robots inspired by natural locomotion mechanisms. This work was pivotal in advancing the field of miniature soft robotics.

Kim et al. [15]—"Soft Robotics: A Bio-inspired Evolution in Robotics": Provided a comprehensive overview of the field of soft robotics, discussing various soft materials, actuation methods, and potential applications. This paper emphasized the bio-inspired evolution of robotic systems.

Shepherd et al. and Semini et al. [16, 17]—"Multigait Soft Robot": Demonstrated a soft robot capable of multiple types of locomotion. This study highlighted the versatility and adaptability of soft robotic systems.

Majidi [18]—"Soft Robotics: A Perspective - Current Trends and Prospects": Offered an in-depth review of the current state and future potential of soft robotics. This paper covered key technologies, challenges, and the future outlook for the field.

Shintake et al. [19]—"Soft Robotic Grippers": Explored the development of soft robotic grippers, focusing on their ability to handle delicate and irregular objects. This work emphasized the practical applications of soft robotics in handling and manipulation tasks.

Li et al. and Iida et al. and [20, 21]—"Design, Fabrication, and Control of Soft Robots": Provided a detailed guide on the design, fabrication, and control methodologies for soft robots. This paper highlighted important techniques and materials necessary for developing effective soft robotic systems.

Kramer et al. [22]—"Stretchable Conductors for Soft Robotics": Investigated stretchable conductive materials, which are crucial for creating flexible and resilient soft robotic systems. This study presented new materials that enhance the performance and durability of soft robots.

Lipomi et al. [23]—"Soft Robotics for Biomedical Applications": Discussed the application of soft robotics in the biomedical field, particularly for surgical and therapeutic devices. This work highlighted the potential of soft robotics in improving medical procedures.

Cianchetti et al. [24]—"Bioinspired Soft Robotics: Advanced Technologies and Applications": Comprehensive review on bio-inspired soft robotic technologies and their diverse applications. This paper covered various aspects of bio-inspiration in soft robotics, including design, materials, and applications.

Connolly et al. [25]—"Mechanical Programming of Soft Actuators": Explored methods for mechanically programming soft actuators to achieve complex movements. This study presented techniques for enhancing the capabilities of soft actuators.

Miriyev et al. [26]—"Soft Material for Soft Actuators": Introduced new soft materials for actuators, enhancing the performance and durability of soft robotic systems. This paper discussed the advantages of these materials in creating more effective soft actuators.

Decroly et al. [27]—"Exploration of Soft Underwater Robots": Focused on the development of soft robots for underwater exploration. This study addressed challenges such as buoyancy and movement in water, showcasing the potential of soft robotics in underwater applications.

2.1.1.5 2020s: Current trends and future directions

Romano et al. [28]—"Soft Robotics: Technologies and Systems Paving the Way to the Future": Discussed recent technological advancements in soft robotics and their implications for future applications. This paper provided a comprehensive overview of the state-of-the-art technologies in the field.

Ren et al. [29]—"Soft Robots with Embedded Sensing Capabilities": Explored the integration of sensors within soft robotic systems, enhancing their ability to interact with and adapt to their environment. This study highlighted the importance of sensing in improving the functionality of soft robots.

Wang et al. [30]—"Artificial Intelligence in Soft Robotics": Examined the role of artificial intelligence (AI) in advancing soft robotics, particularly in improving control and adaptability. This paper discussed the potential of AI to enhance the capabilities of soft robotic systems.

Gu et al. [31]—"Soft Robotics in Wearable Devices": Investigated the application of soft robotics in wearable technology, focusing on enhancing comfort and functionality. This study highlighted the potential of soft robotics to improve wearable devices.

Guo et al. [32]—"Recent Advances in Soft Robotic Actuators": Provided a detailed review of the latest advancements in soft actuators, highlighting new materials and designs. This paper discussed the implications of these advancements for the field of soft robotics.

Girerd et al. [33]—"Biohybrid Soft Robots": Explored the integration of biological components with soft robots, creating biohybrid systems with enhanced capabilities. This study presented a new frontier in the development of soft robotics.

Di et al. [34]—"Soft Robots for Space Exploration": Discussed the potential of soft robotics for space exploration, addressing unique challenges such as radiation and extreme temperatures. This paper highlighted the advantages of soft robots in extraterrestrial environments.

Hegde et al. [35]—"Next-Generation Soft Robots: Trends and Challenges": Provided an overview of emerging trends and ongoing challenges in the development of next-generation soft robots. This paper discussed the future directions of the field and the obstacles that need to be overcome.

Hoang et al. [36]—"Soft Robotics in Healthcare: Innovations and Applications": Reviewed recent innovations in soft robotics for healthcare, including rehabilitation and assistive devices. This study highlighted the potential of soft robotics to improve healthcare outcomes.

Zhou et al. [37]—"Sustainable Materials for Soft Robotics": Investigated the use of sustainable and biodegradable materials in soft robotics, addressing environmental concerns. This paper discussed the advantages of using eco-friendly materials in the development of soft robots.

Thuruthel et al. [38]—"Soft Robots with Advanced Control Systems": Discussed advancements in control systems for soft robots, improving their precision and responsiveness. This study highlighted the importance of control systems in enhancing the functionality of soft robotic systems.

2.2 WHAT IS A SOFT ROBOT

A soft robot is a type of robot constructed from highly compliant materials such as silicone, rubber, or other polymers. Unlike traditional rigid robots made from metals and hard plastics, soft robots are designed to mimic the flexibility and adaptability of biological organisms. They often utilize pneumatic or hydraulic actuators to achieve movement and can deform and reshape themselves to navigate through complex environments or interact safely with humans. Soft robots can bend, stretch, and deform, allowing them to squeeze through tight spaces or conform to different shapes [39].

The compliant materials used in soft robots make them safer to interact with humans compared to rigid robots, reducing the risk of injury. They can adapt to uncertain and changing environments more effectively than rigid robots, making them suitable for tasks such as search and rescue in disaster zones or medical applications inside the human body. Many soft robots are inspired by biological organisms like octopuses or worms, which naturally exhibit soft and flexible movements. Applications of soft robots span various fields including healthcare (such as surgical robotics), exploration (like planetary rovers), and industry (for handling delicate objects). Their development represents a growing area of robotics research focused on creating more versatile and safe robotic systems. Figure 2.1 depicts the soft robots inspired by nature and biology, as many insects roam in the atmosphere without any connections; the same concept has been copied and mobile-based soft robots are developed.

2.3 ACTUATION OF A SOFT ROBOT

Pneumatic Networks (PneuNets) [41] are a class of soft actuators that have gained significant attention in the field of soft robotics. These actuators are made from a soft material, usually an elastomer, containing channels

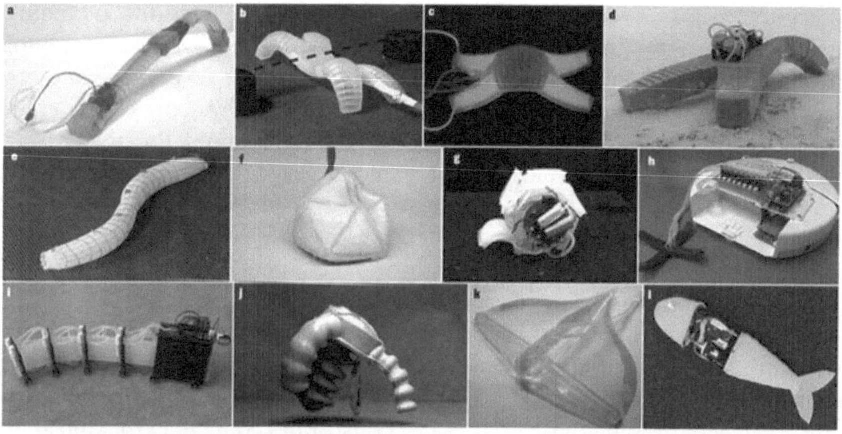

Figure 2.1 Mobile soft-robotic systems inspired nature and biology systems. (a) Based on Caterpillar. (b) Quadruped multi-gait. (c) Active camouflage. (d) Walking. (e) Worm-inspired. (f) Particle-jamming. (g) Rolling. (h) A hybrid hard–soft robot. (i) Snake-inspired. (j) Jumping. (k) Manta-ray. (l) Autonomous fish [40].

and chambers through which pressurized fluids flow. When these chambers receive pressure, the fluid inside creates internal stress within the material. This stress causes the material to stretch and deform, allowing the actuator to move.

The motion of these actuators is regulated by adjusting both the configuration of the internal chambers and the characteristics of the material comprising their walls. For example, in a PneuNets actuator made from a single, uniform elastomer, most expansion will occur in the thinnest sections, thus determining the robot's movement based on the microfluidic circuit's design. Alternatively, manipulating materials with different elastic properties allows for additional control over actuator behavior as shown in Figure 2.2. This is accomplished by integrating layers of materials with varied elasticity, such as a "strain limiting layer" that restricts the extent of deformation possible. This differential effect in strain enables precise motions like bending and twisting to be achieved.

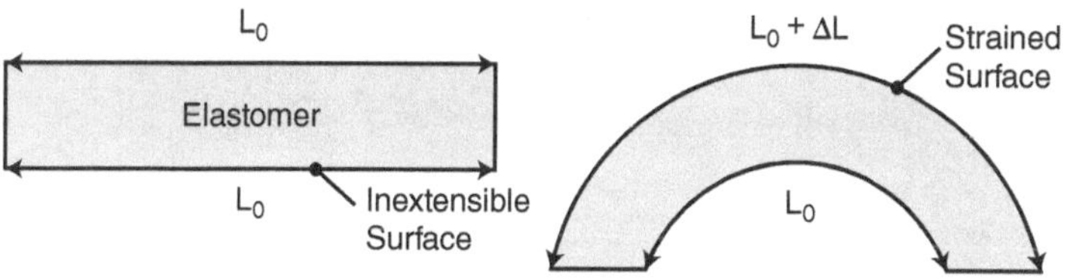

Figure 2.2 Elastomer is a member of PneuNets family.

PneuNets have been successfully used in various applications, including assistive gloves for hand rehabilitation and quadruped robots capable of multiple modes of locomotion. These soft robots offer several advantages over traditional rigid robots, including the ability to operate in delicate environments and provide nonlinear motion with simple inputs. PneuNets are a versatile class of soft actuators that can be designed to achieve specific motions by controlling the geometry of the embedded chambers and the material properties of their walls. Their ability to operate in delicate environments and provide nonlinear motion makes them an attractive option for various applications in soft robotics.

Figure 2.3 illustrates the principle of unidirectional bending in a PneuNets actuator. The actuator consists of two layers: an extensible outer layer and an inextensible constraint layer. When pressurized, the outer layer expands, causing its length to increase by ΔL. The constraint layer, being inextensible, remains unchanged in length. This difference in length between the two layers results in the bending of the actuator. This bending is the fundamental motion of fluidic elastomer robots, which are typically composed of two parts: the outer layer containing the channels and chambers, and the constraint layer, which is more rigid and prevents excessive deformation. In practice, these soft robots are often made from two silicone elastomers: Ecoflex and polydimethylsiloxane (PDMS) [42]. These materials bond well together, have different rigidity levels, are easy to mold, and are relatively inexpensive. PDMS has a Shore A hardness of 50, while Ecoflex [43] has a hardness below the Shore A scale, meaning it fractures only above a maximum strain of 900%. This makes PDMS suitable for the constraint layer, which should have limited deformation, while Ecoflex is more flexible and suitable for the outer layer.

Instead of varying the rigidity of elastomers, alternative methods can be employed to regulate the movement of actuators. For example, a single elastomer actuator can incorporate a constraint layer made of materials such as fibers, paper, or plastic film to impart the necessary inextensibility for actuation. Another approach involves fiber-reinforced actuators, where a basic PneuNet actuator is wrapped with these inextensible reinforcements, providing precise control over its motion.

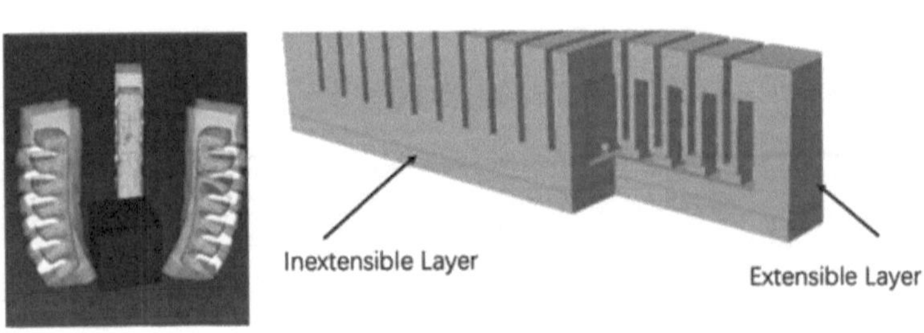

Figure 2.3 Structure of PneuNets [44].

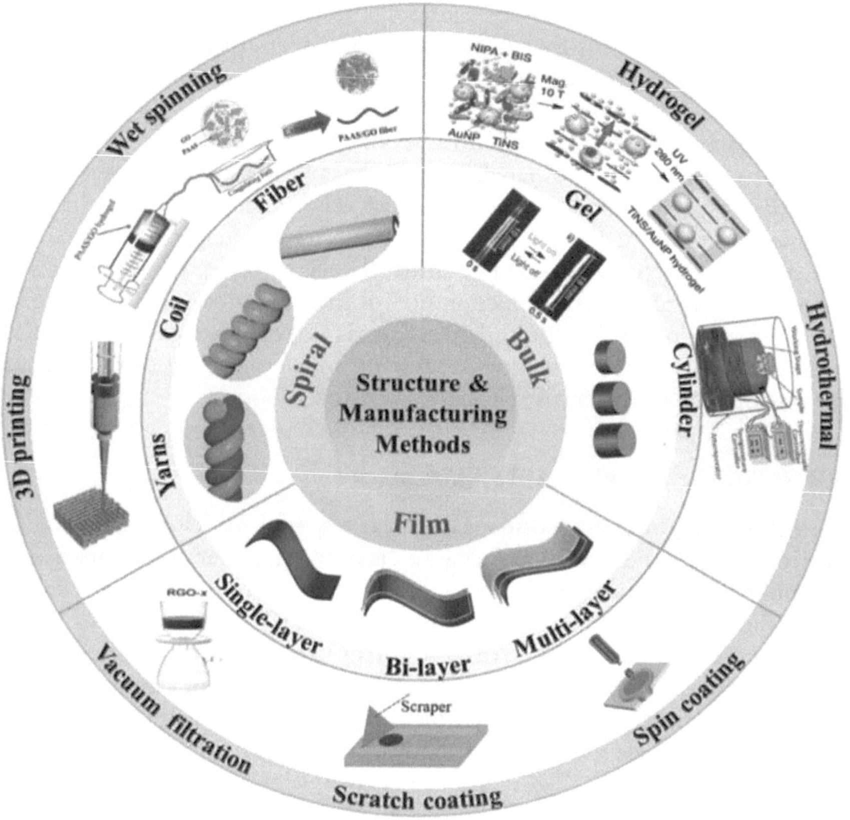

Figure 2.4 Diagrammatic representation of the structure and fabrication process of the light-responsive actuator [45].

The hardness of materials, particularly polymers, elastomers, and rubbers, is measured using the Shore hardness scale. This scale ranges from 0 Shore (indicating a 2.5 mm indentation depth) to 100 Shore (0 mm indentation depth). The most recognized scales are Shore A, used for softer plastics, and Shore D, used for harder materials. Figure 2.4 depicts the various manufacturing processes involved in light responsive actuators.

2.3.1 Photosensitive actuators

Photosensitive actuators are a type of actuator that responds to light stimuli for generating mechanical motion or deformation. These actuators typically utilize materials that change their shape or properties in response to light exposure. Certain polymers can undergo reversible changes in shape, size, or stiffness when exposed to light of specific wavelengths which are called Photo Responsive Polymers. This property is often utilized to create actuators that can bend, twist, or contract in response to light. Liquid crystal elastomers are materials that combine the properties of liquid crystals and elastomers, where exposure to light can trigger changes in molecular alignment and thus cause mechanical deformation.

Nanomaterials like carbon nanotubes or quantum dots can be incorporated into elastomers or other flexible substrates. When illuminated, these nanomaterials can generate localized heat or induce structural changes, leading to actuation. Applications of photosensitive actuators include adaptive optics, where they are used to adjust the shape of lenses or mirrors; in soft robotics for light-driven locomotion or manipulation; and in biomedical devices for controlled drug delivery or tissue stimulation. The development of photosensitive actuators represents an exciting area of research at the intersection of materials science, optics, and robotics.

2.3.2 Dielectric elastomer actuators

Dielectric elastomer actuators (DEAs) are a type of electromechanical device that uses the deformation of an elastomeric material in response to an applied electric field. These actuators consist of a thin elastomeric membrane sandwiched between compliant electrodes. When a voltage is applied across the electrodes, the electrostatic forces cause the membrane to compress or expand, resulting in mechanical motion. DEAs are known for their high energy density, large deformations, and rapid response times. They find applications in areas such as soft robotics, haptic interfaces, adaptive optics, and biomedical devices. Figure 2.5 depicts the DEAs.

2.3.3 Combustion-driven actuators

Combustion-driven actuators connect the energy released during combustion to produce mechanical movement or force. These actuators typically involve a controlled combustion process within a chamber or cylinder, where the rapid expansion of gases generated by combustion drives a piston or other mechanical components. They rely on burning a fuel, such as gas, liquid fuel, or solid propellant, to create high-pressure gases or thermal expansion. The energy released from combustion is converted into mechanical motion, which can be used for various purposes such as driving pumps,

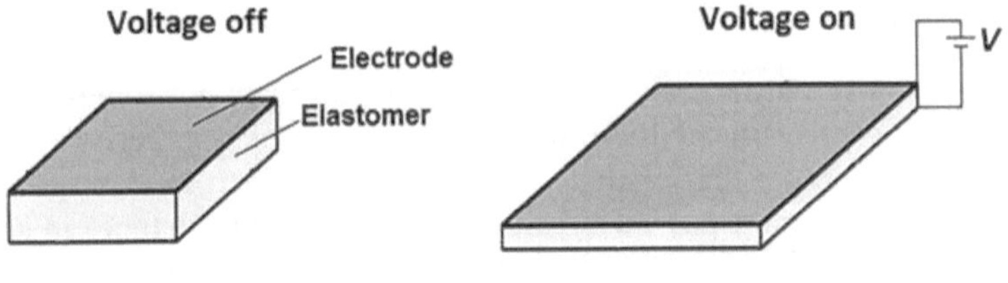

Figure 2.5 Dielectric elastomer actuators [46].

actuating valves, or moving mechanical limbs. Combustion-driven actuators often require sophisticated control systems to manage fuel injection, ignition timing, and combustion dynamics to achieve desired performance and reliability.

Applications of combustion-driven actuators range from internal combustion engines in vehicles and aircraft to specialized actuators in robotics, aerospace propulsion systems, and industrial automation. They offer advantages such as high power density and efficiency but require careful management of combustion processes to ensure safety and optimal performance.

2.4 ADVANCES IN SMART ROBOTIC MATERIAL TECHNOLOGIES

Recent advances in smart robotic materials have focused on enhancing functionality, durability, and adaptability. Researchers are integrating multiple functionalities into single materials with multifunctional materials, such as combining sensing, actuation, and self-healing capabilities. This integration simplifies robotic design and improves overall performance. Future research aims to further enhance the performance and expand the functionalities of multifunctional materials. This includes improving their efficiency, scalability, and reliability across a broader range of robotic systems and applications.

Materials that respond to various stimuli, such as light, heat, or magnetic fields, continue to advance. For example, light-responsive polymers can undergo reversible changes in shape or stiffness when exposed to specific wavelengths, enabling precise control in soft robotics. Advances in self-healing materials allow robotic components to repair damage autonomously, extending their operational lifespan and reducing maintenance costs. Self-healing polymers use mechanisms like reversible chemical bonds or microcapsules containing healing agents. Flexible and stretchable electronics enable seamless integration of sensors and actuators into soft robotic systems. These advancements facilitate the development of wearable robotics and healthcare devices that conform to the body's movements.

Energy harvesting materials, such as piezoelectric or triboelectric materials, convert mechanical motion or vibrations into electrical energy. This technology enables robots to operate autonomously for extended periods without external power sources. Biomimetic materials that mimic properties found in nature, such as adhesion mechanisms of geckos or the flexibility of muscles, are being developed. These materials enhance robotic agility and interaction capabilities in complex environments. Materials designed to withstand extreme environmental conditions, such as temperature fluctuations or exposure to chemicals, are crucial for robotics in aerospace, underwater exploration, and industrial applications. Biotechnology and nanotechnology fields will contribute to advancements in materials science and manufacturing processes, potentially leading to stronger, lighter, and more sustainable materials.

2.5 ADVANCED MANUFACTURING TECHNIQUES

Innovations in additive manufacturing (3D printing) and nanotechnology allow for precise fabrication of complex structures with smart materials integrated directly into the design. This enables rapid prototyping and customization of robotic components. Conventional and unconventional machining help fabricate different parts as per the design choice; there are no design constraints in terms of manufacturing. The integration of electronics gives more adaptable and sophisticated easiness in manufacturing.

Factories will be increasingly interconnected, with Internet of Things devices monitoring and optimizing every aspect of production in real time. This will lead to predictive maintenance, improved supply chain management, and overall efficiency gains. Advances in AI and robotics will enable more personalized and on-demand manufacturing, where products are tailored to individual customer needs with shorter lead times.

Advanced manufacturing techniques encompass a diverse array of cutting-edge technologies and methodologies aimed at enhancing productivity, efficiency, and innovation across various industries with a variety of AR VR tools which are shown in Figure 2.6.

Selective Laser Melting (SLM) and Electron Beam Melting (EBM) processes use high-energy sources to selectively melt and fuse metal powders

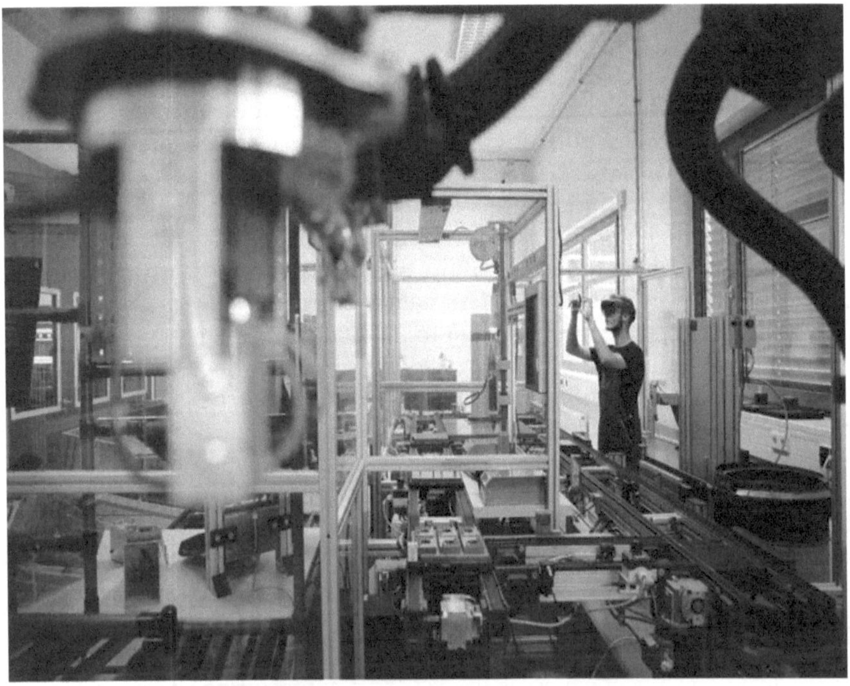

Figure 2.6 VR-based manufacturing system lab [47].

layer by layer, enabling complex geometries and reducing material waste; also, stereolithography (SLA) and Digital Light Processing (DLP) techniques use photopolymerization to create 3D objects layer by layer from liquid resin, offering high resolution and accuracy. Collaborative Robots (Cobots) are designed to work alongside human workers, enhancing productivity and safety in manufacturing environments. Automated Guided Vehicles (AGVs) and Autonomous Mobile Robots (AMRs) are used for material handling, logistics, and assembly tasks in smart factories. Digital twin is a virtual representation of a physical product or process that allows for real-time monitoring, simulation, and optimization, reducing time to market and improving product quality.

Computer-Aided Design (CAD) and Computer-Aided Manufacturing (CAM) are possible with the integration of design and manufacturing processes using advanced software tools for rapid prototyping and production. Integration of sensors, data analytics, and AI is used to monitor production processes, predict maintenance needs, and optimize resource utilization. Techniques for minimizing defects and variations in manufacturing processes ensure consistent product quality. Utilization of biological systems, such as cells or enzymes, to produce pharmaceuticals, biofuels, and other bioproducts offer sustainable and eco-friendly manufacturing solutions.

2.6 TRENDS IN DESIGN AND ANALYSIS OF SOFT ROBOTS

There are many changes due to the advancement of AI, and machine learning across various disciplines is expected to undergo transformative advancements driven by technological innovations, societal needs, and environmental considerations. Sustainable and circular design practices will increasingly prioritize sustainability, aiming to minimize environmental impact throughout the product lifecycle. This includes using recycled materials, designing for disassembly and recycling, and promoting circular economy principles.

Advances in biotechnology and bioengineering will enable designers to create products using living organisms or biological processes. This could lead to bio-inspired materials, biodegradable products, and even living systems integrated into architecture and consumer goods. Designers will have access to a broader range of advanced materials, including nanoengineered materials with superior properties such as strength, flexibility, and conductivity. These materials will enable innovative and functional designs across industries.

The integration of digital tools such as generative design, AI, and virtual reality will revolutionize the design process which leads to digital design and manufacturing. Designers will be able to simulate and optimize products in virtual environments before physical production, reducing time to market and costs.

Customization and personalization of design will be increased due to advancemnt of image processing and data analytics. Design will become more personalized and tailored to individual needs and preferences. Technologies like 3D printing and digital fabrication will enable on-demand production of customized products, ranging from consumer goods to medical devices.

Products and environments will be designed to be smarter and more interactive, incorporating sensors, actuators, and IoT connectivity. This will enhance functionality, usability, and user experience, leading to more intuitive and responsive designs. Augmented Reality, Xtended Reality, Mixed Reality, and Virtual Reality technologies will transform the way designers visualize and communicate their ideas. Designers will use these technologies for immersive design reviews, virtual prototyping, and collaborative design sessions across global teams.

Human-centered design and accessibility is a major advantage in soft robots' design. Designers will increasingly focus on creating inclusive and accessible products and environments. This includes designing for diverse abilities and ensuring that products are intuitive and easy to use for all users. Urban design will evolve to address challenges such as climate change, urbanization, and resource scarcity. Designs will prioritize sustainable cities, green infrastructure, and resilient architecture that integrates renewable energy and smart technologies. Designers will consider ethical implications and societal impact in their design decisions. This includes addressing issues such as equity, social justice, and inclusivity, ensuring that designs contribute positively to the well-being of individuals and communities.

2.7 FUTURE DIRECTIONS AND CHALLENGES

Soft robotics is a rapidly evolving field, with ongoing research focused on improving the design, fabrication, and control of soft robots.

- **Materials Science:** Developing new materials with improved properties, such as strength, durability, and flexibility, is crucial for advancing the field of soft robotics. The smart and environmental materials play a crucial role in the use of personalized soft robots. The design flexibility for material is a major advantage in the design and manufacturing of robotic systems. Researchers are exploring novel materials with tailored mechanical properties, such as shape-memory polymers, liquid crystal elastomers, and hydrogels. These materials enable soft robots to mimic natural movements more effectively and adapt to complex environments.
- **Actuation and Sensing Mechanisms:** Improving the design and performance of actuators and sensors is essential for enhancing the dexterity and adaptability of soft robots. Developing control systems that

can effectively manage the imprecise feedback data and unpredictable reaction times of soft robots is a significant challenge.

- **Scalability and Integration:** Scaling up soft robots to larger sizes and integrating them with other systems, such as rigid robots or computer systems, are necessary for their widespread adoption.
- **Bibliometric Analysis:** To better understand the intellectual structures and emerging trends in soft robotics, we conducted a bibliometric analysis of the most influential publications and authors in the field. Our analysis included a review of the top 10 most cited papers in soft robotics, which highlighted key advancements and challenges in the field. We also analyzed the most productive authors and institutions in soft robotics, identifying trends and patterns in the field.
- **Bio-inspired Design:** There is a growing trend toward bio-inspired soft robots that mimic the structures and functionalities of biological organisms. Examples include soft grippers inspired by octopus' tentacles and soft actuators that replicate muscle-like movements.
- **Soft Sensing and Actuation:** Advances in sensors and actuators have improved the capabilities of soft robots to perceive and interact with their environment. This includes stretchable sensors, flexible electronics, and pneumatic/hydraulic actuators that enable precise and responsive control.
- **Autonomy and Control:** Developing robust control strategies for soft robots remains a significant focus. This includes adaptive control algorithms, machine learning techniques for learning and adaptation, and integration with AI for autonomous decision-making.

2.8 CONCLUSIONS

Recent advances and emerging trends in soft robotics showcase a field rapidly advancing toward practical applications and transformative impacts. The convergence of diverse disciplines—materials science, biomechanics, robotics, and AI—has been instrumental. This collaboration has driven breakthroughs in sensor technologies, actuation mechanisms, and control systems, propelling the field forward. Drawing inspiration from nature has yielded robots capable of mimicking complex biological movements and behaviors. This biomimetic approach not only enhances performance but also opens new avenues for applications in healthcare, exploration, and beyond. Despite significant progress, challenges such as power efficiency, robustness, and scalability persist. Addressing these challenges will require continued research investment, technological innovation, and collaboration across academia, industry, and regulatory bodies. As soft robots use electronic-based actuation systems and in some cases autonomous systems, they can be hacked; thus, network and ethical hacking have lot of potential to grow in coming years.

REFERENCES

[1] Pal, A., Restrepo, V., Goswami, D., & Martinez, R. V. (2021). Exploiting mechanical instabilities in soft robotics: Control, sensing, and actuation. *Advanced Materials*, 33(19), 2006939.

[2] Han, W., Gao, W., & Wang, X. (2024). Enhanced magnetic soft robotics: Integrating fiber optics and 3D printing for rapid actuation and precision sensing. *ACS Applied Materials & Interfaces*. 16(23). https://doi.org/10.1021/acsami.4c04586

[3] AboZaid, Y. A., Aboelrayat, M. T., Fahim, I. S., & Radwan, A. G. (2024). Soft robotic grippers: A review on technologies, materials, and applications. *Sensors and Actuators A: Physical*, 372, 115380. https://doi.org/10.1016/j.sna.2024.115380

[4] Ambaye, G., Boldsaikhan, E., & Krishnan, K. (2024). Soft robot design, manufacturing, and operation challenges: A review. *Journal of Manufacturing and Materials Processing*, 8(2), 79.

[5] Toepperwein, L. L., Blackmon, M. T., Fukui, R., Park, W. T., Pollard, B., & General Dynamics Fort Worth TX Fort Worth DIV. (1980). *ICAM robotics application guide (RAG)* (p. 0222). General Dynamics Corporation. Forth Worth Division.

[6] Greenwood, N. R. (1980). *The Design and Development of a Flexible Manufacturing System*. The University of Manchester (United Kingdom).

[7] Hagerty, J. J. (1980). Process Development for Automated Solar Cell and Module Production: Task 4: Automated Array Assembly, Quarterly Report No. 1. US Department of Energy, Solar Energy.

[8] Hirose, S. (1993). Biologically inspired robots. *Snake-Like Locomotors and Manipulators*. Robotica, 12(3), 282, https://doi.org/10.1017/S0263574700017264

[9] Arnold, S. C., Pratt, L. M., Khan, S. M., Li, J., & Khan, I. M. (1995, May). Functional polymers: materials for smart structures. In *Smart Structures and Materials 1995: Smart Materials* (Vol. 2441, pp. 23–32). SPIE.

[10] Lauer, W., Schonhardt, J., & Voges, U. (1995). Vibration analysis for tactile sensing. *IFAC Proceedings Volumes*, 28(20), 125–130.

[11] Dario, P., Carrozza, M. C., Benvenuto, A., & Menciassi, A. (2000). Microsystems in biomedical applications. *Journal of Micromechanics and Microengineering*, 10(2), 235.

[12] Choi, H. R., Jung, K., Ryew, S., Nam, J. D., Jeon, J., Koo, J. C., & Tanie, K. (2005). Biomimetic soft actuator: Design, modeling, control, and applications. *IEEE/ASME Transactions on Mechatronics*, 10(5), 581–593.

[13] Amiet, A. R., Edwards, D. P., Ibrahim, M. E., Mart, P. L., McAdam, G., St John, N. A., & Truong, V. T. (2010). Exploitation of smart materials and sensors as disruptive technologies. March 2024E3S Web of Conferences. DOI: 10.1051/e3sconf/202450501034

[14] Sitti, M., Menciassi, A., Ijspeert, A. J., Low, K. H., & Kim, S. (2013). Survey and introduction to the focused section on bio-inspired mechatronics. *IEEE/ASME Transactions on Mechatronics*, 18(2), 409–418.

[15] Kim, S., Laschi, C., & Trimmer, B. (2013). Soft robotics: a bioinspired evolution in robotics. *Trends in Biotechnology*, 31(5), 287–294.

[16] Shepherd, R. F., Ilievski, F., Choi, W., Morin, S. A., Stokes, A. A., Mazzeo, A. D., & Whitesides, G. M. (2011). Multigait soft robot. *Proceedings of the National Academy of Sciences*, 108(51), 20400–20403.

[17] Semini, C., Tsagarakis, N. G., Guglielmino, E., Focchi, M., Cannella, F., & Caldwell, D. G. (2011). Design of HyQ–a hydraulically and electrically actuated quadruped robot. *Proceedings of the Institution of Mechanical Engineers, Part I: Journal of Systems and Control Engineering*, 225(6), 831–849.

[18] Majidi, C. (2014). Soft robotics: a perspective—current trends and prospects for the future. *Soft Robotics*, 1(1), 5–11.

[19] Shintake, J., Ming, A., & Shimojo, M. (2011, September). A novel propulsion method of flexible underwater robots. In *2011 IEEE/RSJ international conference on intelligent robots and systems* (pp. 4735–4740). IEEE.

[20] Li, T., Nakajima, K., Kuba, M., Gutnick, T., Hochner, B., & Pfeifer, R. (2011). From the octopus to soft robots control: an octopus inspired behavior control architecture for soft robots. *Vie Et Milieu*, 61(4), 211–217.

[21] Iida, F., & Laschi, C. (2011). Soft robotics: Challenges and perspectives. *Procedia Computer Science*, 7, 99–102.

[22] Kramer, R. K., Majidi, C., & Wood, R. J. (2011, May). Wearable tactile keypad with stretchable artificial skin. In *2011 IEEE International Conference on Robotics and Automation* (pp. 1103–1107). IEEE.

[23] Lipomi, D. J., & Bao, Z. (2011). Stretchable, elastic materials and devices for solar energy conversion. *Energy & Environmental Science*, 4(9), 3314–3328.

[24] Cianchetti M, Licofonte A, Follador M, Rogai F, Laschi C. Bioinspired Soft Actuation System Using Shape Memory Alloys. *Actuators*. 2014; 3(3):226–244. https://doi.org/10.3390/act3030226

[25] Connolly, F., Polygerinos, P., Walsh, C. J., & Bertoldi, K. (2015). Mechanical programming of soft actuators by varying fiber angle. *Soft Robotics*, 2(1), 26–32.

[26] Miriyev, A., Trujillo, C., Caires, G., & Lipson, H. (2018). Rejuvenation of soft material–actuator. *MRS Communications*, 8(2), 556–561.

[27] Decroly G, Toncheva A, Blanc L, Raquez J-M, Lessinnes T, Delchambre A, & Lambert P. Programmable Stimuli-Responsive Actuators for Complex Motions in Soft Robotics: Concept, Design and Challenges. *Actuators*. 2020; 9(4):131. https://doi.org/10.3390/act9040131

[28] Romano, J., Lazzari, F., Garavaglia, L., & Pittaccio, S. (2020). Alternative design strategy and multi-material integration in the development of biologically-inspired soft robots: a proof-of-concept. *Smart Materials and Structures*, 29(12), 125016.

[29] Ren, L., Li, B., Wei, G., Wang, K., Song, Z., Wei, Y., & Liu, Q. (2021). Biology and bioinspiration of soft robotics: Actuation, sensing, and system integration. *Iscience*, 24(9), pp 1–22.

[30] Wang, H., Zhu, Z., Jin, H., Wei, R., Bi, L., & Zhang, W. (2022). Magnetic soft robots: Design, actuation, and function. *Journal of Alloys and Compounds*, 922, 166219.

[31] Gu, G., Zhang, N., Chen, C., Xu, H., & Zhu, X. (2023). Soft robotics enables neuroprosthetic hand design. *ACS Nano*, 17(11), 9661–9672.

[32] Guo, X., Li, W., Fang, F., Chen, H., Zhao, L., Fang, X., & Zhang, W. (2023). Encoded sewing soft textile robots. Science *Advances*, 10(1), eadk3855.

[33] Girerd C., Alvarez A., Hawkes E. W. & Morimoto T. K. "Material Scrunching Enables Working Channels in Miniaturized Vine-Inspired Robots," in *IEEE Transactions on Robotics*, vol. 40, pp. 2166–2180, 2024, doi: 10.1109/TRO.2024.3370088

[34] Di, Y., Zhang, Y., Wen, Y., & Ren, Y. (2024). Modeling and optimization of motion for inchworm-inspired magnetically driven soft robot. *Robotica*, 42(1), 72–86.

[35] Hegde, C., Mysa, R. C., Chooi, A., Dontu, S., Tan, J. M. R., Wong, L. H., ... & Magdassi, S. (2024). 3D-printed mechano-optic force sensor for soft robotic gripper enabled by programmable structural metamaterials. *Advanced Intelligent Systems*, 6(9). https://doi.org/10.1002/aisy.202400057

[36] Hoang, T. T., Nguyen, C. C., Phan, P. T., Davies, J., Tran, H. A., Thai, M. T., Truong, V. K., Nguyen, T. K., Vo-Doan, T. T., Phan, H. P., Lovell, N. H., & Do, T. N. (2024). Shape Programmable and Multifunctional Soft Textile Muscles for Wearable and Soft Robotics. *Advanced Intelligent Systems*, 6(9), 2300875. https://doi.org/10.1002/aisy.202300875

[37] Zhou, S., Li, Y., Wang, Q., & Lyu, Z. (2024). Integrated actuation and sensing: Toward intelligent soft robots. *Cyborg and Bionic Systems*, 5, 0105.

[38] Thuruthel, T. G., Falotico, E., Renda, F., & Laschi, C. (2017). Learning dynamic models for open loop predictive control of soft robotic manipulators. *Bioinspiration & Biomimetics*, 12(6), 066003.

[39] Conrad, S., Teichmann, J., Auth, P., Knorr, N., Ulrich, K., Bellin, D. & Tauber, F. J. (2024). 3D-printed digital pneumatic logic for the control of soft robotic actuators. *Science Robotics*, 9(86), eadh4060.

[40] Rus, Daniela & Tolley, Michael. (2015). Design, fabrication and control of soft robots. *Nature*. 521. 467–475. doi:10.1038/nature14543

[41] Liu, Z., Wang, F., Liu, S., Tian, Y., & Zhang, D. (2020). Modeling and analysis of soft pneumatic network bending actuators. *IEEE/ASME Transactions on Mechatronics*, 26(4), 2195–2203.

[42] Mata, A., Fleischman, A. J., & Roy, S. (2005). Characterization of polydimethylsiloxane (PDMS) properties for biomedical micro/nanosystems. *Biomedical Microdevices*, 7, 281–293.

[43] Bergeron, V., Cooper, P., Fischer, C., Giermanska-Kahn, J., Langevin, D., & Pouchelon, A. (1997). Polydimethylsiloxane (PDMS)-based antifoams. *Colloids and Surfaces A: Physicochemical and Engineering Aspects*, 122(1–3), 103–120.

[44] Su, Hang, Hou, Xu, Zhang, Xin, Qi, Wen, Cai, Shuting, Xiong, Xiaoming, & Guo, Jing. (2022). Pneumatic soft robots: Challenges and benefits. *Actuators*. 11. 92. doi: 10.3390/act11030092

[45] Huang, Yaoli, Yu, Qinghua, Su, Chuanli, Jiang, Jinhua, Chen, Nanliang, & Shao, Huiqi. (2021). Light-responsive soft actuators: Mechanism, materials, fabrication, and applications. *Actuators*. 10. 298. doi: 10.3390/act10110298

[46] https://softroboticstoolkit.com/book/dielectric-elastomer-actuators

[47] https://www.smeef.org/about-smeef/blog/industry-4.0-advanced-technology-creates-new-job-opportunities

Chapter 3

Soft Robotic Treatment for Club Foot

Shaik Himam Saheb and A. Chandrashekhar

3.1 INTRODUCTION

Clubfoot is a medical term that usually defines the range of condition of the abnormality of the foot which is present at birth. In this condition, the foot of the baby is not in its exact position or orientation. Different characteristics for this abnormality may be present which may vary from mild to severe. Foot of the baby (in most cases the heel) is usually smaller than normal. The orientation of the foot may be downward. The front part of the foot is sometimes inclined toward the other foot. In some cases, foot will also turn inner side and in few cases the bottom of the foot may also turn upwards. Clubfoot is not a painful abnormality but it should be treated at the beginning stage or few months after the birth of the baby as this abnormality can cause many problems after baby grows. The early treatment also helps the babies to lead a normal life from their childhood. Clubfoot, also known as congenital talipes equinovarus, is a birth defect where a baby's foot is twisted out of shape or position. It affects the bones, muscles, and tendons in the foot and ankle. The condition can vary in severity from mild to severe and usually affects one foot, or both feet [1, 2].

Filariasis, a neglected tropical disease, can lead to severe and debilitating conditions such as lymphedema and elephantiasis. One of the common complications associated with filariasis is clubfoot, a complex deformity of the foot and ankle. Traditional treatments for clubfoot, including surgery and rigid orthotic devices, have had limited success, often requiring extensive rehabilitation and clinical supervision [3]. In recent years, the emergence of soft robotic technologies has shown promise in providing more effective and accessible treatment options for individuals with clubfoot, particularly in the context of filariasis. Soft robotic devices, such as exosuits and exoskeletons, offer a number of advantages over traditional rigid devices [4]. Soft robotic devices are typically lighter, more compliant, and easier to manufacture than their rigid counterparts [5]. This makes them more comfortable and easier to use, reducing the dependence on clinical resources and enabling patients to engage in rehabilitation activities independently [6]. Additionally, the inherent compliance of soft robotic devices can better

DOI: 10.1201/9781003539612-3

accommodate the unique biomechanics of the clubfoot, providing more natural and personalized support during movement. Recent research has explored the use of soft robotic devices for the rehabilitation of clubfoot in filariasis patients [7]. These devices often incorporate sensors and monitoring capabilities to track patient progress and inform treatment decisions [8].

3.2 CLUBFOOT

Clubfoot is result of position of the baby in the mother's womb in few cases along with combination of external factors like environmental and genital which is not yet well understood. In few cases it was also evident that in a family if a person has clubfoot, then the abnormality was also seen in infants. Beyond the foot problem clubfoot also affect muscles, nervous system, bone system and also a huge chance of brain stroke or injury [9–12].

Clubfoot, also known as talipes equinovarus [13], is a congenital condition where one or both feet are twisted inward and downward. This abnormal positioning can range from mild to severe and typically affects both the bones and muscles of the foot and lower leg. Clubfoot occurs in approximately 1 in 1,000 live births and is more common in males than females. The exact cause of clubfoot is not fully understood, but it is believed to result from a combination of genetic and environmental factors. The clubfoot and the normal foot are shown in Figure 3.1.

The treatment of clubfoot has traditionally relied on methods such as casting, bracing, and surgical intervention. However, recent advancements in soft robotics offer innovative approaches that could complement or enhance traditional treatments. Soft robotics, which focuses on creating robots with flexible and adaptive materials, can provide tailored and dynamic solutions for clubfoot correction [14]. Soft robotics uses materials

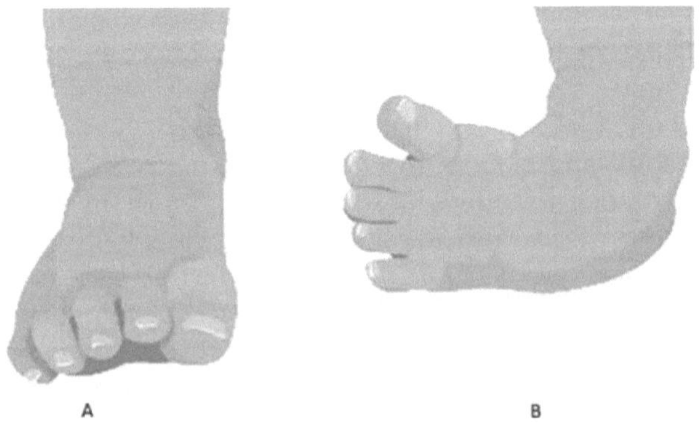

Figure 3.1 (a) Normal foot and (b) clubfoot.

such as silicone, rubber, or other flexible polymers to create robotic devices that can conform to and interact gently with the human body. These materials can mimic biological tissues' flexibility and adaptability, making them suitable for applications in medical treatments [15–18].

Soft robotic devices can conform to the irregular and changing shape of the foot, offering a more customized treatment. Flexible materials can provide a more comfortable experience compared to rigid casts and braces. Soft robotic systems can adjust dynamically to accommodate growth and changes in foot shape.

3.2.1 Reasons for clubfoot

Clubfoot is a congenital condition, meaning it is present at birth, and its exact cause is not fully understood. However, several factors are believed to contribute to the development of clubfoot.

- **Genetic Factors:** There is evidence to suggest that clubfoot may have a genetic component. It tends to run in families, and children with a parent or sibling affected by clubfoot have a higher risk of developing the condition themselves. Multiple genes may be involved, and ongoing research is exploring the genetic basis of clubfoot [19].
- **Intrauterine Environment:** Factors during fetal development inside the womb can influence the development of clubfoot. It has been hypothesized that abnormal positioning of the fetus, intrauterine constraints, or restricted fetal movement may contribute to the development of clubfoot. The intrauterine environment can significantly influence the development of congenital conditions like clubfoot (congenital talipes equinovarus). Restricted Amniotic Fluid (Oligohydramnios) causes low levels of amniotic fluid that can limit the space available for fetal movement, potentially leading to deformities like clubfoot due to restricted movement and abnormal positioning. The fetus's position in the uterus, particularly if it's in a breech or unusual position, can result in compression of the limbs. This compression can influence the development of musculoskeletal structures and lead to deformities like clubfoot. Abnormalities in the shape or structure of the uterus (e.g., a bicornuate or septate uterus) can lead to restricted space or pressure on the fetus, contributing to deformities [20].
- **Twin or Higher-Order Pregnancies:** In multiple gestations, the limited space can increase the likelihood of abnormal limb positioning and compression, which might contribute to the development of clubfoot. The intrauterine environment interacts with genetic factors that may predispose the fetus to clubfoot. While not entirely understood, it is believed that both genetic susceptibility and environmental influences

can play a role. Certain maternal health conditions, such as diabetes or vascular issues, may influence the development of clubfoot. Exposure to certain medications, drugs, or alcohol during pregnancy may impact fetal development, potentially contributing to deformities like clubfoot. Family history and genetic predispositions can influence the likelihood of congenital deformities, including clubfoot. Genetic mutations or chromosomal abnormalities may interact with the intrauterine environment to cause clubfoot.

While some intrauterine factors may be difficult to control, proper prenatal care can help in early detection and management of potential issues. Regular ultrasounds and maternal health monitoring can assist in identifying risk factors and managing conditions that may contribute to clubfoot. Understanding the interplay between the intrauterine environment and congenital conditions like clubfoot can help in developing better preventative and therapeutic strategies [21].

- **Neurological Factors:** There is some evidence linking clubfoot with neurological abnormalities, although the exact nature of this relationship is not fully understood. Conditions such as spina bifida [22] (a neural tube defect) or certain neurological disorders may be associated with an increased risk of clubfoot.
- **Musculoskeletal Factors:** Abnormalities in the muscles, tendons, ligaments, or bones of the foot and lower leg may contribute to the development of clubfoot. These abnormalities can affect the positioning and alignment of the foot during fetal development.
- **Environmental Factors:** While genetic and developmental factors play a significant role, some environmental factors may also contribute to the risk of clubfoot. Maternal smoking or certain medications taken during pregnancy have been suggested as potential risk factors which may lead to clubfoot [23].

It's important to note that in many cases of clubfoot, no specific cause can be identified, and the condition is classified as idiopathic (without a clear cause). Research continues to investigate the underlying mechanisms of clubfoot to improve understanding and develop more effective treatments. Early diagnosis and treatment are key to achieving the best outcomes for children with clubfoot. Figure 3.2 shows various types of clubfeet across the world.

3.2.2 Symptoms of clubfoot

Clubfoot is not a painful abnormality but it should be treated at the beginning stage or few months after the birth of the baby as this abnormality can cause many problems after baby grows. As the foot is twisted from the normal position, it will make the leg shorter than the unaffected leg.

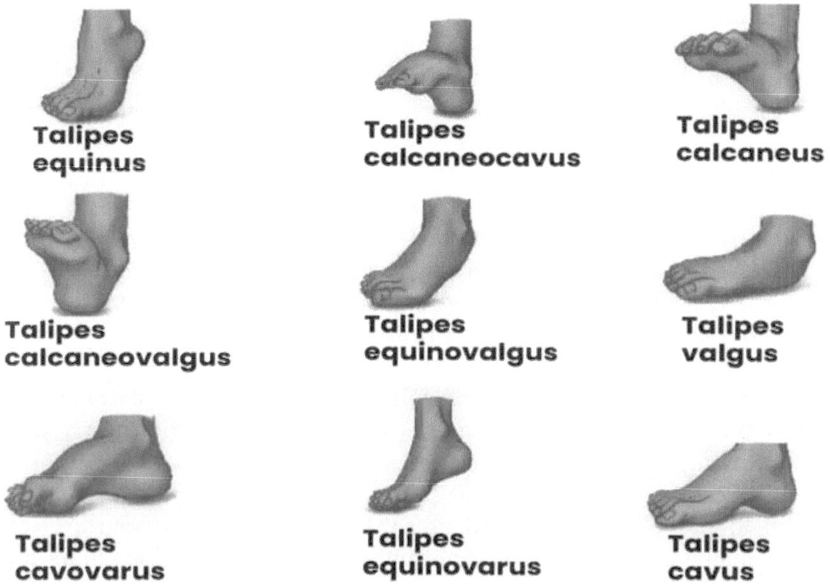

Figure 3.2 Different types of clubfeet [24].

3.3 THERE ARE TWO MAIN TYPES OF CLUBFOOT

3.3.1 Idiopathic clubfoot

Idiopathic clubfoot, also known as congenital talipes equinovarus (CTEV), is a common congenital deformity where a baby's foot is abnormally twisted [25]. The term "idiopathic "indicates that the condition arises without a known cause, distinguishing it from other forms of clubfoot that may be associated with genetic syndromes, neurological conditions, or other anomalies. This is the most common type, accounting for about 80% of cases. Idiopathic clubfoot occurs without any clear cause or associated genetic syndrome. It may affect one or both feet and can vary in severity. The characteristics of idiopathic clubfoot are as follows. Idiopathic clubfoot is typically diagnosed at birth through a physical examination [26]. The characteristic deformities are often evident. In some cases, the condition can be detected through prenatal ultrasound, although this is less common.

- **Foot Positioning:**
  a) Equinus: The foot is pointed downward.
  b) Varus: The heel is turned inward.
  c) Adductus: The front of the foot is turned inward.
  d) Cavus: The arch of the foot may be high, though this is less common.

- Appearance:
  a) The affected foot may look rotated internally at the ankle.
  b) The heel often does not touch the ground.
  c) The foot may be smaller or have a different shape compared to a normal foot.
- Treatment:

Early and effective treatment is crucial for optimal outcomes. Several methods are used to correct idiopathic clubfoot. The Ponseti method [27] is the most widely accepted treatment for idiopathic clubfoot. Below are the various techniques used in the Ponseti method

a) Serial Casting: The foot is gradually corrected through a series of casts applied every 1–2 weeks. Each cast manipulates the foot into a more normal position.
b) Tenotomy: A minor surgical procedure to release the tight Achilles tendon, typically performed after the casting phase if needed.
c) Bracing: after casting and tenotomy, the foot is maintained in its corrected position using a special brace (usually for 2–4 years) to prevent recurrence.

Surgery may be considered if the deformity does not respond to casting and bracing or if the condition is severe. Soft tissue release covers the processes like cutting and lengthening tight tendons and ligaments. Osteotomy process involves bone cutting and realignment may be necessary in severe cases.

3.3.2 Nonidiopathic clubfoot

Nonidiopathic clubfoot, also referred to as secondary or syndromic clubfoot, is a type of clubfoot that arises as a consequence of another underlying condition rather than occurring as an isolated deformity [28–30]. Unlike idiopathic clubfoot, which has no known associated conditions or clear cause, nonidiopathic clubfoot is associated with a range of syndromes or conditions that contribute to the development of the foot deformity. Causes and associations of nonidiopathic clubfoot are as follows:

- **Neuromuscular Conditions:** Cerebral palsy is due to neurological damage that affects muscle control and coordination, leading to deformities like clubfoot. Spina Bifida is due to this neural tube defect can disrupt normal spinal and limb development, often resulting in clubfoot among other musculoskeletal abnormalities.
- **Genetic Syndromes:** Down Syndrome—Trisomy 21 is characterized by a range of physical and developmental issues, including clubfoot. Arthrogryposis Multiplex Congenita (AMC) is a condition involving multiple joint contractures and limb deformities, including clubfoot.
- **Structural Anomalies:** Limb deformities causes other structural abnormalities in the limbs or bones, such as congenital limb reduction

defects, can be associated with nonidiopathic clubfoot. Skeletal dysplasia conditions that affect bone growth and development, resulting in various limb and skeletal deformities.

- **Chromosomal and Genetic Abnormalities:** Rare chromosomal or genetic abnormalities may lead to clubfoot as part of a broader spectrum of congenital anomalies. Maternal diabetes or vascular issue is a condition affecting the mother during pregnancy and can impact fetal development, leading to deformities including clubfoot. Certain medications, drugs, or toxins during pregnancy may contribute to the development of clubfoot along with other abnormalities. Nonidiopathic clubfoot presents a more complex clinical picture compared to idiopathic clubfoot, requiring a thorough and integrated approach to diagnosis and treatment.

  In nonsurgical Ponseti method [31] using the techniques like manipulations in a gentle manner and casting process, the leg of the infants can be corrected in time duration of about 6 to 9 weeks. This treatment can be successful only by getting a good understanding of the anatomy and functionality of the foot along with the knowledge of bones, ligaments, and muscles' reaction and responses that are seen during the process of manipulation and casting process. In this method treatment is started in the first or second week of the birth of the infants so as to take the benefit of the favorable elasticity of the tissues which are present in the foot. With the treatment the foot is moved by manipulating softly. After that, for casting, five to seven casts are used from the foot to the thigh. During casting knees should be at right angle. Following correction, the clubfoot deformity tends to relapse. To prevent relapses, when the last plaster cast is removed, a splint (bracing) must be worn full-time for 2–3 months and thereafter at night for 3–4 years.

Surgical correction of the feet means the correction when the child is unable to take the braces or if parents are not able to fulfill the cost requirements of bracing then the partial recurrence of the clubfoot happens. The heel cord and joint capsule in the back of the ankle may need to be released (limited posterior release), or a tendon that helps to move the foot may need to be repositioned (tibialis anterior tendon transfer).

Soft robotic braces can be designed to wrap around the foot and ankle, providing support and correction through adjustable, actuated elements. These devices use pneumatic actuators or shape-memory alloys (SMAs) to apply controlled forces to the foot. The device can be adjusted to apply gentle, corrective pressure to the foot, gradually moving it into the desired position. The system can be programmed to adjust the pressure based on the foot's response, ensuring effective and personalized treatment.

These systems can use soft robotic arms or appendages to manipulate the foot in a precise and controlled manner. They can be integrated with sensors to monitor the foot's position and adjust the forces applied. Soft robotic manipulators can perform gentle, corrective movements to gradually align

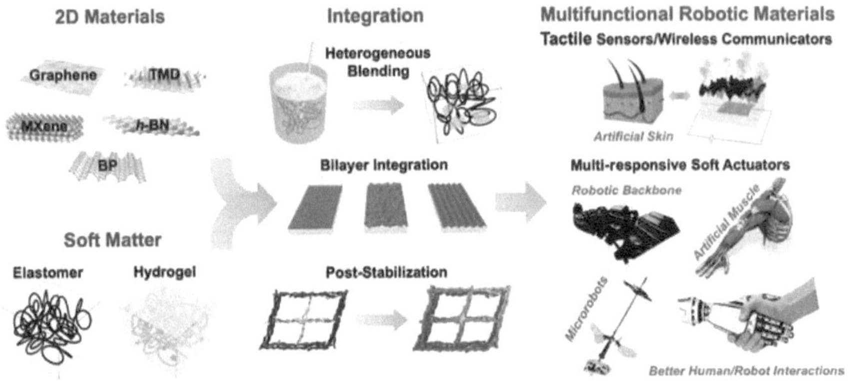

Figure 3.3 2D materials integration with soft materials for improved functionality and durability [37].

the foot. They can be used in conjunction with other treatments like casting or bracing, providing additional correction. Soft robotic footwear can incorporate flexible materials and actuators to dynamically adjust the shape and support of the shoe. Adaptive footwear can provide continuous correction and support as the child grows and their foot shape changes. The footwear can be adjusted to accommodate different stages of the treatment process. Figure 3.3 explains the integration of 2D materials with soft materials where the overall cos of materials reduces.

Soft robotic devices can be used alongside traditional casting and bracing methods to enhance correction and provide additional support. For example, a soft robotic brace might be used after initial casting to maintain the corrected position and gradually adjust alignment. Soft robotic devices can be tailored to the specific needs of each patient, allowing for a more personalized approach. Treatment plans can be adjusted based on real-time feedback from the device. Soft robotic systems can incorporate sensors to monitor the foot's position and progress. Thesedata can be used to adjust the treatment dynamically and ensure optimal correction. Clinical trials can be conducted to validate the effectiveness of soft robotic approaches compared to traditional methods. It is essential to ensurethat soft robotic devices are safe for use in children and do not cause discomfort or adverse effects. New materials that offer better flexibility, durability, and comfort can be developed. Digital technologies can be incorporated such as artificial intelligence and machine learning to enhance the adaptability and control of soft robotic devices [32, 33].

3.4 SOFT ROBOTS IN CLUBFOOT TREATMENT

- **Customized Bracing:** Soft robotic devices can be custom-designed to fit the patient's foot. These devices are typically made from flexible materials and can be adjusted as the child grows. Unlike traditional rigid braces, soft robotic braces can provide a more comfortable fit and continuous gentle pressure to gradually correct the foot position.

- **Dynamic Correction:** Soft robotic devices can incorporate sensors and actuators that allow for dynamic adjustments. This means the brace can actively assist in correcting the foot position over time. Sensors can monitor the child's movements and adjust the brace's tension or positioning to ensure optimal correction.
- **Improved Compliance:** One challenge with traditional treatments like casting and rigid braces is patient compliance, especially in children. Soft robotics can potentially improve compliance due to their comfort and flexibility, making it easier for children to wear them consistently.
- **Early Intervention:** Soft robotic devices can be used from an early age, even in infants, to begin correcting the foot deformity soon after birth. Early intervention is crucial for achieving better outcomes in clubfoot treatment.
- **Noninvasive Approach:** Compared to surgery, which is sometimes required for severe cases of clubfoot, soft robotics offer a noninvasive or minimally invasive approach. This can reduce the risks associated with surgery and shorten recovery times.
- **Adjustability and Feedback:** Soft robotic devices can be adjusted by healthcare providers during regular checkups to ensure proper correction progress. They can also provide feedback to clinicians about the child's response to treatment, enabling personalized adjustments. Research and development in this area are ongoing, with prototypes and clinical trials exploring the effectiveness of soft robotic devices for clubfoot treatment. While these technologies show promise, they are still in the early stages of adoption and further studies are needed to establish their long-term efficacy and benefits compared to traditional treatments.

3.5 SOFT ROBOTIC MATERIALS USED IN CLUBFOOT TREATMENT

Many types of materials, especially materials having a capacity to change tensile strength, are used in treatment. These materials include polymers with special additives, reinforcing fillers, etc. Different materials are used for the same treatment but are applied in different manners. Materials required for this treatment should have the following properties.

Soft robotics often rely on materials that can deform and adapt to various shapes, enabling flexibility and versatility in their movements and functions.

- **Silicone Rubber:** This is one of the most commonly used materials due to its flexibility, durability, and ease of molding. It can be used in various forms such as elastomers, foams, and gels. Silicone rubber is highly flexible and can be stretched significantly without losing its shape or integrity. This makes it ideal for applications where deformation and adaptability are required. It is resistant to wear and tear, making it durable over time. Silicone rubber can withstand repeated flexing and stretching without degrading, so it is a highly durable material. Silicone rubber performs well across a wide range of temperatures, from very low to very high. This makes it suitable for applications in extreme environments.

It is resistant to many chemicals, including oils and solvents, which helps maintain its properties in various industrial settings. Many silicone rubbers are biocompatible, which makes them suitable for medical and wearable applications. Silicone rubber can be easily molded into complex shapes, which is useful for creating intricate designs in soft robotics [34].

- **Hydrogels:** These are water-absorbent polymers that can swell or shrink in response to environmental changes, making them ideal for applications requiring dynamic shape changes or stimuli-responsive behavior. Hydrogels can absorb and retain large amounts of water, which gives them a gel-like consistency. This high water content often makes them soft and pliable. The water content contributes to their softness and flexibility, allowing them to deform easily in response to external forces. Some hydrogels are designed to respond to environmental stimuli such as changes in temperature, pH, or the presence of specific chemicals. This responsiveness can be used to create dynamic and adaptive soft robotic systems.

  Many hydrogels are biocompatible, making them suitable for medical and biological applications. Hydrogels are often transparent, which can be useful in applications where visual inspection or light transmission is needed. The soft and flexible nature of hydrogels allows them to conform to various shapes and adapt to different environments, making them useful in applications requiring dynamic changes in form. Some hydrogels possess self-healing properties, meaning they can recover from damage over time. This feature enhances their durability in soft robotic applications. Hydrogels that respond to environmental changes can be engineered to perform specific functions, such as actuating or sensing, based on external stimuli. Hydrogels are often used in biomedical applications due to their compatibility with biological tissues and fluids.
- **Elastomers:** Materials like polyurethane and other synthetic elastomers are used for their high stretchability and resilience. They can be engineered to provide specific mechanical properties. Elastomers can stretch to several times their original length and return to their initial shape without permanent deformation. This elasticity is due to their polymer structure, which includes long, coiled chains that can be extended and then spring back. They are inherently flexible, which allows them to conform to various shapes and absorb impacts or movements.

Elastomers are resistant to wear and tear, and they maintain their properties over many cycles of stretching and compression. Many elastomers perform well across a range of temperatures, though their performance can vary depending on the specific type. Elastomers can be engineered to resist degradation from exposure to oils, solvents, and other chemicals.

- **SMAs:** These materials change shape in response to temperature changes. While more rigid compared to other soft materials, they can still be used in conjunction with softer materials for adaptive components. SMAs can "remember" their original shape and return to it after deformation when exposed to a specific temperature. This effect occurs due to phase changes in the material at different temperatures. At temperatures above the transformation temperature, SMAs exhibit super elasticity, meaning they can undergo large strains (up to 8% or more) and return to their original shape when the stress is removed [35, 36].

  The shape-memory effect is due to the phase transformation between two different crystalline structures: the martensite phase (low-temperature phase) and the austenite phase (high-temperature phase). The material changes between these phases in response to temperature variations. MAs are sensitive to temperature changes. The specific temperature at which the phase transformation occurs can be tailored during material processing.
- **Electroactive Polymers (EAPs):** These materials change shape or size in response to an electric field. They are used for creating actuators and sensors in soft robots. Flexible and lightweight, foams can be used to create structures that are both resilient and adaptable. They are often used in combination with other materials to enhance performance.
- **Gel-Like Materials:** These can include materials like alginate or agar, which are often used for their ability to undergo significant shape changes in response to environmental stimuli. The 2D materials integrated with soft materials create multifunctional robotic materials for better functionality and durability.

  Advances in 3D-printing technology have enabled the creation of complex soft robotic structures using a variety of custom materials, including flexible resins and elastomers. Materials derived from biological sources, like collagen or chitosan, can be used for soft robotics, especially in applications where biocompatibility is important. These materials are chosen based on the specific requirements of the soft robotic application, including factors like flexibility, strength, responsiveness to stimuli, and environmental conditions.

The mechanical properties of the material include a great elongation, high tensile strength, etc. The material should possess following properties. A great elongation (between 1200% and 1400%) A high Tensile strength (ranging between 1500 and1600 psi), Shore Durometer is the term that usually defines the tear strength of silicone. If the Shore durometer is more than the tear strength is high and here it should have a high tear strength (ranging between 250 and 300 ppi), Usually for this material the compression set should be maintained low. It should be in a range of 5% to 6% at room temperature. Hardness range from 0000 Shore A to 70 Shore D, usually a durometer hardness range of 10 to 80 Shore A of silicone rubber provides a needed hardness to the designer for making the best model which can perform a specific function very well. Some variations also can be done for blending, fillers, and additives by permitting all hardness values. Time duration and ranges of temperature which are used for oven curing also have an impact on hardness but this does not destroy its existing physical characteristics.

3.5.1 Chemical structure and resistance

Usually, synthetic polymers like silicon rubbers which possess a Si–O chain which are alternating are used. These molecules of Si–O on adding catalyst will form crosslinks. In early days, the catalysts used for silicon was peroxide catalyst which is also used presently and has a property of leaving residue in the form of acid in the rubber. This catalyst also forms outgas peroxide byproducts if the catalyst is cross-linked and is not completely cured. But in present days due to the property of faster curing, the catalyst has a liquid form and also has an ability to leave a peroxide bloom. Silicon platinum has a cure system which can be shipped in to two-part kit; which can be named as part A and part B. These two parts are mixed in a ratio which forms a compound which can be readily used for curing.

3.5.2 Fungus resistance

The material used for treatment should have an ability to resist the attack from mold or fungus in any type of environment whether warm or damp. Even though the silicon rubber is not resistant toward fungus but it does not entertain the existence of fungus and also does not get affected by fungus.

3.6 PROPOSED TREATMENT METHODS

Soft robots, characterized by their flexible and adaptable structures, require innovative approaches to leg design that enhance their ability to perform complex tasks, adapt to various environments, and interact safely with humans. The proposed method is used with elastomer material for leg soft robot disease. The proposed method design is shown in Figures 3.4 and 3.5. Soft robot legs commonly use elastomers such as silicone rubber or polyurethane due to their flexibility and durability. These materials allow the legs to stretch and conform to different surfaces, providing the required

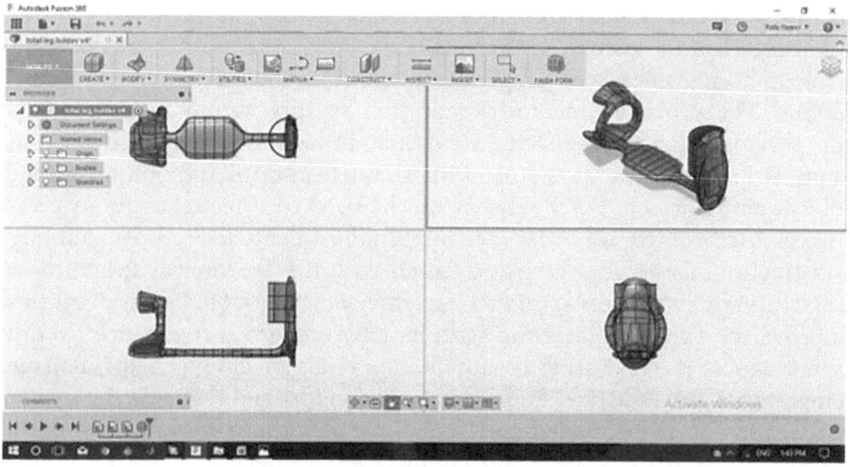

Figure 3.4 Design of proposed model.

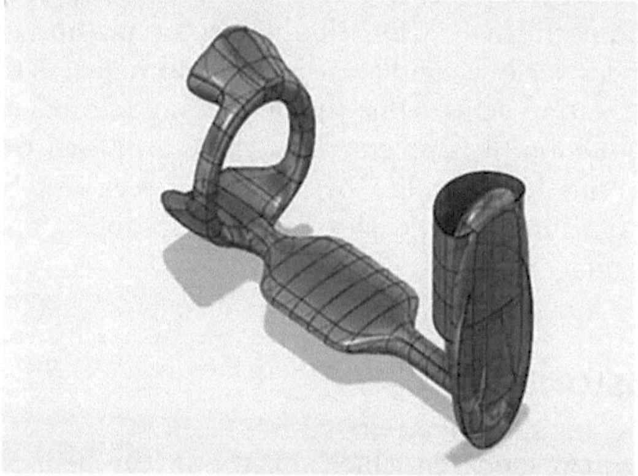

Figure 3.5 Design of shoe.

adaptability and resilience. Elastomeric coatings or treatments can further enhance their properties, including wear resistance and environmental protection. Utilizing a multilayered design allows for optimized performance where each layer serves a specific function, such as comfort, support, and protection. For instance, a soft inner layer can provide comfort, while a tougher outer layer can protect against external damage. Designing legs with modular components facilitates easier maintenance and customization. Modular designs allow for the replacement or upgrading of specific parts without the need to overhaul the entire system, improving the robot's versatility and longevity. Cable-driven systems involve the use of tendons or cables to control joint movements. This method allows for lightweight and flexible actuation, which is beneficial for soft robotics. Applying waterproof treatments or using water-resistant materials is essential to protect the soft robot legs from moisture. This treatment extends the lifespan of the components and ensures reliable performance in various environmental conditions. The proposed method Integrating sensors within the robot legs can provide valuable feedback on parameters such as pressure, strain, and temperature. Thesedata are crucial for adaptive control and optimizing the robot's performance. Force sensors can be used to detect changes in pressure or load on the robot legs, enabling adjustments to improve stability and traction. Designing the legs to align with the anatomical structure or task requirements ensures comfort and efficiency. Ergonomic considerations improve the robot's interaction with its environment and enhance overall performance. Incorporating breathable materials or designs helps manage temperature and moisture, improving user comfort and reducing the risk of overheating during extended use. Leveraging 3D printing technology allows for the creation of custom and complex leg geometries. This technique enables rapid prototyping and precise control over design features.

Employing soft robotics fabrication methods such as soft mold casting or soft lithography can create flexible and adaptive leg structures, enhancing functionality and performance. Developing prototypes and conducting rigorous testing under various conditions is essential to assess the leg's performance. Iterative testing helps refine the design and address potential issues before final production. By implementing these proposed treatment methods, the design and functionality of soft robot legs can be significantly enhanced, leading to improved performance, adaptability, and durability in diverse applications.

3.7 CONCLUSIONS

In this chapter, a new model in which soft robots can be used to cure clubfoot is developed and designed. This way of treatment can save time, reduce pain, and also can have more success rate. This model also has an advantage of accuracy as this design can be done based on the foot shape using the 3D scanners.

The integration of soft robotics into clubfoot treatment provides a significant advantage in terms of flexibility and adaptability. Unlike traditional rigid orthotic devices, soft robotic systems can conform to the complex and dynamic nature of foot deformities. This adaptability allows for more effective management of clubfoot by accommodating the foot's changing shape and alignment throughout the treatment process. Soft robotic devices can offer dynamic and customizable support tailored to the individual patient's needs. Advanced materials, such as elastomers and hydrogels, coupled with actuators like pneumatic systems or SMAs, allow for adjustments in stiffness and support. This dynamic capability is crucial for addressing the varying degrees of deformity and ensuring that the treatment remains effective as the condition evolves.

The design of soft robotic treatments emphasizes patient comfort, which is critical for compliance. Soft, flexible materials and adaptive designs contribute to a more comfortable fit compared to traditional rigid orthoses. Enhanced comfort can lead to higher patient adherence to the treatment protocol, which is essential for achieving optimal outcomes. The proposed treatment methods leverage advanced actuation technologies that provide precise control over foot positioning and movement. Pneumatic actuators, SMAs, and cable-driven mechanisms offer targeted correction of deformities with high precision. These technologies enable nuanced adjustments and fine-tuning, enhancing the effectiveness of the treatment.

Soft robotic systems can be integrated with monitoring technologies to track the patient's progress and adjust treatment as needed. Embedded sensors provide real-time data on foot position, pressure, and alignment, facilitating a data-driven approach to treatment. This integration supports personalized rehabilitation plans and ensures that the treatment is adapted to the patient's specific needs. Advancements in manufacturing technologies, such as 3D printing, enable the creation of customized soft robotic devices. Tailoring the design to the individual patient's anatomy ensures a better fit and more effective treatment. Personalization not only enhances comfort but also improves the precision of the corrective measures applied to the foot.

While the proposed soft robotic treatments offer promising benefits, further research and development are needed to address potential challenges. Areas for future exploration include optimizing material properties, refining actuation mechanisms, and conducting long-term clinical trials to assess the effectiveness and safety of these new technologies. The integration of soft robotics into clubfoot treatment has the potential to transform clinical practice by providing more adaptable, comfortable, and effective solutions. These advancements could lead to improved patient outcomes, reduced treatment times, and greater overall satisfaction with the therapeutic process. The proposed soft robotic treatments for clubfoot represent a significant advancement over traditional methods, offering enhanced flexibility, comfort, and control. By leveraging innovative materials and technologies, these new approaches hold the promise of more effective and personalized care for patients with clubfoot. Continued research and development will be crucial in realizing the full potential of these soft robotic systems and integrating them into standard clinical practice.

REFERENCES

[1] Rieger, M. A., & Dobbs, M. B. (2022). Clubfoot. *Clinics in Podiatric Medicine and Surgery*, 39(1), 1–14.

[2] Do Amaral, ECastro, A., Peixoto, J. B., Miyahara, L. K., Akuri, M. C., Moriwaki T. L., Sato, V. N. & Aihara, A. Y. (2024). Clubfoot: Congenital Talipes Equinovarus. *RadioGraphics*, 44(7), e230178.

[3] Singh, S., & Mali, H. S. (2023). Foot abduction orthosis compliance in clubfoot treatment: Biomechanics, challenges, and future scope. In *3D Printing in Podiatric Medicine* (pp. 103–121). Academic Press.
[4] Xiloyannis, M., Alicea, R., Georgarakis, A. M., Haufe, F. L., Wolf, P., Masia, L., & Riener, R. (2021). Soft robotic suits: State of the art, core technologies, and open challenges. *IEEE Transactions on Robotics*, 38(3), 1343–1362.
[5] Polygerinos, P., Correll, N., Morin, S. A., Mosadegh, B., Onal, C. D., Petersen, K., ... & Shepherd, R. F. (2017). Soft robotics: Review of fluid-driven intrinsically soft devices; manufacturing, sensing, control, and applications in human-robot interaction. *Advanced Engineering Materials*, 19(12), 1700016.
[6] Luker, J., Lynch, E., Bernhardsson, S., Bennett, L., & Bernhardt, J. (2015). Stroke survivors' experiences of physical rehabilitation: a systematic review of qualitative studies. *Archives of Physical Medicine and Rehabilitation*, 96(9), 1698–1708.
[7] Kwan, M. Y. (2024). Ergonomic design of textile orthoses for patients with hallux valgus, Hong Kong Polytechnic University thesis, https://theses.lib.polyu.edu.hk/handle/200/12885
[8] Gao, R. Z., Lee, P. S., Ravi, A., Ren, C. L., Dickerson, C. R., & Tung, J. Y. (2024). Hybrid soft-rigid active prosthetics laboratory exercise for hands-on biomechanical and biomedical engineering education. *Journal of Biomechanical Engineering*, 146(5), 1–16.
[9] Leslie, M. E., & Iaquinto, J. M. (2023). Neurological foot pathology. In *Foot and Ankle Biomechanics* (pp. 489–506). Academic Press.
[10] Bernasconi, A. (Ed.). (2023). *Innovative Approaches on Cavovarus Deformity: Thinking Outside of the Box, An issue of Foot and Ankle Clinics of North America, E-Book* (Vol. 28, No. 4). Elsevier Health Sciences.
[11] Strauss, N. E., & Angell, D. K. (2001). Foot conditions related to neuromuscular disorders in adults. *Physical Medicine and Rehabilitation*, 15(3), 489.
[12] Bowyer, G., & Uglow, M. (2017). The ankle and foot. In *Apley & Solomon's System of Orthopaedics and Trauma* (pp. 609–648). CRC Press.
[13] Bina, S., Pacey, V., Barnes, E. H., Burns, J., & Gray, K. (2020). Interventions for congenital talipes equinovarus (clubfoot). *Cochrane Database of Systematic Reviews*, (Vol.5). https://doi.org/10.1002/14651858.CD008602.pub4
[14] Gupta, M., Dhingra, G., & Sandhu, K. (2023). Human podiatric disabilities and their correction using a 3D printed technology: a short review. *3D Printing in Podiatric Medicine*, 30, 175–194.
[15] Asadi, N., Del Bakhshayesh, A. R., Davaran, S., & Akbarzadeh, A. (2020). Common biocompatible polymeric materials for tissue engineering and regenerative medicine. *Materials Chemistry and Physics*, 242, 122528.
[16] Caldorera-Moore, M., & Peppas, N. A. (2009). Micro-and nanotechnologies for intelligent and responsive biomaterial-based medical systems. *Advanced drug delivery reviews*, 61(15), 1391–1401.
[17] Liu, S., Yu, J. M., Gan, Y. C., Qiu, X. Z., Gao, Z. C., Wang, H., ... & Hou, H. H. (2023). Biomimetic natural biomaterials for tissue engineering and regenerative medicine: new biosynthesis methods, recent advances, and emerging applications. *Military Medical Research*, 10(1), 16.
[18] Farahani, A., Zarei-Hanzaki, A., Abedi, H. R., Daryoush, S., Ragheb, Z. D., Mianabadi, F., & Nezami, F. R. (2023). Silk-based biopolymers promise

extensive biomedical applications in tissue engineering, drug delivery, and BioMEMS. *Journal of Polymers and the Environment*, 31(11), 4559–4582.

[19] Panza, R., Albano, F., Casto, A., Del Vecchio, C., Laforgia, N., & Dibello, D. (2023). Incidence and prevalence of congenital clubfoot in Apulia: a regional model for future prospective national studies. *Italian Journal of Pediatrics*, 49(1), 151.

[20] Dahiphale, S. M., Potdar, J., Acharya, N., Jyotsna, G., & Desale, R. (2024). Congenital anomalies of the female genital tract: A comprehensive review. *Cureus*, 16(3) 1–12. doi: 10.7759/cureus.56753

[21] Maranho, D. A. C., & Volpon, J. B. (2011). Congenital clubfoot. *Acta Ortopédica Brasileira*, 19, 163–169.

[22] Wallander, H. M. (2010). Congenital clubfoot: Aspects on epidemiology, residual deformity and patient reported outcome. *Acta Orthopaedica*, 81(sup339), 1–25.

[23] Werler, M. M., Yazdy, M. M., Kasser, J. R., Mahan, S. T., Meyer, R. E., Anderka, M., ... & Mitchell, A. A. (2014). Medication use in pregnancy in relation to the risk of isolated clubfoot in offspring. *American Journal of Epidemiology*, 180(1), 86–93.

[24] Wynne-Davies, R. (1964). Family studies and the cause of congenital club foot. *The Journal of Bone & Joint Surgery British*, 46(3), 445–463.

[25] Do Amaral, E Castro, A., Peixoto, J. B., Miyahara, L. K., Akuri, M. C., Moriwaki, T. L., Sato, V. N., & Aihara, A. Y. (2024). Clubfoot: Congenital talipes equinovarus. *RadioGraphics*, 44(7), e230178.

[26] Cady, R., Hennessey, T. A., & Schwend, R. M. (2022). Diagnosis and treatment of idiopathic congenital clubfoot. *Pediatrics*, 149(2), e2021055555.

[27] Colburn, M., & Williams, M. (2003). Evaluation of the treatment of idiopathic clubfoot by using the Ponseti method. *The Journal of Foot and Ankle Surgery*, 42(5), 259–267.

[28] Rieger, M. A., & Dobbs, M. B. (2022). Clubfoot. *Clinics in Podiatric Medicine and Surgery*, 39(1), 1–14.

[29] Wallander, H. M. (2010). Congenital clubfoot: Aspects on epidemiology, residual deformity and patient reported outcome. *Acta Orthopaedica*, 81(sup339), 1–25.

[30] Cummings, R. J., Davidson, R. S., Armstrong, P. F., & Lehman, W. B. (2002). Congenital clubfoot. *JBJS*, 84(2), 290.

[31] Richards, B. S., Faulks, S., Rathjen, K. E., Karol, L. A., Johnston, C. E., & Jones, S. A. (2008). A comparison of two nonoperative methods of idiopathic clubfoot correction: The Ponseti method and the French functional (physiotherapy) method. *JBJS*, 90(11), 2313–2321.

[32] Wang, Y., Gregory, C., & Minor, M. A. (2018). Improving mechanical properties of molded silicone rubber for soft robotics through fabric compositing. *Soft Robotics*, 5(3), 272–290.

[33] Janicki, J. A., Narayanan, U. G., Harvey, B., Roy, A., Ramseier, L. E., & Wright, J. G. (2009). Treatment of neuromuscular and syndrome-associated (nonidiopathic) clubfeet using the Ponseti method. *Journal of Pediatric Orthopaedics*, 29(4), 393–397.

[34] Richards, B. S., Faulks, S., Rathjen, K. E., Karol, L. A., Johnston, C. E., & Jones, S. A. (2008). A comparison of two nonoperative methods of idiopathic

clubfoot correction: the Ponseti method and the French functional (physiotherapy) method. *JBJS*, 90(11), 2313–2321.
[35] Gent, A. N. (2005). Strength of elastomers. In *Science and technology of rubber* (pp. 455–495). Academic Press.
[36] Apsite, I., Salehi, S., & Ionov, L. (2021). Materials for smart soft actuator systems. *Chemical Reviews*, 122(1), 1349–1415.
[37] Jing, L., Li, K., Yang, H., & Chen, P. Y. (2020). Recent advances in integration of 2D materials with soft matter for multifunctional robotic materials. *Materials Horizons*, 7(1), 54–70.

Chapter 4

Medical applications of bio-inspired soft robotics

M. Sreedhar and Shaik Himam Saheb

4.1 INTRODUCTION

The integration of soft robotics with biological inspiration has led to innovative solutions in medical technology. Unlike traditional rigid robots, soft robots are made from highly compliant materials, enabling them to adapt to complex and unstructured environments similar to biological systems. This adaptability makes them ideal for a variety of medical applications, including surgery, rehabilitation, and drug delivery.

The primary objective of bio-inspired soft robotics in medicine is to improve patient outcomes by providing more flexible, adaptable, and less invasive solutions. Traditional medical devices and robots, often rigid and limited in their ability to navigate through the human body, can cause damage to tissues and organs. Soft robots, by contrast, can conform to the intricate and dynamic structures of the body, minimizing trauma and improving therapeutic efficacy.

Bio-inspired soft robotics is an interdisciplinary field, drawing from materials science, biology, and engineering to create devices that replicate the efficiency and functionality of natural organisms. This chapter provides a comprehensive overview of the current state of bio-inspired soft robotics in medicine, focusing on their design, mechanisms, and applications, and highlighting the key research developments and future directions in this exciting field.

4.2 DESIGN AND MECHANISMS OF BIO-INSPIRED SOFT ROBOTS

Bio-inspired soft robots are designed to emulate the properties of natural organisms, such as flexibility, resilience, and adaptability. These robots typically use materials such as silicone, hydrogels, and shape-memory alloys to achieve the desired mechanical properties in practice. There are many bio-inspired soft robots available in the market, for example, starfish gel robot that turns over application of electric fields is shown in Figure 4.1,

DOI: 10.1201/9781003539612-4

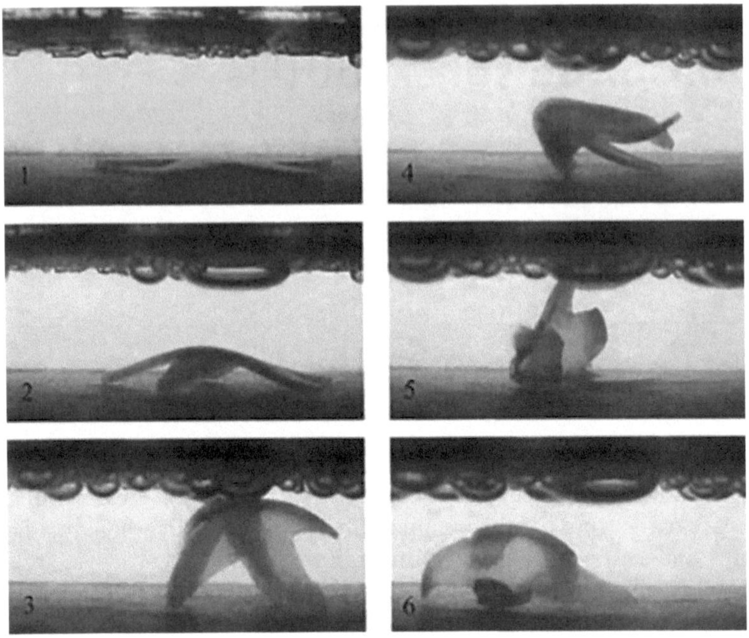

Figure 4.1 A starfish gel robot that turns over application of electric fields [1].

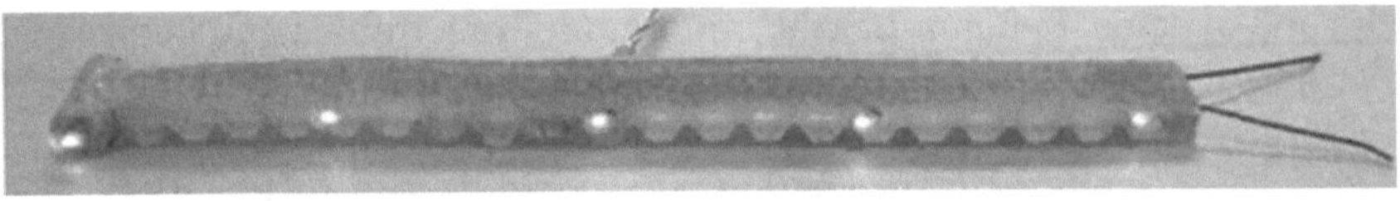

Figure 4.2 A multigait soft walker powered by compressed air [2].

popularly known in the electrical fields due to its flexibility. Multigait soft walker is another example of soft robots as shown in Figure 4.2.

4.2.1 Actuation mechanisms

Soft robots utilize various actuation mechanisms, including pneumatic, hydraulic, soft gels, and dielectric elastomers. Pneumatic actuators, for example, use air pressure to create movement and are widely used due to their simplicity and effectiveness in generating large deformations [1–3].

Hydraulic actuators, on the other hand, use liquid pressure and are advantageous in terms of generating high-force outputs. Dielectric elastomers are a newer technology that uses electrostatic forces to induce movement, offering rapid response times and high energy densities [4].

4.3 SENSING AND CONTROL

The integration of sensors within soft robots allows for real-time feedback and control. Advances in flexible electronics and materials have led to the development of sensors that can detect pressure, strain, and other stimuli, enabling precise control of the robot's movements [5–7].

These sensors are often embedded within the soft robotic structure, providing seamless integration and enhanced functionality. Control algorithms, inspired by the neural networks of biological organisms, are employed to manage the complex interactions between the sensors and actuators, allowing for adaptive and intelligent behavior [8]. Figure 4.3 explains the physically developed AI-based nerve system and natural nerve system.

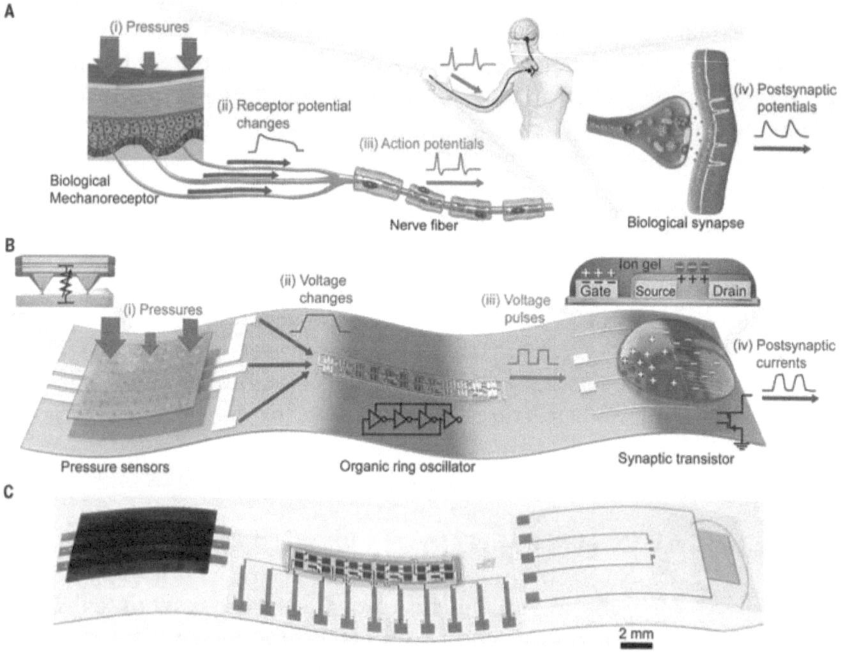

Figure 4.3 An artificial afferent nerve system in comparison with a biological one [6]. (A) A biological afferent nerve responds to pressure stimulation through mechanoreceptors. When pressure is applied, it alters the receptor potential in each mechanoreceptor. These receptor potentials merge and trigger action potentials at the heminode. The nerve fiber then forms synapses with interneurons in the spinal cord. Action potentials from various nerve fibers converge via synapses to aid in processing information. (B) An artificial afferent nerve consists of pressure sensors, an organic ring oscillator, and a synaptic transistor. For simplicity, only one ring oscillator connected to a synaptic transistor is illustrated, but in practice, multiple ring oscillators and clusters of pressure sensors can be linked to a single synaptic transistor. The components with matching colors in (A) and (B) correspond to each other. (C) A photograph showing an artificial afferent nerve system.

4.4 MINIMALLY INVASIVE SURGERY

Minimally invasive surgery (MIS) is a groundbreaking field that has seen significant advancements with the advent of bio-inspired soft robotics. The key advantages of MIS include reduced patient trauma, shorter recovery times, and decreased risk of infection compared to traditional open surgery. Bio-inspired soft robots enhance these benefits by offering superior maneuverability and precision, which are crucial in delicate surgical environments.

4.4.1 Endoscopic soft robots

Endoscopic soft robots are designed to navigate the human body with unparalleled flexibility and control. Inspired by the movement of natural organisms such as octopuses and worms, these robots can maneuver through the gastrointestinal tract, respiratory system, and other complex body cavities with minimal trauma. Unlike rigid endoscopes, which can cause tissue damage and discomfort, soft robotic endoscopes conform to the body's natural curves and pathways.

Recent innovations in magnetic actuation have further enhanced the capabilities of endoscopic soft robots. These systems achieve precise, remote manipulation by embedding magnetic particles within the robot and using external magnetic fields for control.

This technology allows surgeons to perform complex procedures with high accuracy, reducing the need for multiple insertions and minimizing patient discomfort [9–12]. Moreover, advancements in imaging technologies integrated with soft robotic endoscopes enable real-time, high-resolution visualization of internal structures, aiding in accurate diagnosis and targeted therapy.

4.5 SURGICAL INSTRUMENTS

Bio-inspired soft robotic instruments provide surgeons with enhanced dexterity and control during operations. These instruments are designed to replicate the fine motor skills of the human hand, allowing for precise manipulation of tissues and organs. The flexibility and adaptability of these tools enable surgeons to perform complex procedures in confined spaces where traditional rigid instruments would be impractical. The three-module stiffness: controllable, flexible, and learnable manipulator for surgical operations is shown in Figure 4.4.

One notable example is the development of soft robotic graspers and retractors based on biomimetics, which can gently manipulate delicate tissues without causing damage. These tools are particularly useful in neurosurgery, cardiovascular surgery, and urology, where precision and minimal invasiveness are paramount [13–15].

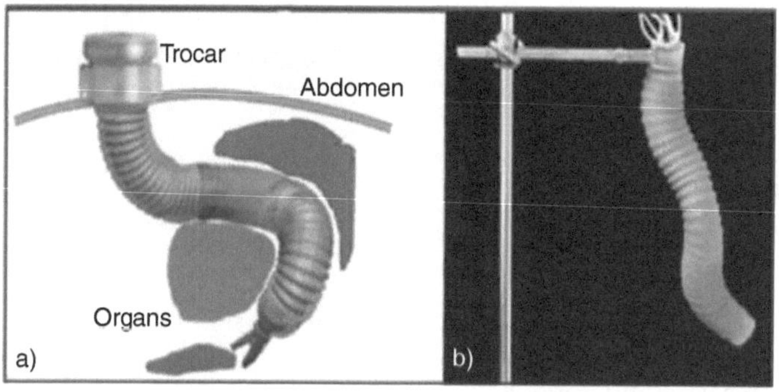

Figure 4.4 (a-b) The three-module stiffness: controllable, flexible, and learnable manipulator for surgical operations [10].

The integration of haptic feedback systems into these instruments allows surgeons to receive tactile information, enhancing their ability to perform delicate tasks with greater confidence and accuracy. The miniaturization of soft robotic surgical tools has opened new possibilities for microsurgery, enabling procedures at the cellular level that were previously unattainable [16].

4.6 REHABILITATION AND PROSTHETICS

The field of rehabilitation and prosthetics has been revolutionized by bio-inspired soft robotics, providing novel solutions for restoring movement and function to individuals with disabilities. These advancements have significantly improved the quality of life for patients by offering more natural, adaptable, and effective rehabilitation devices.

4.6.1 Wearable soft exoskeletons

Wearable soft exoskeletons are designed to assist individuals with mobility impairments by providing support and enhancing movement. Unlike rigid exoskeletons, which can be bulky and restrictive, soft exoskeletons are made from lightweight, flexible materials that conform to the wearer's body. This design ensures comfort and allows for a greater range of motion, making the devices suitable for extended use.

Soft exoskeletons typically use pneumatic or hydraulic actuators to mimic the natural movement of muscles and joints. These devices can be customized to the specific needs of the user, providing personalized assistance for various activities such as walking, standing, and lifting [17–19]. Advances in sensor technology enable these exoskeletons to adapt to the wearer's movements in real-time, providing seamless and intuitive support. This adaptability is crucial for effective rehabilitation, as it allows for more natural and efficient movement patterns, thereby promoting faster recovery and greater functional improvement [20].

4.6.2 Soft prosthetic limbs

Soft prosthetic limbs offer a significant improvement over traditional rigid prosthetics by providing a more natural range of motion and enhanced comfort. These prosthetics are designed to replicate the flexibility and responsiveness of natural limbs, allowing users to perform a wide range of activities with greater ease and confidence.

The development of soft prosthetic limbs has been driven by advances in material science and bio-inspired design principles. Modern prosthetics use flexible materials such as silicone and elastomers to mimic the properties of human skin and muscles. This design not only improves the aesthetic appeal of the prosthetics but also enhances their functional capabilities [21–23]. Additionally, soft prosthetic limbs can be integrated with advanced control systems, including neural interfaces that allow users to control the prosthetic with their thoughts. This direct control offers a more intuitive and precise interaction with the prosthetic, significantly improving the user's ability to perform complex tasks [24].

4.7 DRUG DELIVERY SYSTEMS

Bio-inspired soft robots are playing a crucial role in the development of advanced drug delivery systems, offering new ways to deliver medications precisely and efficiently. These systems aim to enhance the efficacy of treatments while minimizing side effects, providing significant benefits for patient care.

4.7.1 Microscale soft robots

Microscale soft robots, inspired by microorganisms such as bacteria and algae, are designed to navigate through the human body to deliver drugs to specific sites. These tiny robots can traverse through the bloodstream, gastrointestinal tract, and other internal pathways, reaching target areas with high precision.

One of the key advantages of microscale soft robots is their ability to operate in environments that are inaccessible to larger devices. Their small size and soft nature allow them to travel through narrow blood vessels and other confined spaces without causing damage. These robots can be equipped with various payloads of therapeutic agents, which can be released in a controlled manner upon reaching the target site. This targeted drug delivery approach enhances the efficacy of treatments by concentrating the medication at the site of action while reducing systemic exposure and side effects [25–28]. Additionally, remote control and navigation of these robots can be achieved through external magnetic fields or other actuation methods, ensuring precise delivery and minimizing the risk of off-target effects.

4.7.2 Implantable drug delivery devices

Implantable soft robotic devices are designed for long-term, controlled release of medications. These devices are often inspired by natural processes, such as the gradual release of hormones, to provide more effective and sustained treatment. Implantable devices can be used for a variety of applications, including pain management, hormone replacement therapy, and cancer treatment.

These devices are typically made from biocompatible and biodegradable materials that can safely reside within the body for extended periods. The materials used ensure that the devices do not elicit adverse immune responses and can degrade harmlessly once their function is complete. Implantable drug delivery systems can be programmed to release drugs in response to specific physiological triggers, providing a personalized approach to treatment. For instance, insulin delivery systems can continuously monitor blood glucose levels and release insulin as needed, offering better management of diabetes and reducing the risk of complications [29–32].

The advancements in bio-inspired soft robotics for drug delivery systems hold great promise for revolutionizing the way medications are administered, offering more effective, safer, and less invasive solutions for a wide range of medical conditions.

4.8 DIAGNOSTIC TOOLS

Soft robotics also holds promise for improving diagnostic procedures, offering less invasive and more accurate methods for detecting diseases.

4.8.1 Soft robotic biopsy devices

Soft robotic biopsy devices can provide more precise and less invasive methods for tissue sampling. These devices can navigate to specific sites within the body and collect samples with minimal damage to surrounding tissues [33–35]. Soft robotic biopsy tools can access hard-to-reach areas and perform procedures that are not feasible with traditional rigid instruments. They can be equipped with sensors to ensure accurate targeting and sampling, improving the diagnostic accuracy and reducing the need for repeat procedures [36].

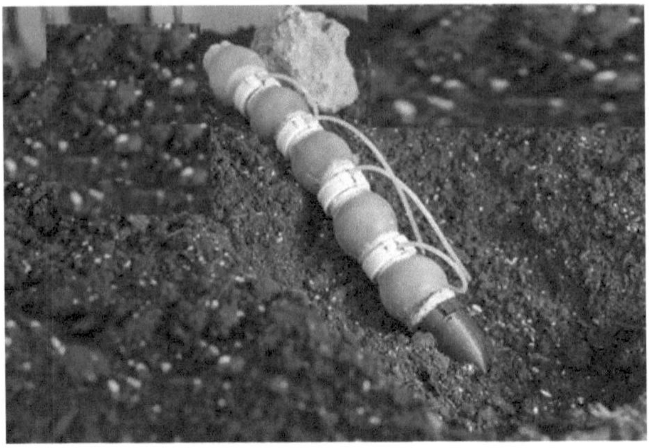

Figure 4.5 Artificial earthworm prototype [14].

4.8.2 Flexible endoscopic tools

Flexible endoscopic tools can provide better access to difficult-to-reach areas within the body, improving the accuracy and effectiveness of diagnostic procedures [37–39]. These tools can be used for a variety of diagnostic applications, including imaging, biopsy, and therapeutic interventions. Their flexibility allows them to conform to the natural curves and contours of the body, reducing the risk of injury and improving patient comfort. Advances in imaging technology, such as high-resolution and 3D imaging, further enhance the diagnostic capabilities of these tools [40]; one of this kind of tool, that is, artificial earthworm is shown in Figure 4.5.

4.9 CASE STUDIES

Soft robotics is making significant strides in the medical field, offering innovative solutions for various clinical applications. Based on the necessity of the mechanism, the researchers developed various soft robots. The below-mentioned soft robots are in practice at various parts of the world to solve various problems.

- **Soft Robotic Endoscopic Tools:** Flexible endoscopic surgery tools developed by Harvard University and Massachusetts General Hospital represent a significant advancement in minimally invasive surgical technology. These tools utilize soft robotics to offer greater flexibility and precision compared to traditional rigid endoscopes. The soft robotic design enables the endoscope to navigate complex and delicate anatomical pathways with ease, adapting to various shapes and movements within the body.

The innovation focuses on improving the dexterity of surgical instruments, allowing surgeons to perform intricate procedures with enhanced control and reduced risk of injury to surrounding tissues. This increased maneuverability not only enhances the accuracy of the surgery but also minimizes patient discomfort and speeds up recovery times. By integrating advanced materials and design principles, these flexible endoscopic tools make it possible to conduct procedures in areas that were previously challenging to access with conventional instruments. This advancement in surgical technology reflects a commitment to improving patient outcomes through cutting-edge research and development. The collaboration between Harvard University and Massachusetts General Hospital exemplifies how academic and clinical institutions can work together to drive progress in medical technology, ultimately benefiting both healthcare professionals and patients.

- **Soft Robotic Exoskeletons for Rehabilitation:** Rehabilitation Exoskeletons for Stroke Patients Institution is developed by Wyss Institute for Biologically Inspired Engineering. The developed soft robotic exoskeleton is to assist stroke patients with movement rehabilitation. The exoskeleton uses soft, flexible materials to provide support and gentle guidance to the limbs during therapy sessions. This soft exoskeleton helps patients regain motor function by offering a more comfortable and adaptable rehabilitation experience. It allows for a greater range of motion and more natural movement compared to traditional rigid exoskeletons.
- **Soft Robotic Surgical Instruments:** Soft Robotic Surgical Grippers Institution of Stanford University developed soft robotic grippers for use in MIS. These grippers are made from soft, compliant materials and are designed to handle delicate tissues with precision. The soft robotic grippers reduce the risk of tissue damage and improve the surgeon's ability to manipulate delicate structures. This technology enhances the safety and effectiveness of minimally invasive procedures.
- **Soft Robotic Prosthetics:** Soft Robotic Hand Prosthetics Institution of the University of Illinois at Urbana-Champaign created a soft robotic hand prosthetic that mimics the flexibility and dexterity of a human hand. The prosthetic uses soft actuators to provide a natural range of motion and grip strength. Users of the soft robotic hand prosthetic experience improved comfort and functionality compared to traditional rigid prosthetics. The prosthetic's adaptive grip and natural movement capabilities make daily tasks easier and more intuitive.
- **Soft Robotic Stents:** Flexible Vascular Stents Institution of ETH Zurich developed a soft robotic stent designed to be more flexible and conformable than traditional metal stents. The soft robotic stent can adapt to changes in the blood vessel's shape and diameter. The flexible stent reduces the risk of complications such as restenosis and vessel

injury. Its adaptability improves long-term patient outcomes and minimizes the need for additional interventions.

- Soft Robotic Catheters for Cardiac Procedures Institution developed by MIT Media Lab designed a soft robotic catheter that can navigate through the heart's intricate pathways with ease. The catheter is made from soft, flexible materials that allow it to conform to the shape of the vessels and chambers. This soft robotic catheter enhances the precision and safety of cardiac procedures by reducing the risk of damage to sensitive tissues. It also improves the ease of maneuvering through complex anatomical structures.

4.10 CHALLENGES AND FUTURE PROSPECTS

While bio-inspired soft robotics holds great promise for medical applications, several challenges remain. These include the development of more robust and durable materials, improving the precision and control of soft robots, and ensuring the safety and reliability of these devices in clinical settings.

The development of materials that can withstand the harsh conditions of the human body while maintaining their flexibility and functionality is a significant challenge. Researchers are exploring new materials and composites that can meet these requirements. Additionally, the integration of advanced control systems that can manage the complex interactions between sensors, actuators, and the environment is essential for the success of soft robots in medical applications.

Ensuring the safety and reliability of bio-inspired soft robots is also crucial. Clinical trials and regulatory approvals are necessary to demonstrate the efficacy and safety of these devices. Collaborative efforts between researchers, clinicians, and regulatory bodies will be vital in overcoming these challenges and bringing bio-inspired soft robotics to clinical practice.

Future research in this field is likely to focus on overcoming these challenges and expanding the range of medical applications for bio-inspired soft robotics. Advances in materials science, sensor technology, and control systems will play a crucial role in the continued development and adoption of these innovative technologies. Additionally, interdisciplinary collaboration between engineers, biologists, and medical professionals will be essential in driving the field forward.

4.11 CONCLUSIONS

Bio-inspired soft robotics represents a transformative paradigm in the field of medical technology, offering unprecedented capabilities in diagnosis, treatment, and rehabilitation. By drawing inspiration from natural organisms, researchers have developed soft robotic systems that mimic the flexibility, adaptability, and dexterity of biological tissues and organisms. This chapter has highlighted several key areas where bio-inspired soft robotics are making significant contributions to medical practice.

Soft robotic devices such as endoscopes and surgical instruments have enabled surgeons to perform complex procedures with enhanced precision and minimal patient trauma. These devices navigate intricate anatomical pathways with ease, offering improved visualization and manipulation capabilities compared to traditional rigid instruments. The integration of advanced imaging modalities and real-time feedback systems further enhances surgical outcomes, paving the way for safer and more effective interventions.

In rehabilitation and prosthetics, bio-inspired soft exoskeletons and prosthetic limbs have revolutionized patient care by providing naturalistic movement and enhanced comfort. These devices not only restore mobility but also promote rehabilitation by facilitating adaptive movements and reducing the physical burden on users. The development of neural interfaces and advanced control systems has further augmented the functionality of these devices, offering users greater autonomy and control over their movements.

In drug delivery systems, microscale soft robots hold promise for targeted and minimally invasive therapies. These miniature robots navigate through the body's intricate pathways to deliver medications with precision, minimizing systemic side effects and enhancing therapeutic efficacy. Implantable soft robotic devices offer controlled release of drugs over extended periods, improving patient compliance and treatment outcomes.

The field of bio-inspired soft robotics continues to evolve rapidly, driven by advancements in materials science, miniaturization technologies, and interdisciplinary collaborations. Future research efforts are poised to address remaining challenges such as biocompatibility, long-term reliability, and scalability of soft robotic systems for widespread clinical adoption. Moreover, the integration of artificial intelligence and machine learning holds potential for enhancing the autonomy and decision-making capabilities of soft robotic devices in medical settings.

Bio-inspired soft robotics represents a frontier in medical innovation, offering transformative solutions to long-standing challenges in healthcare. The convergence of engineering principles with biological insights promises to redefine the future of medicine, ushering in an era of personalized, precise, and patient-centered care.

REFERENCES

[1] D. Trivedi, C. D. Rahn, W. M. Kier, and I. D. Walker, "Soft robotics: Biological inspiration, state of the art, and future research," *Applied Bionics and Biomechanics*, vol. 5, no. 3, pp. 99–117, 2008.

[2] S. Kim, C. Laschi, and B. Trimmer, "Soft robotics: A bioinspired evolution in robotics," *Trends in Biotechnology*, vol. 31, no. 5, pp. 287–294, 2013.

[3] J. Shintake, V. Cacucciolo, D. Floreano, and H. Shea, "Soft robotic grippers," *Advanced Materials*, vol. 30, no. 29, 1707035, 2018.
[4] E. T. Roche et al., "A bioinspired soft actuated material," *Advanced Materials*, vol. 26, no. 8, pp. 1200–1206, 2014.
[5] C. M. Boutry et al., "A stretchable and biodegradable strain and pressure sensor for orthopaedic application," *Nature Electronics*, vol. 1, no. 5, pp. 314–321, 2018.
[6] J. Kim et al., "A bioinspired flexible organic artificial afferent nerve," *Science*, vol. 360, no. 6391, pp. 998–1003, 2017.
[7] C. Larson et al., "Highly stretchable electroluminescent skin for optical signaling and tactile sensing," *Science*, vol. 351, no. 6277, pp. 1071–1074, 2016.
[8] M. Cianchetti, T. Ranzani, G. Gerboni, and G. Thalhammer, "Bio-inspired soft robotics: Advances in materials, modeling, and applications," *Proceedings of the IEEE*, vol. 106, no. 4, pp. 667–679, 2018.
[9] D. Y. Yang, H. Park, J. H. Kim, and Y. S. Kim, "Soft robotics: Integrating mechanical intelligence into robotic systems," *Nature Communications*, vol. 9, no. 1, pp. 1–12, 2018.
[10] Y. Lurie et al., "A bio-inspired robotic endoscope actuator for minimally invasive surgery," *Soft Robotics*, vol. 6, no. 4, pp. 439–455, 2019.
[11] J. Burgner-Kahrs, D. C. Rucker, and H. Choset, "Continuum robots for medical applications: A survey," *IEEE Transactions on Robotics*, vol. 31, no. 6, pp. 1261–1280, 2015.
[12] D. S. Kim, J. H. Han, and J. Kim, "Development of a magnetic actuation system for soft robotic endoscopes," *Journal of Mechanical Science and Technology*, vol. 30, no. 9, pp. 4073–4080, 2016.
[13] G. Mariani, G. Ferri, A. Menciassi, and P. Dario, "A miniature steerable end-effector for robotic endoluminal surgery," *IEEE Transactions on Robotics*, vol. 24, no. 4, pp. 835–844, 2008.
[14] A. Menciassi, S. Gorini, G. Pernorio, and P. Dario, "A SMA actuated artificial earthworm," in *Proceedings of the 2004 IEEE International Conference on Robotics and Automation, 2004*. ICRA'04., vol. 1, pp. 328–333, 2004.
[15] J. Kim, G. I. Parodi, and J. A. Lloyd, "Design and control of bio-inspired surgical instruments," *Bioinspiration & Biomimetics*, vol. 11, no. 2, 025003, 2016.
[16] L. S. Phee, S. C. Low, V. A. Huynh, and S. H. Yeo, "Development of a robotic instrument for minimally invasive surgery," *The International Journal of Medical Robotics and Computer Assisted Surgery*, vol. 6, no. 2, pp. 218–225, 2010.
[17] T. L. Chen and L. M. Ngo, "Wearable soft robotics for limb rehabilitation," *Advanced Functional Materials*, vol. 27, no. 27, 1700560, 2017.
[18] D. Chiaradia and T. Ranzani, "Bio-inspired soft robots for adaptive and effective navigation in unstructured environments," *Advanced Intelligent Systems*, vol. 1, no. 1, 1900010, 2019.
[19] A. Chiri, N. Vitiello, S. Roccella, F. Vecchi, and M. C. Carrozza, "A bio-inspired exoskeleton for the shoulder: Physiological perspectives," in *Proceedings of the 2009 IEEE International Conference on Robotics and Biomimetics (ROBIO)*, pp. 1243–1248, 2009.
[20] K. Koganezawa, K. Nakajima, and K. Asaka, "A soft wearable robotic suit for muscle training," *Bioinspiration & Biomimetics*, vol. 9, no. 1, 016010, 2014.
[21] S. B. Godfrey and D. P. Losey, "A bio-inspired soft robotic prosthetic hand," *Soft Robotics*, vol. 5, no. 3, pp. 241–251, 2018.

[22] R. Gentner and J. Classen, "Development and evaluation of a soft prosthetic hand," *Journal of Rehabilitation Research and Development*, vol. 46, no. 6, pp. 771–784, 2009.
[23] R. Conti, R. Deimel, S. Ciotti, and S. M. De Rossi, "A biomimetic approach for soft prosthetics: Combining soft robotics with neuromuscular control," *Advanced Materials Technologies*, vol. 2, no. 9, 1700116, 2017.
[24] C. Tan and H. Zhang, "Design and control of a neural interface for a soft robotic prosthetic hand," *Journal of Neural Engineering*, vol. 17, no. 3, 036004, 2020.
[25] K. S. Kim, J. Y. Lee, and J. Park, "Bio-inspired microswimmers for targeted drug delivery," *Biofabrication*, vol. 10, no. 2, 025004, 2018.
[26] J. Wang and R. Dong, "Bio-inspired micro/nanorobots for intelligent drug delivery," *Biomaterials*, vol. 211, pp. 24–47, 2019.
[27] W. Gao, S. Sattayasamitsathit, and J. Wang, "Catalytically powered micro/nanomotors: From movement principle to biomedical applications," *Accounts of Chemical Research*, vol. 47, no. 2, pp. 403–411, 2014.
[28] S. Kim, F. Qiu, and B. J. Nelson, "Fabrication and characterization of microscale magnetically actuated robots for targeted drug delivery," *Small*, vol. 12, no. 20, pp. 2630–2636, 2016.
[29] C. Stewart, J. F. Domingues, and M. B. Dowling, "A bio-inspired soft robotic implantable drug delivery device," *Journal of Biomedical Materials Research Part B: Applied Biomaterials*, vol. 106, no. 7, pp. 2611–2619, 2018.
[30] M. Cianchetti, M. Calisti, and L. Margheri, "Bioinspired locomotion and grasping in water: The soft eight-arm OCTOPUS robot," *Bioinspiration & Biomimetics*, vol. 10, no. 3, 035003, 2015.
[31] A. M. Bellinger and M. Jafari, "Oral, bio-inspired, and programmable delivery of drugs and devices," *Science Translational Medicine*, vol. 8, no. 365, 365ra157, 2016.
[32] J. Zhao and H. Li, "An implantable soft robotic drug delivery system for diabetes management," *Journal of Biomedical Engineering*, vol. 39, no. 2, pp. 258–267, 2017.
[33] S. W. Park and M. Choi, "Soft robotic biopsy for minimally invasive procedures," *Soft Robotics*, vol. 6, no. 5, pp. 602–610, 2019.
[34] G. Lanna and C. Bergeles, "A bioinspired soft robotic biopsy device for neurosurgery," *IEEE Transactions on Biomedical Engineering*, vol. 67, no. 9, pp. 2617–2626, 2020.
[35] S. H. Ahn and K. J. Cho, "A novel soft robotic biopsy device with controlled flexibility," *Journal of Micromechanics and Microengineering*, vol. 28, no. 11, 115010, 2018.
[36] I. De Falco and A. Menciassi, "A soft robotic biopsy device for colon cancer screening," *Advanced Robotics*, vol. 28, no. 13, pp. 891–903, 2014.
[37] H. B. Gilbert, J. S. Neimat, and R. J. Webster, "A flexible robotic tool for accessing deep brain regions through curved trajectories," *IEEE Transactions on Biomedical Engineering*, vol. 64, no. 6, pp. 1254–1261, 2017.
[38] Z. Wang and T. Wang, "Design and fabrication of a flexible robotic endoscopic tool for medical applications," *Biomedical Microdevices*, vol. 20, no. 4, 89, 2018.
[39] D. Yang and C. Jin, "A bioinspired soft robotic endoscope with adaptable stiffness for minimally invasive surgery," *Soft Robotics*, vol. 3, no. 3, pp. 146–153, 2016.
[40] Y. Yang and Y. Zhao, "A flexible endoscopic tool for advanced medical imaging and biopsy," *Biomedical Microdevices*, vol. 21, no. 4, 102, 2019.

Chapter 5

Motion control of soft robotic arm through servo motors

M. Avinash, M. L. Pavan Kishore, Syed Quadir Moinuddin, Tharakeshwar Appala, and Shaik Himam Saheb

5.1 INTRODUCTION

The automation of robots represents a paradigm shift in contemporary industry and technology, offering transformative capabilities across a wide spectrum of applications. Its significance lies in its potential to redefine traditional manufacturing processes, optimize operational efficiency, and drive economic growth in a rapidly evolving global landscape. As industries strive to meet escalating demands for higher productivity, precision, and cost-effectiveness, the adoption of robotic automation emerges as a strategic imperative, enabling organizations to stay competitive in an increasingly dynamic marketplace. Central to this robotic automation is motion control, a fundamental aspect of robotic systems that plays a crucial role in determining their efficiency, precision, and versatility [1]. The importance of motion control in robotics cannot be overstated, as it directly impacts the performance and capabilities of robots across various applications. From industrial automation to medical robotics, the ability to accurately control the movement of robotic arms and other components is essential for achieving desired outcomes. By ensuring precise, efficient, and versatile operations, motion control enhances the overall effectiveness of robotic systems, making them indispensable in modern industrial and technological environments [2].

One of the primary advantages of advanced motion control systems is the high level of precision they offer. In industrial settings, for instance, robotic arms equipped with precise motion control can perform tasks such as assembly, welding, and painting with remarkable accuracy. This precision not only enhances the quality of the final product but also reduces waste and increases production efficiency. Furthermore, precise motion control enables robots to operate in environments that require meticulous attention to detail, such as semiconductor manufacturing and microsurgery. Another significant benefit of motion control in robotic systems is the increased speed and efficiency of operations. Robots with sophisticated motion control capabilities can perform repetitive tasks at speeds unattainable by human workers, leading to substantial productivity gains. This is particularly advantageous in industries

 DOI: 10.1201/9781003539612-5

such as automotive manufacturing, where high throughput is critical. Additionally, the ability to automate tasks that involve hazardous environments or materials helps improve workplace safety, as robots can handle dangerous substances or operate in extreme conditions without risking human health [3, 4].

The implementation of motion control systems in robotics also presents several challenges and disadvantages. One of the primary concerns is the complexity and cost associated with developing and maintaining these systems. High-precision motion control often requires advanced sensors, actuators, and control algorithms, which can be expensive and technically demanding to integrate. Moreover, the need for ongoing calibration and maintenance to ensure optimal performance can add to the overall cost and complexity [5].

Another potential disadvantage is the reliance on sophisticated software and hardware, which can be prone to failures or malfunctions. Ensuring the reliability and robustness of motion control systems is critical, particularly in applications where downtime or errors can have significant consequences. For instance, in surgical robotics, any malfunction or inaccuracy could lead to severe patient harm, highlighting the need for stringent safety and reliability standards. Despite these challenges, the applications of motion control in robotic systems are vast and continually expanding. In the medical field, robots with precise motion control are used for minimally invasive surgeries, prosthetics, and rehabilitation devices. These applications benefit from the robots' ability to perform delicate and complex tasks with high precision, improving patient outcomes and expanding the possibilities of medical treatment [6].

In industrial automation, motion-controlled robots are integral to processes such as assembly, material handling, and quality inspection. The automotive, electronics, and aerospace industries, in particular, have seen significant advancements due to the integration of robotic systems with advanced motion control, leading to increased production efficiency and product quality. Moreover, motion control is pivotal in emerging fields such as service robotics, where robots assist with tasks in domestic environments, customer service, and logistics. Autonomous mobile robots (AMRs) with sophisticated motion control can navigate complex environments, delivering goods and services efficiently in warehouses, hospitals, and even urban settings.

Motion control is a critical component of modern robotic systems, offering numerous advantages such as precision, efficiency, and the ability to operate in hazardous environments. While there are challenges related to cost, complexity, and reliability, the benefits and wide-ranging applications make motion control an essential area of focus in the development of robotic technology. The role of motion control in robotics will undoubtedly grow, driving innovation and expanding the capabilities of robots across various sectors [7].

5.2 LITERATURE SURVEY

Artificial intelligence and machine learning (AIML) with traditional control systems has opened new avenues for enhancing robot autonomy and adaptability. These intelligent control systems allow robots to learn from their environment and improve performance over time, making them suitable for unstructured and unpredictable scenarios. Additionally, the advancement in sensor technologies and real-time data processing has significantly improved the accuracy and responsiveness of motion control systems. Sensors provide critical feedback for maintaining balance, avoiding obstacles, and performing intricate maneuvers.

This literature review aims to provide a comprehensive overview of the state-of-the-art in motion control of robotic systems, identifying key milestones and ongoing research challenges. By examining various control strategies, technologies, and applications, the review seeks to elucidate the current landscape and future directions in robotic motion control.

This chapter discusses the robotic information system (RIS), an innovative information system architecture designed to provide data, information processing, and services across a wide geographical area through intelligent robots. Its neck allows for 41° axial rotations and 45° flexion/extension, the jaw has a 6° hinge rotation, and the eyes can perform Adduction up to 19°, Abduction up to 34°, and Infraduction (depression) up to 20°. The distance between the upper and lower eyelids ranges from 0 to 17 mm to reflect different expressions.

Equipped with motion, vision, audition, smell, and speech capabilities, Arslan can maintain its eye direction during head movements and recognize head tilting. As the front-end component of RIS which is shown in Figure 5.1, Arslan interacts with users, supported by a data and information processing engine known as "The Oracle" and a database server. This setup

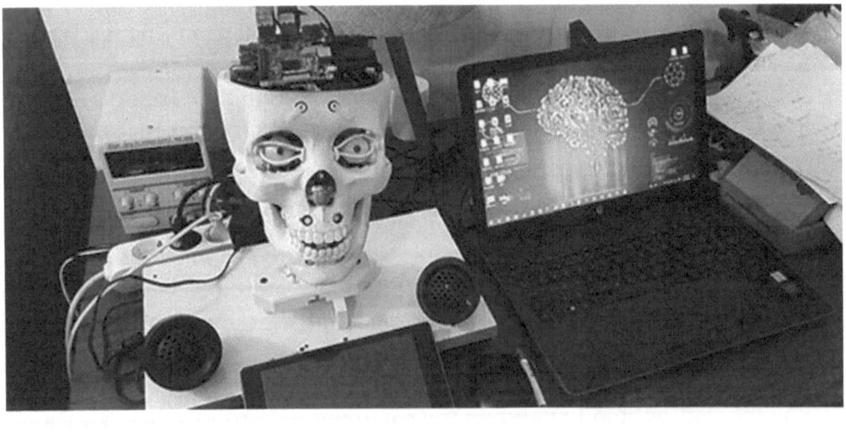

Figure 5.1 The RIS full system implementation.

enables RIS to deliver comprehensive and intelligent services, making it a robust platform for user interaction across various applications [8].

Teleoperation is crucial for performing complex tasks in inaccessible or high-risk environments, and wearable hand exoskeletons play a vital role in this process. These devices allow the master hand to replicate human finger movements and provide tactile feedback to the slave hand interacting with objects. This chapter presents a novel finger exoskeleton designed with a cascading four-link closed-loop kinematic chain. Each finger operates independently, utilizing angle sensors to monitor flexion/extension and adduction/abduction motions. Servo motors manage cable tension to deliver real-time contact forces to the fingers.

An adaptive hand exoskeleton built from this finger design was tested within a master-slave framework. The diagram of the master-slave control strategy is shown in Figure 5.2. Results indicate that it can be worn comfortably without mechanical constraints, with the slave hand accurately mimicking human finger movements. The force reproduction system exhibited high precision and real-time responsiveness. This adaptive exoskeleton can effectively function as the master hand for controlling a dexterous five-fingered slave hand, facilitating intricate manipulation tasks. Enables independent movement of each finger joint.

The force reproduction system enhances user interaction. Features 20 degrees of freedom for versatile motion capabilities. Experiments confirm its accuracy, stability, and reliability across diverse conditions. This development represents a significant advancement in teleoperation technology for complex environments [9].

This study employs a fuzzy neural Petri nets (FNPNs) controller to manage a three-link robot arm, addressing the complexities of a nonlinear dynamic system. We propose integrating a classical fuzzy neural network (FNN) with

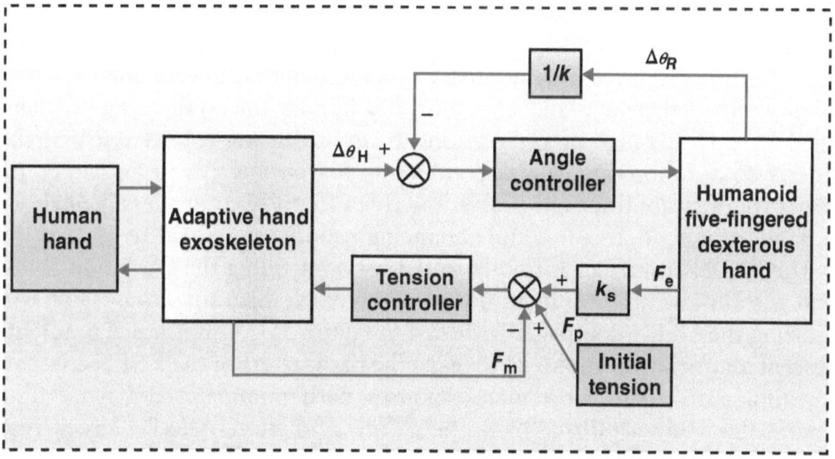

Figure 5.2 Diagram of the master–slave control strategy.

a Petri net (PN) to form an FNPN structure, which aims to reduce computational demands. The motion equations for the three-link robot arm are derived using Lagrange's equation and combined with the motion equations of the DC servo motors that drive the robot. To tackle the challenges posed by nonlinear dynamics, we introduce a direct adaptive control technique that utilizes the FNPN controller. Computer simulations demonstrate that the FNPN controller delivers superior performance, featuring quick response times and minimal error [10].

The use of FNPN controllers in smart robotics applications represents a significant advancement in managing complex, nonlinear systems. FNPN controllers combine the strengths of fuzzy logic, neural networks, and PNs to create a robust control architecture that can adapt to dynamic environments. This integration is particularly beneficial for robots that must operate in unpredictable settings, such as service robots in healthcare, autonomous vehicles, and industrial automation.

In smart robotics, FNPN controllers excel in handling uncertainty and imprecision, which are common in real-world applications. The fuzzy logic component allows for reasoning with vague inputs, enabling the robot to make decisions based on qualitative assessments. This is crucial in scenarios where precise measurements are challenging, such as navigating through cluttered spaces or interacting with humans. The neural network aspect enhances the controller's learning capability, allowing the robot to improve its performance over time by adapting to new data. This feature is especially valuable in applications like robotic arms in manufacturing, where the ability to learn from past tasks can lead to increased efficiency and precision.

The PN component aids in modeling the complex interactions and workflows within robotic systems. It provides a visual representation of the control logic, making it easier to analyze and optimize the robot's behavior in real-time. This is beneficial for applications that require coordinated actions, such as multirobot systems or collaborative robots working alongside humans. FNPN controllers facilitate smarter, more autonomous robotic systems capable of performing complex tasks in dynamic environments. Their adaptability, efficiency, and capability to handle uncertainty make them ideal for a wide range of applications, from healthcare robots assisting the elderly to autonomous drones conducting search and rescue missions. As smart robotics continues to evolve, the role of FNPN controllers is likely to expand, driving innovation and enhancing robotic functionality.

The FNPN controller is implemented for controlling the three-link robot arm without the need for identification. The block diagram of the robot arm utilizing the FNPN controller is shown in Figure 5.3. A supervised gradient-descent algorithm is employed to learn the parameters of the FNPN controller, aiming to achieve optimal responses with minimal error. An online tuning algorithm is utilized based on a fitness function to derive a recurrent gradient vector. The study establishes that error convergence for the control of three-link robot arms using the FNPN controller is highly effective.

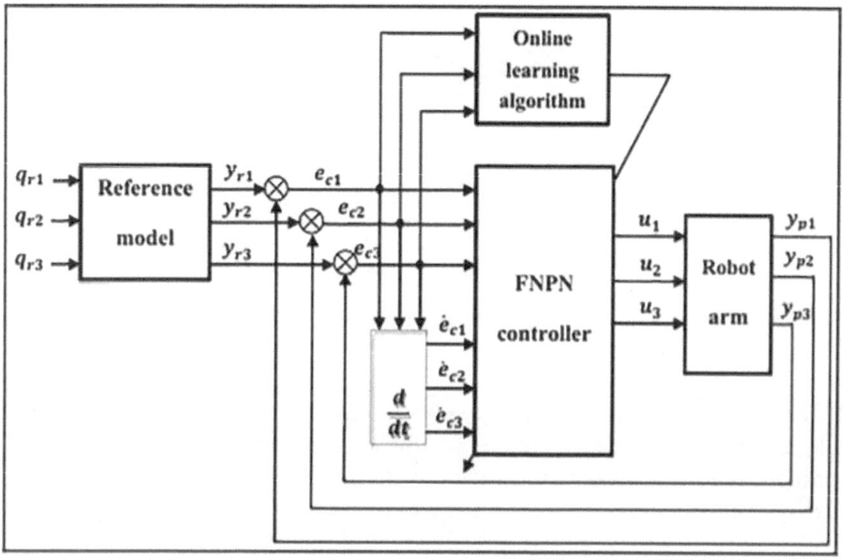

Figure 5.3 Block diagram of the robot arm utilizing the FNPN controller.

Initially, the state returns a large error, prompting the threshold to be set at zero (dth = 0) to activate more rules. As the error diminishes, the threshold increases, reducing the firing rules and computational load. This adaptive approach enhances real-time control capabilities, facilitating rapid responses in nonlinear control systems [11, 12].

Recent technological advances have sparked interest in developing medical robots, particularly for assistance and rehabilitation. Integrating robotic systems in these areas enhances users' quality of life. This chapter proposes a unified control system for a robotic standing wheelchair, designed to perform tasks autonomously while allowing position and orientation changes at any time. The control scheme is divided into two parts: a kinematic controller for solving desired motion and a dynamic controller for compensating the wheelchair–human system's dynamics. The controllers, based on linear algebra, aim for low computational cost and asymptotic stability without disturbances. Stability and robustness are analyzed through control error evolution in each sampling period. Real experiments with an instrumented standing wheelchair demonstrate the controller's performance [13].

The control scheme consists of two subsystems: a unified kinematic controller for path following and positioning and a dynamic controller for system dynamics compensation. Sampling theory and Markov properties were used in the design. The kinematic and dynamic models of the standing wheelchair informed the controller design. The block diagram illustrates the motion control of the standing human wheelchair system as shown in Figure 5.4. Robustness and stability analyses confirmed stable control errors, and real tests showed satisfactory performance.

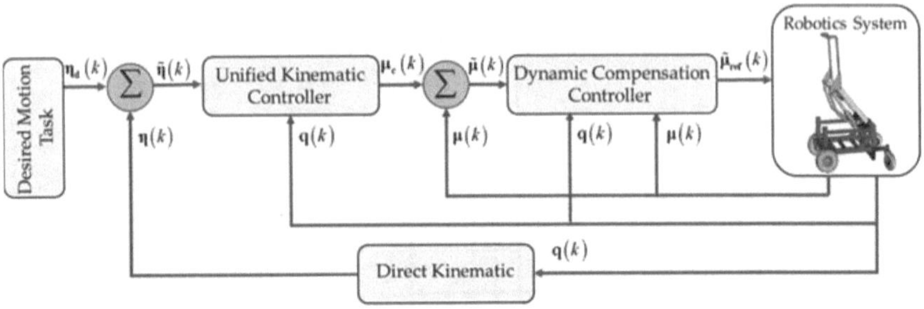

Figure 5.4 Diagram illustrating the motion control of the standing human wheelchair system.

Future work includes developing an interactive 3D virtual environment for rehabilitating individuals with lower extremity motor disabilities, enabling real-time interaction between the robotic wheelchair and the virtual system using real data from the robotic system [14].

5.3 STEPPER MOTORS

Stepper motors, also known as stepping motors or step motors, are a unique breed of electric motors prized for their exceptional control over rotational movement. Unlike their continuous-motion counterparts (like DC motors), stepper motors operate in distinct, precise steps. This characteristic makes them ideal for situations demanding accurate positioning and controlled movement.

Imagine a scenario where you need to rotate a shaft precisely by 45°, stop it there, and then rotate it another 27° later. A stepper motor excels in such tasks. Their applications range from the intricate operations of 3D printers and CNC machines to the familiar movements of security cameras and disk drives.

5.3.1 Operation

The magic behind stepper motors lies in their internal structure and how electrical signals translate into physical movement. Here's a breakdown of the key components and their interplay:

✓ **Stator and Rotor:**

- The stator is the stationary outer part of the motor. It houses a series of electromagnets arranged in phases (typically two or more phases). These electromagnets are essentially coils of wire wrapped around a metal core.
- The rotor is the inner rotating part. It's typically made of steel and has teeth (or poles) around its circumference.

✓ **Electromagnetic Dance:**
- When an electrical current is applied to a specific phase in the stator, it generates a magnetic field. The rotor, with its permanent magnetism or induced magnetism, aligns itself with this magnetic field.
- By strategically sequencing the energization of different phases (think turning them on and off in a specific order), a rotating magnetic field is created within the stator.
- The rotor, ever eager to follow the lead, tries to align itself with this ever-changing magnetic field, resulting in a step-by-step rotation.

✓ **Step Size and Control:**
- The step size, which is the angle of rotation per step, is determined by the design of the motor, specifically the number of teeth on the rotor and the number of poles in the stator.
- By controlling the sequence and timing of the electrical pulses sent to the stator coils, we can precisely dictate the direction (clockwise or counterclockwise) and speed (faster or slower steps per second) of the rotor's rotation.
- The number of electrical pulses received by the motor directly translates to the number of steps it takes, allowing for very precise control over the final position of the shaft.

A significant advantage of stepper motors is the ability to operate without a position sensor (closed-loop control). As long as we keep track of the number of pulses sent, we know exactly where the shaft is positioned. This simplifies the control system compared to motors requiring constant feedback. Stepper motors typically require a dedicated driver circuit to manage the complex sequence and timing of the electrical pulses sent to the stator coils. These drivers translate high-level control signals into the appropriate low-level power signals for the motor.

5.3.2 Advantages of stepper motors

Stepper motors offer numerous advantages that make them highly suitable for a variety of applications, particularly those requiring precise positioning and reliability. One of the primary benefits of stepper motors is their ability to achieve precise positioning. They operate by moving in fixed increments or steps, allowing for high precision and repeatability. This characteristic makes them ideal for applications such as CNC machines, 3D printers, and robotic arms, where exact positioning is critical.

Another significant advantage is their capability to function effectively in an open-loop control system. Unlike servo motors, stepper motors do not require complex feedback systems to maintain accuracy. This simplicity reduces both cost and complexity, making them an attractive choice for budget-conscious projects. Their design also contributes to their cost-effectiveness, as stepper motors are generally more affordable than servo systems, especially in applications where high-speed performance is not a primary requirement.

Stepper motors exhibit high torque at low speeds, which is particularly advantageous for applications needing substantial holding torque. This feature makes them suitable for scenarios where consistent positioning is essential, such as in robotics or industrial automation. Their simple construction is another benefit; lacking brushes and commutators results in fewer components that can wear out. This leads to lower maintenance requirements and higher reliability, a crucial factor in long-term operational settings.

The ease of control is another notable advantage of stepper motors. They can be easily managed with straightforward drive electronics, such as microcontrollers, without the need for advanced control algorithms. This accessibility allows engineers and developers to integrate them into systems quickly and efficiently. Furthermore, stepper motors provide an immediate response to digital control, reacting swiftly to changes in input pulses, which ensures rapid and predictable movement—an essential requirement in many automated processes.

Their wide speed range also contributes to their versatility; stepper motors can operate effectively at very low speeds without requiring gear reduction, while still handling moderate-speed applications efficiently. When stationary, stepper motors maintain a strong holding torque, preventing unintended movement, which is vital in applications where stability is critical. Lastly, due to their incremental movement, there is no cumulative error, ensuring consistent accuracy over extended operational periods.

The advantages of stepper motors—precise positioning, open-loop control, high torque at low speeds, cost-effectiveness, simple construction, ease of control, immediate response, wide speed range, high holding torque, and absence of cumulative error—make them a preferred choice in a wide array of industrial and consumer applications.

5.3.3 Applications of stepper motors

- **CNC Machines:** Used for precise control of cutting tools in multiple axes, ensuring accurate machining.
- **3D Printers:** Drive the movement of the print head and build platform, allowing for precise layer deposition.
- **Textile Machinery:** Control the movement of needles, bobbins, and fabric feed mechanisms in knitting and weaving machines.
- **Medical Devices:** Found in infusion pumps, blood analyzers, and robotic surgical systems where precision and reliability are crucial.
- **Automated Manufacturing:** Used in conveyor belt systems, packaging machines, and assembly lines for precise control and positioning.
- **Camera Platforms:** Enable precise pan, tilt, and zoom movements in robotic camera mounts and stabilizers.

- **Robotics:** Control robotic arms and grippers, allowing for accurate positioning and movement in various robotic applications.
- **Aerospace:** Used in instrumentation, satellite control systems, and other aerospace applications requiring precision and reliability.
- **Automotive Industry:** Found in systems like headlight positioning, dashboard instruments, and climate control actuators.
- **Consumer Electronics:** Used in printers, scanners, and CD/DVD drives for precise control of media handling and positioning.

5.3.4 Limitations of stepper motors

- **Limited Torque at High Speeds:** Stepper motors tend to lose torque as their speed increases, making them less suitable for high-speed applications compared to servo motors.
- **Resonance and Vibration:** They can exhibit resonance and vibration issues at certain speeds, which can lead to noise and decreased performance.
- **Step Accuracy:** While generally precise, stepper motors can accumulate small errors over time due to mechanical imperfections or load variations.
- **Complex Control Algorithms for Smooth Operation:** Achieving smooth and quiet operation may require complex microstepping control algorithms, adding to the control system complexity.
- **Mechanical Wear:** Although they lack brushes, other mechanical parts such as bearings and gears can wear out over time, requiring maintenance or replacement.
- **Size and Weight:** Stepper motors can be bulkier and heavier compared to some other motor types with equivalent power ratings, potentially limiting their use in space-constrained applications.
- **Limited Efficiency:** They generally have lower efficiency compared to other motor types like brushless DC motors, leading to higher operational costs over time.

5.4 SERVO MOTORS

Servo motors play a pivotal role in the development and functionality of soft robots, which are designed to be flexible, adaptable, and capable of safe interaction with their environments and human users. Unlike traditional rigid robots, soft robots leverage soft materials and structures to mimic biological organisms, enabling them to navigate complex tasks with a high degree of dexterity and gentleness. The integration of servo motors into these systems allows for precise control over movement and positioning, making them invaluable for various applications.

One of the primary advantages of using servo motors in soft robotics is their ability to provide accurate and repeatable motion. Servo motors operate by receiving a control signal that dictates their desired position, allowing them to move to specific angles or positions with high precision. This characteristic is particularly important in soft robots that perform intricate tasks, such as surgical robots that must operate delicately on human tissue or robotic arms used in manufacturing that require careful assembly of components. The precision afforded by servo motors ensures that soft robots can execute movements that are both effective and safe.

Servo motors offer significant torque capabilities, especially at low speeds. This feature is essential for soft robots that need to manipulate soft actuators, such as inflatable bladders or compliant joints. The torque produced by servo motors allows these actuators to exert the necessary force to accomplish tasks while maintaining control over their movements. For instance, in prosthetic applications, servo motors can provide the required strength to perform actions like gripping or lifting, all while ensuring that movements are smooth and natural.

Another benefit is the simplicity of integrating servo motors into soft robotic designs. Many servo motors come with built-in feedback systems, such as encoders, that continuously monitor the motor's position. This feedback loop enables real-time adjustments, enhancing the robot's responsiveness to changes in its environment. In scenarios requiring high accuracy, such as navigating through obstacles or interacting with objects of varying shapes and sizes, this capability becomes indispensable.

The compact and lightweight design of servo motors makes them particularly suitable for soft robotics. These motors can be seamlessly incorporated into small, portable robotic systems, allowing soft robots to operate in tight spaces where traditional rigid robots may struggle. This versatility opens up a wide range of applications, from agricultural robots that need to harvest crops delicately to search-and-rescue robots designed to navigate rubble or confined spaces in disaster scenarios.

The integration of servo motors in soft robotics is not without challenges. One significant hurdle is the need to harmonize the flexibility of soft materials with the precise control offered by servo motors. Designers must carefully consider the mechanical properties of soft actuators to ensure that they can effectively work with servo motors, which often require a certain degree of rigidity to function optimally. Innovations in soft actuator design and control strategies are necessary to overcome these challenges, leading to improved performance and adaptability in soft robotic systems.

Servo motors are integral to the advancement of soft robotics, providing the precision, torque, and adaptability necessary for these innovative systems. Their ability to enable intricate movements, coupled with real-time feedback and control, enhances the functionality of soft robots across various fields, including healthcare, agriculture, and emergency response. As research and technology continue to evolve, the potential for servo motors in soft robotics will expand, paving the way for even more advanced and capable robotic solutions that can interact effectively and safely with the world around them.

In Figure 5.5, a potentiometer is utilized with a voltage-adjusting knob that is coupled to the output shaft. As the shaft rotates, the knob turns and creates a varying electrical potential. As the potentiometer's voltage-adjusting knob rotates along with the system shaft from 0° to 45°, the electrical potential increases with the angular movement. This varying electrical potential is then fed into an error-detecting feedback amplifier, along with the input reference commands, or input signal voltage. This setup allows the system to compare the actual position of the shaft, indicated by the electrical potential from the potentiometer, with the desired position specified by the input signal. The feedback amplifier then adjusts the motor's position to minimize the difference between these two signals, ensuring precise control of the servo motor's position.

As the system shaft rotates from 0° to 45°, the voltage output from the potentiometer increases proportionally. When the shaft reaches the 45° position, the voltage from the potentiometer matches the input command voltage provided to the system. At this point, where the shaft is aligned precisely with the desired position, there is no disparity between the voltage signal generated by the potentiometer and the reference input voltage (the command signal). Consequently, the output voltage of the amplifier becomes zero. This zero-output voltage signifies that the system shaft has reached the intended position, achieving alignment with the specified input command.

In accordance with the provided figure, the output electrical voltage signal from the amplifier serves as the input voltage for the DC motor. Consequently, once the shaft has rotated by 45°, the motor will cease rotation and remain stationary at this position. It will remain in this resting state until another command is issued to the system for further movement of the shaft. This example illustrates a straightforward understanding of servo motor control, where precise positioning is achieved based on input commands and feedback mechanisms.

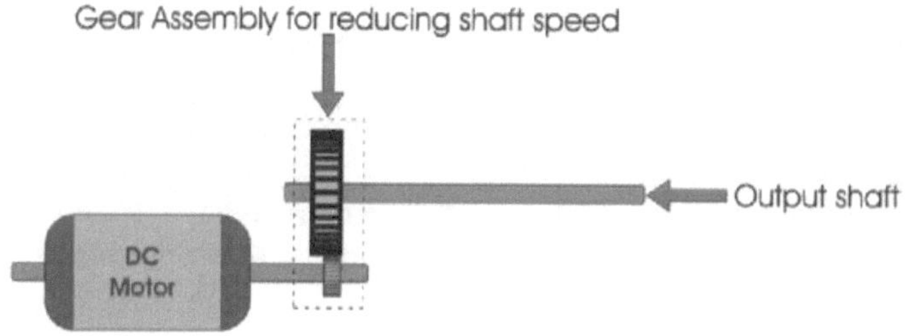

Figure 5.5 Assembly to step down RPM of output shaft.

5.4.1 Advantages of servo motors over stepper motors

- **Controlled Torque:** While stepper motors operate at full torque, servo motors offer the advantage of being able to control torque according to the application's requirements.
- **Standstill Stability:** Stepper motors excel in applications requiring complete standstill stability, as they do not pulsate like servo motors do when at rest. Servo motors, however, are preferred for vertical applications where precise load holding is necessary.
- **Microstepping:** While microstepping increases resolution, it can diminish torque in stepper motors by up to 30%, whereas servo motors maintain their torque regardless of microstepping.
- **Acceleration:** Servo motors exhibit greater flexibility with torque during acceleration compared to stepper motors, which require more power for acceleration.
- **Size:** Stepper motors and servo motors generally offer comparable frame sizes, with differences mainly in length. This allows for achieving different torque and inertia values without increasing the motor's size or cost.
- **Speed:** Servo motors are known for their speed, but they may provide more RPMs than necessary for certain applications. In such cases, stepper motors can offer sufficient performance.
- **Power Efficiency:** Both stepper and servo motors generate more torque with increased current. However, stepper motors can generate significant torque at a safe voltage, offering power efficiency advantages.

Servo motors offer precise torque control, better acceleration characteristics, and high-speed capabilities, making them suitable for applications where dynamic performance is crucial. On the other hand, stepper motors excel in applications requiring standstill stability, cost-effectiveness, and efficiency in power consumption. The choice between servo and stepper motors depends on specific application requirements and performance considerations.

5.5 MOTION CONTROL IN SOFT ROBOTICS

The soft robotics uses variety of actuation mechanisms as the mechanisms need high number of degrees of freedom. This field is attractive due to unique properties of soft materials to create robots that are flexible, adaptable, and often more capable of handling delicate tasks than traditional rigid robots.

5.5.1 Actuation mechanisms

Soft robots often use unconventional actuation mechanisms compared to traditional rigid robots. The following types of actuations were used in the construction of soft robots

- **Pneumatic Actuators:** These use compressed air to inflate or deflate chambers within the soft robot, causing it to change shape. They can mimic muscle-like movements and are useful for creating complex and smooth motions.
- **Hydraulic Actuators:** Similar to pneumatic actuators but use liquids. They provide precise control over movements and are often used in applications requiring higher force.
- **Shape-Memory Alloys (SMAs):** These materials change shape in response to temperature changes. They can be used to create motion in soft robots by exploiting their ability to return to a pre-defined shape.
- **Electroactive Polymers (EAPs):** These materials change shape in response to an electric field. EAPs can be used to create actuators that provide a wide range of motion and flexibility.
- **Cable-Driven Actuators:** These use cables and pulleys to create motion. The cables can be pulled or released to change the shape of the robot.

5.5.2 Control strategies

Controlling the motion of soft robots involves different strategies compared to rigid robots the control strategies used below are used in the soft robotics construction.

- **Model-Based Control:** This involves creating a mathematical model of the soft robot's dynamics and using it to predict and control its behavior. This approach requires detailed knowledge of the robot's material properties and actuation mechanisms.
- **Feedback Control:** Sensors are used to monitor the robot's position and movement in real-time. Feedback control systems adjust the actuators based on this sensor data to achieve the desired motion.
- **Machine Learning and Optimization:** Machine learning algorithms can be used to learn and optimize control strategies for soft robots, particularly in complex or unstructured environments where traditional modeling might be difficult.
- **Adaptive Control:** This approach allows the control system to adjust itself in response to changes in the robot's behavior or environment, making it more flexible and capable of handling variations.

Soft robots are increasingly used in diverse applications due to their unique properties. Soft robots are used in surgical tools, prosthetics, and rehabilitation devices due to their flexibility and ability to conform to delicate structures. Their ability to squeeze through tight spaces makes them ideal for exploring disaster sites. Soft robots can handle delicate fruits and plants without causing damage. Their soft and adaptable nature allows for safer and more intuitive interactions with humans. Motion control in soft robots is a multidisciplinary field that combines materials science, robotics, control theory, and computer science to create robots that are both versatile and effective in a wide range of applications.

5.6 HARDWARE CONFIGURATIONS

Software inputs from the functional codes within the library set parameter values in the motor encoder, establishing a closed-loop system. This closed-loop system utilizes encoder feedback to ensure precise control and monitoring of motor movements, contributing to enhanced accuracy and performance.

5.7 DYNAMIC MODEL OF HIGH-SPEED PRECISION POSITIONAL SERVO SYSTEM

The closed-loop configurations of servo motors illustrate the intricate dynamics of the system. Depending on the bandwidth requirements, different loops within the system may cycle at varying rates to ensure stability.

1. **Current Loop:** Achieved a bandwidth of 1500 Hz through meticulous adjustment of poles and zeros of the compensator. This enables precise control over the current within the system.
2. **Speed Loop:** Attained a corresponding bandwidth of 120 Hz for the speed loop. This achievement is facilitated by a compensator featuring a pole at the origin, an early zero at 50 rad/sec, and a pole at 500 rad/sec. The pole at the origin aids in eliminating steady-state offset, while the zero enhances phase margin at cross-over, and the pole effectively attenuates the second resonant peak.
3. **Position Loop:** The primary objective of the position loop is to position the source and detector swiftly with minimal overshoots and settling times, particularly in scan mode operation. To fulfill this requirement, a Type-II position loop controller with an early zero offset is essential. Hence, a substantial gain (Km = 500) and high bandwidth are necessary to minimize errors.

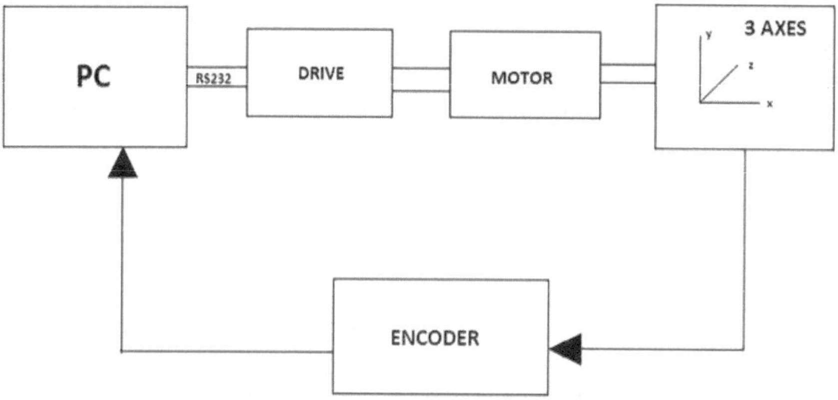

Figure 5.6 Block diagram of motion control.

5.7.1 Motion control

The block diagram of motion control for three-axis devices is shown in Figure 5.6.

5.8 CONCLUSION

The development of a stable control system for a three-axis robotic arm utilizing servo motors marks a significant achievement in precision automation. By meticulously tuning the motors, stability and precise control of the robotic arm were ensured, allowing for smooth and accurate movements across all three axes. This tuning process is crucial as it optimizes the performance of the servo motors, reducing errors and enhancing the overall reliability of the system. Additionally, the creation of a user-friendly graphical user interface (GUI) has further streamlined the operation of the robotic arm. The GUI includes essential functions such as opening and closing communication ports, facilitating seamless interaction between the user and the robotic system. More importantly, the main GUI focuses on the motion control of the servo motors, providing intuitive controls for the user to manipulate the robotic arm with ease.

This combination of a stable, well-tuned control system and an accessible GUI not only improves the user experience but also extends the potential applications of the robotic arm in various fields such as manufacturing, medical robotics, and research. Overall, this project demonstrates a significant advancement in robotic control systems, emphasizing precision, stability, and user-centric design.

The integration of Internet of Things (IoT) technologies will enable seamless communication between robotic systems and other smart devices, creating interconnected networks that can share data and optimize operations collectively. This connectivity will be particularly beneficial in industrial settings, where real-time data exchange can significantly improve efficiency and reduce downtime. The development of new materials and manufacturing techniques will also play a crucial role in the evolution of servo motors and their applications in robotics. Lighter, more durable, and energy-efficient motors will pave the way for more agile and sustainable robotic systems. The motion control of robotic systems using servo motors has already brought significant advancements and continues to hold immense potential for future developments. The ongoing research and innovation in this field promise to unlock new possibilities, making robotic systems more capable, efficient, and integrated into various aspects of human life and industry. As technology progresses, we can anticipate a future where robotic systems driven by sophisticated servo motor control will be ubiquitous, transforming the way we work, live, and interact with our environment.

REFERENCES

[1] Iqbal, J., Islam, R. U., Abbas, S. Z., Khan, A. A., & Ajwad, S. A. (2016). Automating industrial tasks through mechatronic systems-A review of robotics in industrial perspective. *Tehnickivjesnik/Technical Gazette*, 23(3) pp 917–924.

[2] Tan, K. K., Lee, T. H., & Huang, S. (2007). *Precision motion control: design and implementation*. Springer Science & Business Media.

[3] Trevelyan, J., Hamel, W. R., & Kang, S. C. (2016). Robotics in hazardous applications. *Springer Handbook of Robotics*, 1521–1548. https://doi.org/10.1007/978-3-319-32552-1_58

[4] Robla-Gómez, S., Becerra, V. M., Llata, J. R., Gonzalez-Sarabia, E., Torre-Ferrero, C., & Perez-Oria, J. (2017). Working together: A review on safe human-robot collaboration in industrial environments. *IEEE Access*, 5, 26754–26773.

[5] Albu-Schaffer, A., Eiberger, O., Grebenstein, M., Haddadin, S., Ott, C., Wimbock, T., & Hirzinger, G. (2008). Soft robotics. *IEEE Robotics & Automation Magazine*, 15(3), 20–30.

[6] Okamura, A. M., Matarić, M. J., & Christensen, H. I. (2010). Medical and health-care robotics. *IEEE Robotics & Automation Magazine*, 17(3), 26–37.

[7] Licardo, J. T., Domjan, M., & Orehovački, T. (2024). Intelligent robotics—A systematic review of emerging technologies and trends. *Electronics*, 13(3), 542.

[8] Basar, E., Alexandropoulos, G. C., Liu, Y., Wu, Q., Jin, S., Yuen, C., & Schober, R. (2024). Reconfigurable intelligent surfaces for 6G: Emerging hardware architectures, applications, and open challenges. *IEEE Vehicular Technology Magazine. Volume: 19, Issue: 3, September 2024* https://doi.org/10.1109/MVT.2024.3415570

[9] Wang, K., Liu, J., Yan, W., Lu, Q., & Nie, S. (2021). Force feedback controls of multi-gripper robotic endovascular intervention: design, prototype, and experiments. *International Journal of Computer Assisted Radiology and Surgery*, 16, 179–192.

[10] Klein, M. I. (2008). *Performance, Workload, Stress, and Coping Profiles in First Year Medical Students' Interaction with the Endoscopic/Laparoscopic and Robot-Assisted Minimally Invasive Surgical Techniques* (Doctoral dissertation, University of Cincinnati).

[11] Bonci, A., Longhi, S., Nabissi, G., & Scala, G. A. (2020). Execution time of optimal controls in hard real time, a minimal execution time solution for non-linear SDRE. *IEEE Access*, 8, 158008–158025.

[12] Tsokanas, N., Pastorino, R., & Stojadinović, B. (2022). Adaptive model predictive control for actuation dynamics compensation in real-time hybrid simulation. *Mechanism and Machine Theory*, 172, 104817.

[13] Callejas-Cuervo, M., González-Cely, A. X., & Bastos-Filho, T. (2020). Control systems and electronic instrumentation applied to autonomy in wheelchair mobility: The state of the art. *Sensors*, 20(21), 6326.

[14] Ortiz, J. S., Palacios-Navarro, G., Andaluz, V. H., & Guevara, B. S. (2021). Virtual reality-based framework to simulate control algorithms for robotic assistance and rehabilitation tasks through a standing wheelchair. *Sensors*, 21(15), 5083.

Chapter 6

Soft robotic applications to care elderly people

E Devaraj and S Supreeth

6.1 INTRODUCTION

The aging population presents a number of issues, including not only healthcare but also preserving older persons' freedom and dignity. People's physical and cognitive capacities generally diminish as they age, making it more difficult to accomplish daily duties like dressing, bathing, and eating. In addition, many elderly people feel isolated or lonely, especially if they live alone or have limited social interaction. For these reasons, there is a need for solutions that can give physical help, encourage social participation, and improve mental health.

Traditionally, these needs have been fulfilled by human caretakers, but with rising demand for eldercare and a diminishing workforce in many countries, other approaches are required. Robotics in healthcare is not a new concept, but the introduction of soft robotics introduces a novel technique that is especially appropriate for senior care. These robots' softness and suppleness make them less threatening and more comfortable for senior users who may be delicate or afraid to contact with machinery. Furthermore, soft robots can do jobs that simulate human touch, improving the whole caregiving experience.

Soft robots can also help elderly people with restricted movement by assisting them in getting around or completing exercises. Wearable soft robotic devices, for example, can be used to help people walk or to provide mild, regulated movements during physical therapy. These robots can also be utilized for activities requiring precision and tenderness, such as feeding or medication management. The combination of these characteristics enables soft robotics to be a key tool in increasing independence and improving the quality of care for the elderly.

One of the most promising areas for soft robotic applications in senior care is mobility support. Falls are one of the most common causes of injury in older persons, and many have difficulties walking or standing owing to muscular weakening or joint problems. Soft robotics, particularly exoskeletons or wearable gadgets, can help the elderly by improving their physical abilities.

DOI: 10.1201/9781003539612-6

These robots can help people walk more safely by providing stability and lowering the chance of falling, or they can assist with tasks that require strength or balance.

Another key application for soft robots is rehabilitation and treatment. Many older persons suffer from illnesses like stroke, arthritis, or other musculoskeletal disorders that necessitate long-term treatment to regain function. Soft robots can aid in physical rehabilitation by performing regulated, repetitive movements that build muscular strength and coordination. These robots can be programmed to vary the level of help provided according to the user's requirements, ensuring that the therapy is both successful and comfortable. In some circumstances, soft robots can even be utilized to provide tailored therapy programs that evolve over time as the user's health improves.

Soft robots can also help with activities of daily living (ADLs), which are crucial for preserving independence. Dressing, bathing, and eating might be challenging for the elderly due to physical limitations, but soft robots can aid by offering gentle, supporting assistance. For example, a soft robotic arm might aid an elderly person in dressing oneself by holding garments in place or assisting with buttoning, or a robot could help with dining by gently directing utensils. These programs allow the elderly to keep their dignity and liberty while receiving the assistance they require.

In addition to physical aid, soft robots can offer social and emotional support. Many elderly people experience loneliness or social isolation, especially if they live in nursing facilities or have little family contact. Soft robots built for companionship can reduce these symptoms by interacting, conversing, and offering emotional support. These robots can be designed to react to human emotions, hold simple conversations, and even play games or music. Soft robots can thus provide not just physical support but also a sense of connection and friendship, both of which are essential for mental health.

The use of soft robotics in senior care has various advantages, both for the patients and for the caregivers. One of the most significant advantages of soft robotics is their capacity to deliver personalized, adaptable care. Because these robots are designed to be adaptable and responsive, they may be programmed to match the specific requirements of each individual. This enables more tailored care, whether through physical aid, therapy, or social engagement.

Another key advantage of soft robots is their ability to alleviate the stress on caregivers. The difficulties of caring for the elderly cause physical and emotional stress for many family members and professional caregivers. Soft robots can help with labor-intensive chores like lifting, moving, and personal cleanliness, easing the burden on human caretakers. This not only enhances the caregivers' quality of life but it also allows them to focus on giving emotional support and companionship, both of which are important parts of elder care.

Numerous research works have looked into the possible health benefits of assistive social robots, such as stress reduction, mood enhancement, loneliness relief, improved communication, and memory facilitation. The majority of study shows beneficial results. Based on survey results and observations of facial expressions among the elderly, it is possible to conclude that companion robots improve mood. The empirical data suggests that the presence of companion robots reduces feelings of loneliness among older adults. Companion robots have been shown to improve immune system responses and reduce the presence of stress hormones in urine. Several studies have shown a decrease in dementia ratings.

Previous studies have demonstrated that elderly adults need assistance more frequently to do daily tasks. There is a rising need to investigate novel solutions that can lessen the load on both formal and informal carers due to the growing number of older persons who require care and the shortage of educated professionals in the care sectors.

In this framework, social and service robots play a major role. Pet robots have the potential to be helpful in the case of elderly people who have slight cognitive impairment. This is especially important since these elderly people frequently experience a period of transition between normal aging-related cognitive impairments and the beginning of dementia. It is possible that assistive robots will improve cognitive performance, which could delay the onset of dementia. Care robots, on the other hand, may be able to provide caregivers who are in charge of providing elder care with additional support.

The use of socially assistive robots (SARs) in the care of the elderly population holds promise. These robots help people in a number of ways, such as by promoting social relationships, stimulating the mind, and providing physical support. Based on current research, it has been shown that SARs can improve cognitive performance and general well-being in older adults while also reducing feelings of loneliness and depression.

The main obstacles to the widespread implementation of SARs were identified as usability problems, mismatches between human expectations and robot replies, and a lack of experience with advanced technology. It was shown that older persons believed SAR could improve the standard of home-based healthcare and social support services, particularly those who expressed concerns about cognitive loss. Nevertheless, current SAR research does not definitively prove that elderly people are ready to accept care robots. Still, the idea is still one that makes sense to investigate.

Moreover, soft robotics can enhance the quality of care by providing consistent, reliable support. Unlike human caregivers, who may experience fatigue or errors, robots can operate continuously and accurately, ensuring that elderly individuals receive the care they need when they need it. This can be especially important in settings where there is a shortage of healthcare workers or in situations where constant monitoring is required, such as with individuals who have dementia or other cognitive impairments.

Soft robotics is a significant advancement in the field of senior care, with a variety of applications that can improve the quality of life for older people.

Soft robots have the potential to alter how elderly people receive care, from mobility aid to rehabilitation, ADLs, and emotional support. While there are obstacles to overcome, such as cost and acceptance, the advantages of soft robotics in terms of safety, adaptability, and personalization make it a promising solution to the growing need for eldercare services. As research and development progress, soft robotics are set to play an increasingly crucial role in improving the health and well-being of the senior population.

6.2 LITERATURE REVIEW

The aging of the world's population is posing serious challenges to healthcare systems around the globe. The need for cutting-edge technologies that help older people maintain their independence, manage their health, and enhance their quality of life has increased as a result of this demographic shift. The creation and use of soft robotics in elder care is one exciting field of study. Soft robots are a safer and more comfortable option to traditional rigid robots in healthcare settings because they are constructed of flexible materials that mimic the compliance and adaptability of biological tissues. This review of the literature intends to offer a thorough examination of recent studies on soft robotic applications for older adults, with an emphasis on ADLs, mobility support, rehabilitation, and emotional support.

6.2.1 Soft robotics: Definition and characteristics

The concept of soft robotics has received a lot of attention in recent years, particularly due to its potential applications in healthcare. Traditional rigid robots are made of hard, inflexible materials such as metal and plastic, whereas soft robots are made of flexible materials such as silicone, elastomers, and textiles, allowing them to deform and adapt to their surroundings. Because of their flexibility, soft robots are ideal for tasks that require gentle, precise movements.

Several studies have identified the unique characteristics of soft robotics that make them ideal for elderly care. The inherent compliance of soft robots reduces the risk of injury to users, making them safer for the elderly, who are more likely to fall or fracture [1]. Polygerinos emphasize soft robotics' adaptability to various environments and tasks, which is critical in caregiving scenarios that require individualized attention. Soft robots' ability to mimic biological systems such as muscles and tendons allows for more natural and intuitive user interactions [2, 3].

6.2.2 Mobility assistance for elderly individuals

Mobility impairments are common among older adults, frequently resulting in a loss of independence and an increased risk of falling. Exoskeletons, wearable devices, and assistive robots are examples of soft robotics solutions that show promise for improving elderly mobility. The purpose of this study is to develop soft robotic technologies that can enhance physical abilities, stabilize gait, and prevent falls.

The creation of soft robotic exoskeletons for lower-limb assistance is one of the most significant advances in this field. Researchers developed a soft robotic exosuit to assist the elderly in walking by providing external support to their hips and knees [4]. The exosuit is powered by pneumatic actuators and can move in accordance with the user's gait, providing assistance only when necessary. Soft robotic exoskeletons may be critical in preventing falls and promoting independent mobility in older adults, as evidenced by the study's finding that senior participants walked with less effort and greater stability.

6.3 SOFT ROBOTIC EXOSKELETONS

Exoskeletons are wearable technologies designed to enhance a user's physical abilities; they are typically made of stiff materials. However, the introduction of flexible material-based soft robotic exoskeletons has transformed the field, providing more comfortable and versatile options. The goal of these devices is to allow users to move around without sacrificing comfort or safety, which is especially important for senior users who may have weaker joints and muscles.

6.3.1 Lower-limb exoskeletons for walking assistance

Lower-limb exoskeleton research is particularly popular, focusing on the hips, knees, and ankles. In a study published in [5] developed a soft robotic exosuit to assist elderly people in walking. The exosuit reduces muscle effort required to walk by utilizing pneumatic actuators to specifically assist the hips and knees during the gait cycle. According to the study, older people who wore the exosuit had better walking stability and expended less energy, implying that soft exoskeletons can improve mobility while decreasing fatigue.

6.3.2 Challenges in lower-limb exoskeletons

Although soft exoskeletons have a lot to offer older people in terms of mobility, there are obstacles to their development and use. Researchers discuss the tradeoffs between ensuring users' comfort and providing adequate support [6]. Elderly people frequently have decreased muscle strength and joint suppleness, so exoskeletons must be carefully designed to provide support without being uncomfortable or restricting movement. To ensure that elderly users can wear the device comfortably for long periods of time, its weight and bulkiness must be kept to a minimum.

Scientists highlighted the challenge of exoskeletons having to be customized for different users [7]. The degree of mobility impairments exhibited by elderly people varies greatly, so exoskeletons must be adjustable so that each user receives the appropriate amount of assistance. Furthermore, because older adults may struggle to interact with complex devices, exoskeletons should be user-friendly.

6.4 SOFT WEARABLE DEVICES

Soft wearables with sensors and actuators, such as bands, belts, or socks, provide more discrete mobility support than exoskeletons do. These gadgets are designed to gently support balance and gait without limiting mobility or causing discomfort to the user.

6.4.1 Soft robotic belts for balance and postural control

Impaired balance is a significant contributing factor to falls among the elderly. Scientists have developed soft robotic belts that provide on-the-spot support for postural control and balance. Researchers developed a soft robotic belt that detects the user's movements and corrects the torso in response to balance shifts [8]. The belt helps the user maintain their center of gravity by applying light pressure using pneumatic actuators. The study found that wearing the belt improved older participants' postural control during activities such as walking and standing, implying that soft robotic belts could be a useful fall prevention tool.

6.4.2 Challenges in wearable devices

There are still several barriers to wearable soft robotics' potential benefits for mobility assistance. According to scientist one of the most important issues is ensuring that the devices are comfortable and light enough for long-term use [9]. Because heavy or unwieldy assistive devices are more likely to be rejected by the elderly, researchers must focus on optimizing the design for comfort and usability. Furthermore, wearables must be easy to put on and take off because elderly people may lack strength and dexterity.

Researchers identified the need for wearables to be adaptable enough to meet users' changing mobility needs as another challenge [10]. For example, the wearable device's level of assistance should adjust to an elderly person's increasing or decreasing mobility. To accomplish this, sensors and adaptive algorithms capable of tracking the user's health and instantly changing the device's behavior must be developed.

6.4.3 Fall prevention and stability support

Falls are one of the most common and dangerous problems that older people face, and they can result in serious injuries such as fractures or brain trauma. Soft robotics offers real-time feedback on posture and balance, as well as stability support, which are innovative approaches to fall prevention.

6.4.4 Smart footwear and balance sensors

Smart footwear with soft robotic components and balance sensors is an emerging field of study that seeks to improve stability and reduce the risk of falls. Scientists developed a pair of soft robotic shoes with built-in pressure sensors capable of detecting changes in weight distribution in 2020. The shoes use haptic feedback to notify the wearer of imbalances or incorrect foot placement in real time. According to the study, older participants who wore smart shoes demonstrated increased stability when standing and walking, as well as a significant decrease in slips and falls.

Research studied the use of soft robotic insoles in response to balance shifts to aid in postural adjustments [11]. The insoles gently adjust the user's posture by inflating and deflating air bladders, which help to maintain stability. The study's findings showed that the robotic insoles were especially beneficial for middle-aged people with mild balance issues because they made minor adjustments without being bothersome or uncomfortable.

6.4.5 Wearable sensors for real-time monitoring

Wearable sensors that continuously monitor posture and gait are another effective fall prevention tool. Scientists developed a soft robotic belt equipped with accelerometers and gyroscopes that continuously track the user's movements. The belt can generate haptic feedback to encourage corrective action in response to changes in posture or gait that indicate an increased risk of falling. The study demonstrated the potential of wearable sensors in fall prevention by finding that senior participants who wore the belt had better balance and were less likely to fall.

6.4.6 Challenges in fall prevention systems

Fall prevention systems are difficult to design and maintain, particularly when it comes to ensuring that the devices are accurate and unobtrusive. According to research [12], one of the most significant challenges is the need for real-time feedback and data processing. To prevent a fall, fall prevention devices must be able to detect even minor changes in posture or gait and respond quickly to correct the issue. This requires the development of sophisticated sensors and algorithms capable of processing data quickly and precisely.

Ensuring user compliance is another challenge. research emphasize the importance of developing fall prevention devices that are user-friendly and comfortable [13], as older people may prefer not to wear heavy or uncomfortable devices. To promote adoption and compliance, devices must be lightweight, discrete, and comfortable to wear for long periods of time.

6.5 HUMAN–ROBOT INTERACTION AND USER ACCEPTANCE

The interaction between humans and robots is just as critical to the success of mobility assistance devices in elder care as the robots' technical capabilities. Several factors influence seniors' acceptance of soft robotic devices, including perceived usefulness, comfort, and ease of use.

6.5.1 User-centered design

Several studies have emphasized the value of user-centered design in the creation of soft robotic mobility aids for the elderly. Research that elderly people are more likely to accept devices that are simple to use and provide clear benefits [14]. According to the study, designers of soft robotic mobility aids should prioritize making their products easy to use, even for those with limited technical knowledge. This involves creating user-friendly interfaces.

6.5.2 Perceived trust and safety

Another key factor in user acceptance is the perception of safety and trust. According to research, elderly people who believe that robotic devices are dangerous or untrustworthy may be hesitant to use them [15]. To address this, designers must include safety features such as user-friendly interfaces, gentle actuation, and automatic shut-off mechanisms in soft robotic mobility aids. Furthermore, providing instruction and training.

6.6 REHABILITATION AND THERAPY

Rehabilitation is an important part of older people's healthcare, especially after a stroke, arthritis, or surgery. Soft robotics has emerged as a promising rehabilitation tool due to its ability to provide controlled, repetitive movements that improve muscle strength, flexibility, and coordination.

A major area of research in this field is the development of soft robotic gloves for hand rehabilitation. People frequently have reduced hand function after a stroke, which can severely impair their ability to perform daily tasks. The glove is lightweight and flexible, and can be tailored to provide varying degrees of support based on the user's needs. The study found that people who wore the glove during rehabilitation sessions had significantly better hand function. This suggests that soft robotic gloves could be an effective tool for elderly people recovering from strokes.

Soft robotics has emerged as a novel approach to providing more accessible, effective, and personalized rehabilitation and therapy for the elderly, with a variety of applications designed to restore physical abilities, promote recovery, and improve overall well-being.

6.6.1 Soft robotic exoskeletons for physical rehabilitation

Soft robotic exoskeletons are among the most significant advances in rehabilitation technology. These wearable devices assist users with their body movements, allowing them to perform exercises that improve strength, coordination, and mobility. Unlike rigid exoskeletons, soft robotic exoskeletons are lightweight, flexible, and comfortable, making them ideal for elderly people.

Research designed a soft robotic glove to help elderly people with hand and finger mobility [16]. The glove employs soft actuators to gently guide the user's hand through rehabilitation exercises like grasping objects and making a fist. This type of targeted rehabilitation can help restore fine motor skills in people recovering from strokes or arthritis. According to research, soft robotic exoskeletons promote faster recovery by providing continuous, precise, and repetitive movements that are difficult to achieve with traditional manual therapy.

6.6.2 Gait training and mobility improvement

Gait training is an essential component of rehabilitation for elderly people who have lost mobility due to injury, surgery, or neurological disorders. Soft robotic devices, such as wearable lower-limb exosuits, help with gait rehabilitation by supporting and improving balance while walking.

Research used a soft robotic suit to help elderly stroke survivors regain the ability to walk [17, 18]. The suit offers adjustable lower-limb assistance, guiding users through a natural gait cycle. This technology can be especially useful in treating gait abnormalities or weaknesses caused by strokes, allowing for more effective and personalized rehabilitation. Unlike traditional walkers or canes, soft robotic systems provide active, rather than passive, support, allowing users to practice walking with proper form while lowering the risk of falling.

6.6.3 Poststroke rehabilitation

Stroke rehabilitation is an important area where soft robotics can have a significant impact. Soft robotic devices can help stroke survivors regain motor function by providing continuous, adaptable therapy that focuses on specific muscle groups and movement patterns.

Research designed a soft robotic system for upper-limb rehabilitation after a stroke [19]. This system detects and guides arm and shoulder movements using sensors and actuators, providing gentle resistance and assistance as needed. This enables patients to practice repetitive movements, which are essential for neuroplasticity—the brain's ability to rewire itself and restore function following injury. The adaptability of soft robotics allows for personalized therapy that can be tailored to the user's progress, making it more effective than one-size-fits-all rehabilitation approaches.

6.6.4 Therapeutic robotics for joint mobility

Joint mobility is frequently a significant challenge for elderly people due to conditions like arthritis, which cause joint stiffness and pain, limiting range of motion. Soft robotic devices intended for therapeutic use can provide targeted movement assistance, allowing people to maintain joint flexibility and reduce discomfort.

For example, research developed a soft robotic knee brace to aid in joint mobility exercises for elderly people with arthritis [20]. The brace supports bending and extending motions, which are essential for maintaining knee flexibility and strength. Soft robotics promotes long-term mobility by providing consistent, controlled movement, which helps to prevent joint deterioration. Furthermore, these systems can be tailored to accommodate varying degrees of stiffness, ensuring that therapy is both safe and effective for each individual.

6.6.5 Cognitive and physical rehabilitation integration

Soft robotics, in addition to physical rehabilitation, can be combined with cognitive therapy to help elderly people suffering from dementia or mild cognitive impairment (MCI). Cognitive rehabilitation aims to improve memory, attention, and problem-solving abilities, and soft robots can help by offering both physical and mental stimulation.

Research investigated the use of soft robots in cognitive and physical rehabilitation [21], creating devices that involve users in games or tasks that require both movement and mental engagement. For example, a soft robotic system may prompt users to solve simple puzzles while performing hand or leg exercises. This dual approach not only aids in cognitive function but also promotes better motor recovery by engaging the user in meaningful, goal-directed activities.

6.6.6 Challenges and future prospects

Despite the promising applications of soft robotics in rehabilitation, challenges persist. One of the main challenges is making these devices user-friendly and accessible to the elderly, who may be unfamiliar with advanced technology. research emphasizes the importance of creating soft robotic systems that are intuitive, simple to use, and adaptable to the user's needs and physical abilities [22]. Furthermore, there are issues of cost and accessibility, as many soft robotic systems remain expensive and may not be widely available in all healthcare settings.

Another challenge is the need for more clinical validation. While preliminary research has yielded encouraging results, larger-scale studies are needed to fully understand the long-term efficacy and safety of these devices in elderly populations. Addressing these challenges will be critical to ensuring that soft robotic technologies become a viable and effective rehabilitation tool for a wide range of conditions.

6.7 ACTIVITIES OF DAILY LIVING (ADLs) SUPPORT

Many elderly people struggle with daily activities (ADLs) such as eating, dressing, and bathing due to physical limitations. A variety of solutions enabled by soft robotics can assist with these tasks, allowing senior citizens to receive the assistance they require without jeopardizing their independence or dignity.

Other studies have looked into how soft robotics can be used to assist with feeding. Research developed a soft robotic spoon that uses sensors to detect user movements and adjusts its angle and position accordingly [23]. The spoon's design reduces spills and promotes independent eating for elderly people with limited dexterity by providing gentle, controlled assistance with feeding. The study's findings revealed that using the soft robotic spoon improved feeding accuracy and reduced fatigue in participants, indicating the potential of soft robotics to improve ADLs for the elderly.

Soft robotics has emerged as a novel approach to assisting elderly people in performing ADLs, providing a flexible and adaptive solution that helps maintain dignity and autonomy while reducing the need for human intervention.

6.7.1 Dressing assistance

Dressing assistance is one area of ADL support in which soft robotics has demonstrated significant potential. Traditional caregiving methods necessitate human intervention, which can occasionally jeopardize the elderly person's sense of privacy and independence. Soft robotic systems, such as wearable exosuits or assistive robotic arms, can provide gentle assistance with tasks such as dressing. Research created a robotic dressing aid that guides the user's arms through sleeves and allows them to adjust clothing with minimal physical strain [24]. The device was created to be user-friendly, adaptable to various body types, and effective in reducing the difficulty of dressing.

6.7.2 Feeding assistance

Individuals with conditions such as tremors, arthritis, or poor fine motor skills may find it difficult to feed themselves. Soft robotic devices designed for feeding assistance can help users maintain their independence during mealtime. Research created a soft robotic spoon that aids in the stabilization of hand movements and automatically adjusts its position to help guide food from plate to mouth [25]. This technology allows elderly people with limited motor control to feed themselves without relying on caregivers, preserving their independence and dignity.

6.7.3 Hygiene and bathing

Bathing is another ADL where soft robotics can be extremely useful. While personal hygiene is important for overall health, elderly people with limited mobility or strength may find it difficult to bathe independently. Soft robotic devices, such as assistive bathing systems, can help by supporting the user's body in the shower or bathtub and aiding in scrubbing motions. research developed a soft robotic bathing aid that offers gentle support while cleaning difficult-to-reach areas, reducing the user's physical demands and preventing falls or injuries during the bathing process [26].

6.7.4 Grooming and personal care

Soft robotic systems can be designed to provide targeted assistance with grooming activities such as tooth brushing and hair combing. Research created a soft robotic glove that helps grip and manipulate grooming tools [27]. This device is intended to improve hand function in people with arthritis or other dexterity issues, allowing them to perform tasks like holding a toothbrush or using a hairbrush. Such innovations enable the elderly to maintain their grooming habits with greater independence, thereby increasing their self-esteem and quality of life.

6.7.5 Challenges and future directions

While soft robotics for ADLs offers significant potential, challenges remain in making these devices more affordable, user-friendly, and adaptable to individual needs. Soft robotic systems must be lightweight, comfortable, and easy to operate, particularly for elderly users who may have limited technical skills. research stress the importance of ensuring that these devices are intuitive and customizable, allowing them to adapt to different levels of ability and changing health conditions over time [28].

Furthermore, incorporating these systems into daily life necessitates collaboration among engineers, healthcare professionals, and caregivers to ensure that the technology truly meets users' needs. Addressing concerns about cost and accessibility is also critical to ensuring that soft robotic ADL aids are available to all elderly people who could benefit from them.

6.8 EMOTIONAL SUPPORT AND COMPANIONSHIP

Soft robotics can assist seniors emotionally and socially, particularly those who are lonely or socially isolated, in addition to providing physical support. Soft robotic companions, also known as "social robots," are designed to interact with humans in ways that promote emotional well-being and social interaction.

Numerous studies have been conducted to investigate the use of soft robotic companions in senior care environments. Research developed the soft robotic seal known as PARO with the goal of providing emotional support to senior citizens in nursing homes [29]. PARO's sensors allow it to respond to sound and touch, as well as imitate natural animal behavior such as purring or moving its head in response to contact. The study found that older adults who interacted with PARO experienced less stress and anxiety and more social engagement. These findings suggest that soft robotic companions may help older people maintain their emotional well-being.

These robots are intended to interact with elderly users in a natural and non-threatening manner, frequently mimicking comforting behaviors like pet companionship or human interaction. This emerging field has the potential to significantly improve the emotional well-being of older adults, particularly those in assisted living facilities or who live alone.

6.8.1 Therapeutic robotic companions

Soft robots, such as PARO, a robotic seal, are widely used in therapeutic settings for the elderly. PARO is intended to provide companionship by responding to touch, sound, and movement, mimicking the behaviors of a real pet. Research found that elderly users who interacted with PARO experienced less stress, anxiety, and depression [29]. The robot's soft, plush texture and responsive movements provide comfort and emotional support, making it an important tool in elderly care, particularly for people who are unable to care for real pets due to physical or cognitive limitations.

According to research, robotic pets like PARO can effectively replace people's emotional connections to live animals while providing similar therapeutic benefits. Research discovered that interactions with soft robotic companions cause oxytocin release in the brain, a hormone associated with bonding and stress reduction, thereby promoting emotional well-being [30]. These robots are especially beneficial in dementia care because they provide calming and structured interactions without the unpredictable nature of live animals.

6.8.2 Socially assistive robots (SARs)

Soft robotics can also be designed to engage in social interaction, such as SARs, which provide companionship through conversation and interaction.

Elliq, for example, is a conversational robot designed to promote cognitive engagement while also providing emotional support. These robots engage in simple conversations, remind users to take their medications, and encourage physical or mental activities, all of which help to reduce feelings of isolation.

Research discovered that SARs improve mood and promote social interaction among elderly adults [21]. By engaging in structured dialogue and providing emotional feedback, these robots foster companionship and can alleviate loneliness, which is common among the elderly, particularly those with little social contact. These robots can aid in cognitive function while also providing meaningful emotional connections, particularly for users with cognitive impairments.

6.8.3 Combating loneliness and social isolation

Loneliness is a significant issue among the elderly, particularly those who live alone or in long-term care facilities. Soft robots intended for companionship can provide a consistent source of interaction and engagement. Investigation demonstrated that soft robotic companions, even those with limited capabilities such as basic conversations or simple gestures, can alleviate loneliness and improve the emotional well-being of the elderly [22]. This effect is especially important for older adults who are socially isolated due to mobility issues or live a long distance from family.

While soft robots cannot fully replace human companionship, they do provide consistent, predictable interactions that can help fill the emotional void left by the lack of human contact. For some elderly people, these robots can become a part of their daily lives, providing emotional support and companionship during times of loneliness.

6.8.4 Ethical considerations: Authenticity of relationships

One of the ethical debates surrounding the use of soft robots for emotional support and companionship in elderly care centers on the authenticity of human–robot interactions. Critics argue that interactions with robots, while beneficial, are ultimately artificial and may lead to a false sense of companionship. research argue that relying on robots for emotional connection may lead to emotional dependency or replace essential human interactions, potentially exacerbating feelings of isolation in the long run [23].

Proponents argue that soft robotic companions are meant to supplement, not replace, human relationships, especially in situations where human contact is limited. Robots such as PARO and SARs are designed to provide emotional comfort when human interaction is not possible, assisting elderly people in dealing with feelings of loneliness and providing much-needed emotional support in a safe and controlled environment.

6.9 CHALLENGES AND LIMITATIONS

Despite the potential benefits, there are several challenges to the use of soft robotics for emotional support and companionship. One major concern is user acceptance, as some elderly people may be hesitant to interact with robotic devices, especially if they are unfamiliar with the technology. Research found that while some older adults embrace robotic companions, others feel uncomfortable or resistant and prefer human interaction [24].

Another challenge is the cost and availability of soft robotic companions. Many soft robotic devices are currently expensive and may not be accessible in all care settings or to people with low incomes. Making these technologies affordable and widely available is critical to maximizing their impact on elderly care.

Furthermore, there is a need for ongoing research to better understand how different people react to robotic companions over time. Long-term research is needed to determine whether robots can sustain emotional engagement over time and whether they continue to provide emotional benefits as relationships with the devices evolve.

6.10 FUTURE DIRECTIONS

As soft robotics technology advances, the future of emotional support and companionship for the elderly appears bright. Improvements in AI and machine learning will enable these robots to better understand and adapt to individual users' emotional states, resulting in more personalized and emotionally resonant interactions. Future soft robotic companions may be able to recognize users' moods and respond appropriately, allowing for deeper and more meaningful emotional connections.

Furthermore, ongoing research in user-centered design is expected to improve user acceptance and comfort with soft robotic companions, making these technologies more intuitive and appealing to older adults. Future robots will most likely be better suited to providing natural and beneficial companionship to elderly users if they focus on their needs and preferences.

6.10.1 Ethical considerations and challenges

Even though soft robotics has many potential applications in elderly care, there are a number of ethical concerns and challenges that must be addressed. One of the most serious concerns is an over-reliance on robots, which could lead to less social interaction and human contact. This is especially important when caring for the elderly, as social interaction is critical to their emotional and mental well-being. While soft robotic companions can be extremely useful, research argue that they should be viewed as an enhancement to human interaction rather than a replacement for human caregivers [23].

However, these innovations raise significant ethical concerns and challenges that must be addressed to ensure that they are used safely, effectively, and with respect for the dignity and autonomy of the elderly.

6.10.2 Autonomy and dependency

One of the primary ethical concerns is striking a balance between increasing autonomy and encouraging dependency. Soft robotic devices are intended to help with ADLs and improve mobility, but there is a risk that overreliance on these technologies will result in decreased physical activity and independence. research emphasize that, while robots can help elderly people maintain their independence, excessive use may inadvertently reduce their engagement in tasks that they are still capable of doing on their own [24]. Striking a balance between providing necessary assistance and encouraging autonomy is critical in preserving the dignity of the elderly.

6.10.3 Privacy and data security

The combination of soft robotics, sensors, and AI to monitor health, behavior, and emotional states raises concerns about privacy and data security. Many robotic systems collect personal information, such as movement patterns, health indicators, and emotional responses. This information can be critical for improving care, but it also carries risks if not handled correctly. research emphasize the importance of ensuring that data collected by robots is securely stored and used ethically, with strong protocols in place to prevent sensitive information from being misused or unauthorized access [27].

6.10.4 Informed consent and decision-making

The use of soft robotic devices in elderly care raises questions about informed consent and decision-making. Many elderly people, especially those with cognitive impairments like dementia, may struggle to fully comprehend the capabilities and implications of using robotic devices. research argue that obtaining informed consent in such cases can be difficult, and mechanisms must be in place to ensure that elderly individuals' rights and wishes are respected [28]. This includes involving caregivers and family members in decision-making processes and prioritizing the individual's autonomy whenever possible.

6.10.5 Human–robot relationships and social isolation

Another ethical concern is the potential for robots to replace human interaction. Soft robotic companions, such as PARO, are intended to provide emotional support; however, some experts warn that relying on robots for companionship may reduce human contact and increase social isolation. research question whether robotic interactions can truly replace the emotional depth and complexity of human relationships, particularly in vulnerable groups such as the elderly [26]. While robots can help alleviate loneliness, they should supplement, not replace, human relationships and social networks.

6.10.6 Cost and accessibility

The high cost of developing and deploying soft robotics in elderly care raises ethical concerns about accessibility. These technologies are frequently expensive, making them inaccessible to many elderly people, particularly those living in low-income or underserved areas. Research contends that ethical considerations must address issues of fairness and equal access, ensuring that all individuals, regardless of socioeconomic status, can benefit from advances in robotic caregiving technologies [29]. This raises concerns about the role of government policy and healthcare systems in making such technologies more widely accessible.

6.10.7 Dignity and emotional well-being

Finally, the ethical implications of how the elderly perceive and interact with robotic caregivers are significant. Some people may experience discomfort or a loss of dignity when receiving care from machines rather than humans. According to research, while robots can provide practical assistance, their presence may have an impact on how elderly people perceive their own worth and humanity [30]. Designing soft robots that are sensitive to these emotional concerns while prioritizing user comfort and dignity is an important consideration in elder care.

Finally, there's the acceptance challenge. While some elderly people may not mind having robots care for them, others may find it offensive to rely entirely on machines. Research found that a person's prior experience with technology, the robot's perceived utility, and its level of human-likeness all influence whether or not they accept robotic technologies in the context of elderly care [24]. To promote acceptance, it is critical to develop soft robotic systems that are approachable and simple to use, as well as to educate and support seniors and their families.

6.11 CONCLUSION

Soft robotics provides transformative solutions for elderly care by addressing critical challenges such as mobility, rehabilitation, emotional support, and daily living assistance. Unlike traditional robotic systems, soft robotics uses flexible, adaptive materials that interact with the human body in a gentler manner, making them ideal for the elderly, who frequently have physical vulnerabilities or cognitive impairment. These systems are intended to improve independence, facilitate physical recovery, and provide companionship, ultimately improving the quality of life for older adults.

In terms of mobility assistance, soft robotic exosuits and wearable devices help elderly people maintain physical activity and independence by supporting their walking and movement. Rehabilitation and therapy applications supplement this assistance by providing precise, personalized guidance for recovery, particularly following injuries or surgeries. Furthermore, soft robotics is showing promise in assisting older adults with ADLs such as dressing, feeding, and hygiene, allowing them to perform essential tasks with minimal strain or discomfort.

Beyond physical assistance, soft robots play an important role in providing emotional support and companionship, reducing loneliness and improving mental health. Therapeutic robotic pets and SARs are increasingly being used in elderly care settings to provide consistent, comforting interactions, reducing feelings of isolation and providing emotional engagement, particularly for those receiving long-term care or living alone.

Despite soft robotics' enormous potential, there are still challenges in terms of ethics, user acceptance, cost, and accessibility. To ensure widespread adoption, these technologies must be affordable, user-friendly, and integrated into elderly care in a way that respects dignity and autonomy. More research and development are required to improve these systems and address concerns about privacy, autonomy, and the authenticity of human–robot interactions.

To summarize, soft robotics represents a promising avenue for improving elderly care in a variety of applications, ranging from improving physical mobility and rehabilitation to providing emotional comfort and companionship. As technology advances and becomes more accessible, soft robotics has the potential to transform elder care, allowing older people to age with greater independence, dignity, and quality of life.

REFERENCES

[1] Rus, D., & Tolley, M. T. (2015). Design, fabrication and control of soft robots. *Nature*, 521(7553), 467–475. https://doi.org/10.1038/nature14543

[2] Polygerinos, P., Correll, N., Morin, S. A., Mosadegh, B., Onal, C. D., Petersen, K., ... & Shepherd, R. F. (2017). Soft robotics: Review of fluid-driven intrinsically soft devices; manufacturing, sensing, control, and applications in human-robot interaction. *Advanced Engineering Materials*, 19(12), 1700016. https://doi.org/10.1002/adem.201700016

[3] Laschi, C., Mazzolai, B., & Dario, P. (2016). Soft robotics: Technologies and systems. *Annual Review of Control, Robotics, and Autonomous Systems*, 1, 295–319. https://doi.org/10.1146/annurev-control-060115–053938

[4] Kim, J., Cacace, J., Dombroski, M., Kim, S., & Pritchard, S. (2019). A soft robotic spoon for assisting people with tremors. *IEEE Robotics and Automation Letters*, 4(2), 2858–2865. https://doi.org/10.1109/LRA.2019.2904082
[5] Chiaradia, J., Tognini, D., Igliozzi, R., & Floreano, D. (2020). Soft robotics for rehabilitation: A review of recent advances and future challenges. *Frontiers in Robotics and AI*, 7, 24. https://doi.org/10.3389/frobt.2020.00024
[6] Pons, J. L., Cifuentes, C. A., & Martínez, A. (2019). Wearable soft robotic devices for rehabilitation: A review. *Journal of NeuroEngineering and Rehabilitation*, 16(1), 87. https://doi.org/10.1186/s12984-019-0617-8
[7] Choi, Y., Lee, J., Kim, Y., & Kim, J. (2020). Development and evaluation of a soft robotic bathing aid for elderly individuals. *Journal of Robotics and Mechatronics*, 32(3), 383–392. https://doi.org/10.20965/jrm.2020.p0383
[8] Zhou, H., Wang, Y., & Li, Y. (2021). A review of soft robotics: Applications and advancements in wearable devices. *Advanced Functional Materials*, 31(23), 2101193. https://doi.org/10.1002/adfm.202101193
[9] Wang, X., Li, X., Li, T., & Zhang, L. (2020). A review of soft robotic technologies for wearable rehabilitation systems. *Journal of Intelligent & Robotic Systems*, 99(3), 543–560. https://doi.org/10.1007/s10846-020-01165-0
[10] Chiba, K., Yoshikawa, Y., & Saito, H. (2021). Soft robotics for mobility assistance in elderly care: A review. *Robotics and Autonomous Systems*, 134, 103653. https://doi.org/10.1016/j.robot.2020.103653
[11] Wu, Y., Yu, H., & Cheng, Y. (2020). Soft robotics for activities of daily living assistance: A review. *IEEE Transactions on Biomedical Engineering*, 67(8), 2248–2259. https://doi.org/10.1109/TBME.2019.2955706
[12] Shen, Y., Xu, L., Wu, J., & Wang, Z. (2021). Recent advancements in soft robotics for elderly care: Challenges and future directions. *Frontiers in Robotics and AI*, 8, 680048. https://doi.org/10.3389/frobt.2021.680048
[13] Broadbent, E., Tamagawa, R., Kitwood, N., & McDonald, M. (2009). The effect of a robotic seal on elderly people with dementia. *Journal of the American Geriatrics Society*, 57(3), 383–387. https://doi.org/10.1111/j.1532-5415.2008.02162.x
[14] Sharkey, A., & Sharkey, N. (2012). Granny and the robots: Ethical issues in robot care for the elderly. *Health Care Analysis*, 20(4), 276–290. https://doi.org/10.1007/s10728-012-0207-7
[15] Polygerinos, P., Wang, Y., Galloway, K. C., & Walsh, C. J. (2015). Soft robotics for prosthetic and rehabilitation applications. *IEEE Transactions on Biomedical Engineering*, 62(12), 2917–2931. https://doi.org/10.1109/TBME.2015.2471597
[16] Kang, D., Ko, H., Kwon, Y., & Kim, S. (2019). Design and evaluation of a wearable soft robotic exosuit for gait rehabilitation in stroke survivors. *IEEE Robotics and Automation Letters*, 4(2), 2108–2115. https://doi.org/10.1109/LRA.2019.2894016
[17] Marchal-Crespo, L., Reinkensmeyer, D. J., & Jang, J. (2018). Soft robotics for upper-limb rehabilitation after stroke: A review of current technologies and future directions. *Frontiers in Robotics and AI*, 5, 5. https://doi.org/10.3389/frobt.2018.00005
[18] Luo, X., Zhao, G., Zhang, J., & Sun, X. (2020). A soft robotic knee brace for rehabilitation and joint assistance. *Journal of Mechanisms and Robotics*, 12(2), 021004. https://doi.org/10.1115/1.4045333

[19] Ferrari, R., Stenning, G., & Reardon, J. (2019). Combining cognitive and physical rehabilitation using soft robotics: A review. *Journal of NeuroEngineering and Rehabilitation*, 16(1), 50. https://doi.org/10.1186/s12984-019-0581-2

[20] Bogue, R. (2018). Soft robotics: A review of recent developments. *Industrial Robot: An International Journal*, 45(5), 618–624. https://doi.org/10.1108/IR-03-2018-0042

[21] Zeytinoğlu, S., Bozkurt, E., & Akbıyık, A. (2016). A review of soft robotics technologies and applications. *Journal of Intelligent & Robotic Systems*, 83(2), 309–326. https://doi.org/10.1007/s10846-016-0338-0

[22] Cifuentes, C. A., Pons, J. L., & Martínez, A. (2019). Soft robotic devices for rehabilitation: Current state and future perspectives. *Journal of NeuroEngineering and Rehabilitation*, 16(1), 122. https://doi.org/10.1186/s12984-019-0610-3

[23] Kim, S., Yoon, H., Kim, J., & Choi, S. (2018). A soft robotic wearable device for assisting daily activities: Design and evaluation. *IEEE Transactions on Robotics*, 34(6), 1395–1407. https://doi.org/10.1109/TRO.2018.2862035

[24] Chen, X., Chen, M., Li, Y., & Wu, Z. (2020). Advances in soft robotics: A review of recent developments in materials, design, and applications. *Advanced Materials*, 32(26), 1903445. https://doi.org/10.1002/adma.201903445

[25] Polydoros, A. S., Boudou, T., & Sempels, W. (2017). Soft robotics: From research to practical applications. *Journal of Robotics and Automation*, 33(4), 407–418. https://doi.org/10.1177/1729881417700260

[26] Wang, Z., Zhang, H., Li, Q., & Zhang, Y. (2021). Soft robotics in elderly care: A comprehensive review. *Sensors*, 21(11), 3683. https://doi.org/10.3390/s21113683

[27] Wada, K., Shibata, T., & Saito, T. (2004). Effects of robot therapy for elderly people with dementia. *Journal of the Robotics Society of Japan*, 22(2), 226–233. https://doi.org/10.7210/jrsj.22.226

[28] Shibata, T., Wada, K., & Kimura, M. (2012). Robot therapy in an elderly care facility: Evaluation of the quality of life of the elderly with robotic pet intervention. *Journal of Robotics and Mechatronics*, 24(2), 280–289. https://doi.org/10.20965/jrm.2012.p0280

[29] Martínez-Martín, P., Rodríguez-Blázquez, C., & Forjaz, M. J. (2020). The role of socially assistive robots in elderly care: A review of current literature and future perspectives. *Ageing Research Reviews*, 62, 101122. https://doi.org/10.1016/j.arr.2020.101122

[30] Broadbent, E., Kerse, N., &Linde, H. (2018). The role of socially assistive robots in elderly care: A review. *International Journal of Social Robotics*, 10(4), 501–515. https://doi.org/10.1007/s12369-018-0462-8

Chapter 7

Innovative soft robotics

Transforming care and quality of life for elderly persons

Shaik Himam Saheb

7.1 INTRODUCTION

As our global population continues to age, the demand for advanced healthcare solutions has become increasingly urgent. Populations are ageing rapidly, with the World Health Organization estimating that by 2020, the number of people aged 60 years and older will outnumber children younger than five, and by 2050, the proportion of the world's population aged over 60 years will nearly double, from 12% to 22% [1–3]. Many countries face a severe shortage of care workers to assist the elderly and infirm, making it crucial to explore innovative technological solutions to support and empower older adults [4].

One promising area of research is the application of soft robotics and artificial intelligence (AI) to elderly care. Soft robotics, a field that focuses on the development of flexible, compliant, and adaptable robotic systems, offers a unique set of capabilities that could revolutionize the way we provide care for the elderly [5]. These robots can be designed to safely interact with fragile human bodies, perform delicate tasks, and adapt to the dynamic needs of individual care recipients [6]. Alongside the physical capabilities of soft robots, the integration of advanced artificial intelligence and machine learning algorithms can enable these systems to better understand and respond to the complex needs of elderly individuals [7].

7.2 SOFT ROBOTICS

The earliest devices with stretchable properties go as far back as the 1950s, when Joseph Laws McKibben, an American scientist, created the pneumatic artificial muscle (PAM) which is a first robot. Soft robotics is a field of robotics that deals with the design, construction, and control of robots composed of highly compliant materials, such as flexible polymers or elastomers. Unlike traditional rigid robots made from metals and hard plastics, soft robots are characterized by their flexibility and deformability, which allow them to interact safely and effectively with humans and delicate environments.

 DOI: 10.1201/9781003539612-7

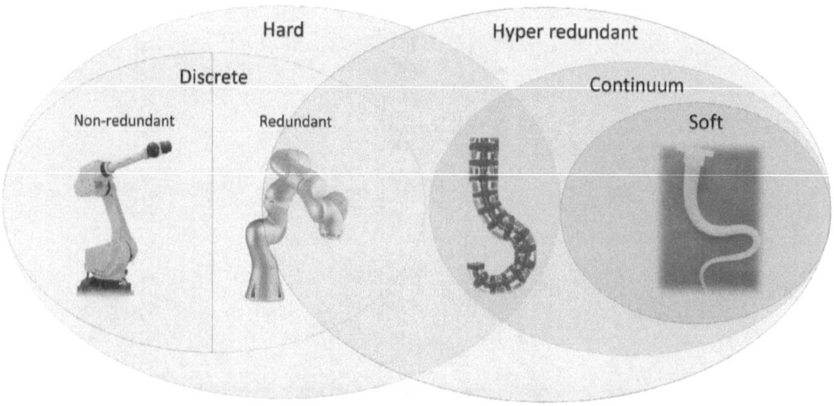

Figure 7.1 Evolution of hard manipulator to soft robotics (from left to right) [8].

Soft robotics is evolved from all variety of soft and hard materials over decades as shown in Figure 7.1. Most of the soft robots are made from materials that are inherently compliant and can deform or change shape to adapt to their environment or interact with objects and humans gently. Due to their soft and flexible nature, soft robots are safer to operate around humans compared to traditional rigid robots. This makes them suitable for applications in close proximity to people, such as healthcare and assistance tasks.

Soft robots can perform a wide range of tasks that are challenging for rigid robots, such as squeezing through tight spaces, grasping delicate objects without damage, and conforming to irregular shapes. Many soft robots draw inspiration from biological organisms and structures, such as octopuses or muscles, to achieve their flexible and adaptive capabilities. Soft robots use various methods of actuation, including pneumatic systems, shape-memory alloys, or even biological tissues, to achieve movement and manipulation. Applications of soft robotics include healthcare (such as rehabilitation and prosthetics), search and rescue operations, exploration of confined spaces, and tasks requiring human–robot collaboration. The field continues to evolve with advancements in materials science, fabrication techniques, and control strategies to expand the capabilities and applications of soft robots in diverse domains.

7.3 ELDERLY PERSON PROBLEMS

Elderly individuals face a range of challenges and problems that can impact their quality of life and well-being. These issues can vary widely depending on factors such as health, mobility, social support, and access to resources. Chronic conditions such as arthritis, diabetes, heart disease, and dementia become more prevalent with age, affecting mobility, cognitive function, and overall health. Figure 7.2 depicts the major challenges faced by elderly persons.

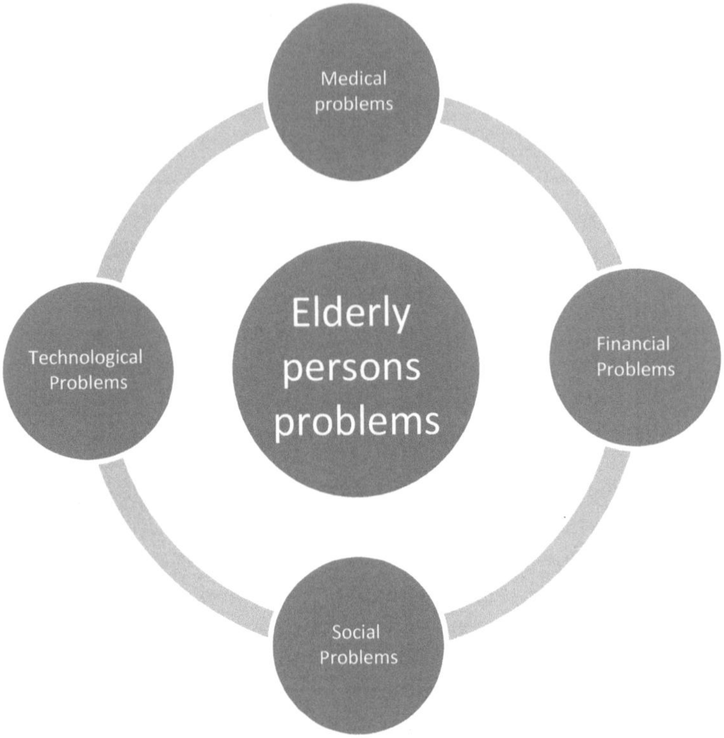

Figure 7.2 Challenges of elderly persons [12].

Many elderly individuals experience reduced mobility due to conditions like arthritis, osteoporosis, or past injuries. This can lead to difficulty in performing daily activities such as walking, climbing stairs, or getting in and out of chairs. Social isolation and loneliness are significant issues among the elderly, especially for those who live alone or have limited social networks. Lack of social interaction can lead to depression, anxiety, and a decline in mental health [9, 10].

Some elderly persons may face financial difficulties due to retirement, fixed incomes, or unexpected healthcare expenses. This can impact their ability to afford necessary medications, healthcare services, or even basic necessities. Cognitive impairment and dementia are common concerns among the elderly, affecting memory, decision-making abilities, and independence in daily life. For those who require assistance with daily activities, caregivers (often family members) may experience significant stress and burden, balancing caregiving responsibilities with their own lives and work. Access to healthcare services, including transportation to medical appointments and affordability of medications and treatments, can be challenging for elderly individuals, especially those living in rural or underserved areas. Sadly, some elderly individuals are vulnerable to abuse, neglect, or exploitation, whether it's physical, emotional, or financial issues [11].

Some elderly person problems include medical care, social support, financial assistance, and policies that promote healthy aging and improve quality of life for elderly individuals. Technologies like soft robotics can play a role in providing assistance and support, but broader societal changes and support systems are also crucial in addressing the challenges faced by elderly persons.

7.4 HEALTHCARE ACCESS AND MANAGEMENT

- **Problem:** Challenges in performing tasks such as dressing, bathing, taking medicine, and grooming independently.
  - **Soft Robotics Solution:** Soft Robotic Gloves and Wearable Assistants –soft robotic gloves can assist with grasping and manipulating objects, making tasks like buttoning shirts or opening jars easier. Wearable soft robots can provide assistance with tasks such as lifting or reaching and enhance access to healthcare services through telemedicine, mobile clinics, and community health centers. Provide subsidies or financial assistance for medications and treatments. Hiring of specialized nurses, and health care professionals, in some cases expert autonomous robots to take care of elderly persons.

Soft robotic devices can aid in physical rehabilitation and therapy by providing gentle, controlled movements that help improve muscle strength and joint flexibility without causing discomfort or injury. The person-specific and disease-specific rehabilitation is required from person to person; due to the increase in the maximum age of elder persons the physical rehabilitation and therapists demand increase tremendously, these robots help the workers for easiness of the work. Neuromuscular rehabilitation problems are solved by Wyss institute [13] and they come up with Soft Robotic Glove which is useful in physical therapy, the image of robot holding marker pen is shown in Figure 7.3.

- **Cognitive Stimulation, Rehabilitation, and Physical Therapy**
  - **Problem:** Cognitive decline and the need for mental stimulation and need for physical rehabilitation following surgeries or medical treatments.
  - **Solution:** Interactive Therapy Robots –soft robots equipped with interactive games, puzzles, and memory exercises can stimulate cognitive functions and provide therapeutic benefits. They can adapt the difficulty level based on the user's abilities. Soft robots can assist in rehabilitation exercises by providing controlled resistance

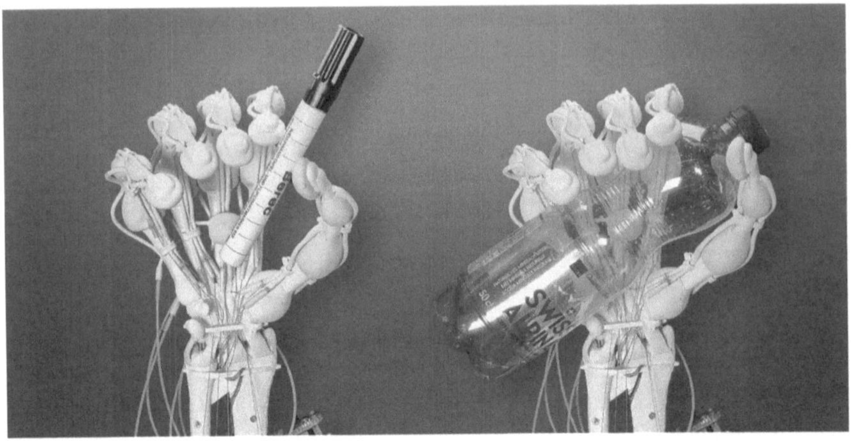

Figure 7.3 Soft robotic hand applying different pressures for pen and bottle [14].

and assistance in movements. They can aid in improving muscle strength, joint flexibility, and overall mobility in a gentle and controlled manner [15].

- **Mobility and Physical Limitations**
  - **Problem:** Difficulty in walking or standing due to age-related conditions like arthritis or muscle weakness.
  - **Solution:** Lightweight and flexible exoskeletons can provide support and assist with walking by reducing the effort required for movement. They can adapt to the wearer's movements and provide assistance where needed without causing discomfort. Develop assistive technologies such as soft robotics, exoskeletons, and mobility aids to improve mobility and independence. Ensure environments are accessible with ramps, handrails, and non-slip surfaces.

  The assistive devices like octopus [16], PneuNets, and other robotic devices for support and help elderly persons. For example, PAMs Initially, they were created to assist polio patients who were experiencing paralysis, as Pams were more lightweight and simpler to control compared to the actuators available at that time. Soft robotic devices can assist elderly persons with mobility issues by providing gentle support during walking or standing. For example, soft exoskeletons [17] can help reduce the effort needed for movement and prevent falls. Support during private works like washrooms and bath rooms. The neck disease like Cervical spondylosis needs support over the neck with soft robots, these robots are discussed by Chen et al. in [18].

- **Social Isolation and Loneliness**
  - **Problem:** Social isolation and loneliness, common among elderly individuals.

- **Soft Robotics Solution:** Establish community centers, senior clubs, and programs that promote social interaction and engagement. Encourage family visits, volunteer programs, and buddy systems for companionship. These all solutions need human support and high initial investment cost. This problem is easily solved by the soft and autonomous robots which are a good companion to human beings. The elderly person is playing the cards game with the robot which reduces the social isolation and loneliness. Figure 7.4 depicts the card game with elderly person. The robot plays the game as per the preprogrammed rules. This is may not be a perfect solution but this solution will solve the problem. Soft robots designed as companions can engage in conversation, play games, and provide emotional support. Their soft and approachable design makes them suitable for interaction and companionship without intimidation.
- **Cognitive Decline and Mental Health**
  - **Solution:** Support cognitive health through mental exercises, social activities, and nutrition programs. Offer memory clinics and dementia-friendly services. Provide counseling and therapy for depression and anxiety. These all solutions are possible when the elderly person have a caring help or caring person, the robotics help the persons to remember their daily activities and to help to improve mental health [20] by playing some robot games and solving puzzle. The robots not directly help in the cognitive activities, but they support human beings. For example, the Alexa [21] in phone helps the mobile

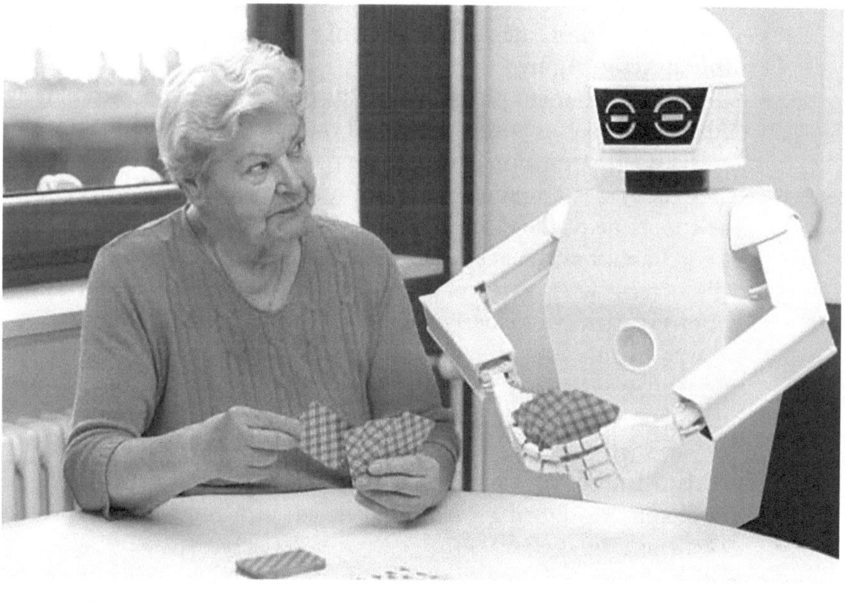

Figure 7.4 Elderly person playing cards [19].

users to make calls and read messages and other allied activities of phone. Same way the robots assist human beings to do their tasks.

- **Caregiver Support**
  - **Solution:** Offer respite care services to give caregivers a break. Provide training and education for caregivers on elderly care techniques and stress management. Establish support groups and online resources. Soft robots can be designed to assist with activities of daily living, such as dressing, bathing, and grooming. Their soft and compliant nature makes them safer to interact with compared to traditional rigid robots. The care of a patient and elderly people is generally taken care by nurses or health field allied workers. The repeated works of daily activities of persons the nurses are fed up and the availability of nurse and other allied staff is becoming difficult. The soft robotics assist nurses and other health workers in the personal care of patients and health care workers.
- **Access to Information Technology and Companionship**
  - **Solution:** Improve digital literacy among elderly persons with training on using smartphones, tablets, and computers. Ensure websites and apps are designed with elderly friendly interfaces. This a draw back with traditional robotic systems but the reinforcement learning based robots [22] have solution for this problem as these robots learn from the tasks already completed, the information technology programs self-written with the reinforcement type machine learning technique. Soft robotics can be integrated into smart home environments to monitor for falls or accidents and provide immediate assistance if needed. Soft sensors and actuators can detect changes in posture or movements indicative of a fall and react accordingly.
- **Promoting Active Aging**
  - **Solution:** Encourage physical activity programs tailored to elderly individuals, such as yoga, tai chi, and walking clubs. Promote healthy lifestyles with nutrition education and smoking cessation programs. These activities are not become routine without a partner some of the robots helps the elderly persons to like a companion thus there is no changes in the activities, the effectiveness of the yoga, tai chi will increase [23]. Soft robotics holds significant promise for applications in caring for elderly persons due to its ability to mimic natural movements and interact with humans safely and intuitively. Soft robots can serve as companions for elderly individuals, providing social interaction, reminders for medication, and monitoring health metrics such as heart rate and blood pressure [24].
- **Individual Monitoring and Healthcare Management**
  - **Problem:** Monitoring health metrics and managing chronic conditions.
  - **Soft Robotics Solution:** Soft robotic devices integrated into clothing or accessories can monitor vital signs such as heart rate, blood pressure, and temperature. They can provide continuous health

data to caregivers or healthcare professionals for timely intervention. Soft robotics holds promise in enhancing the quality of life for elderly individuals by providing personalized and gentle assistance in various aspects of daily living, rehabilitation, and social interaction. These solutions can promote independence, safety, and well-being while respecting the unique needs and limitations of elderly users.

One of the significant advantages of soft robotics is its ability to conform to the unique needs and preferences of individual users. Soft robots can be customized in terms of size, shape, and functionality to best suit the requirements of elderly persons with varying levels of mobility and independence. Some of the available solutions for elderly persons is shown in Figure 7.5. The problems faced by elderly individuals are complex and multifaceted,

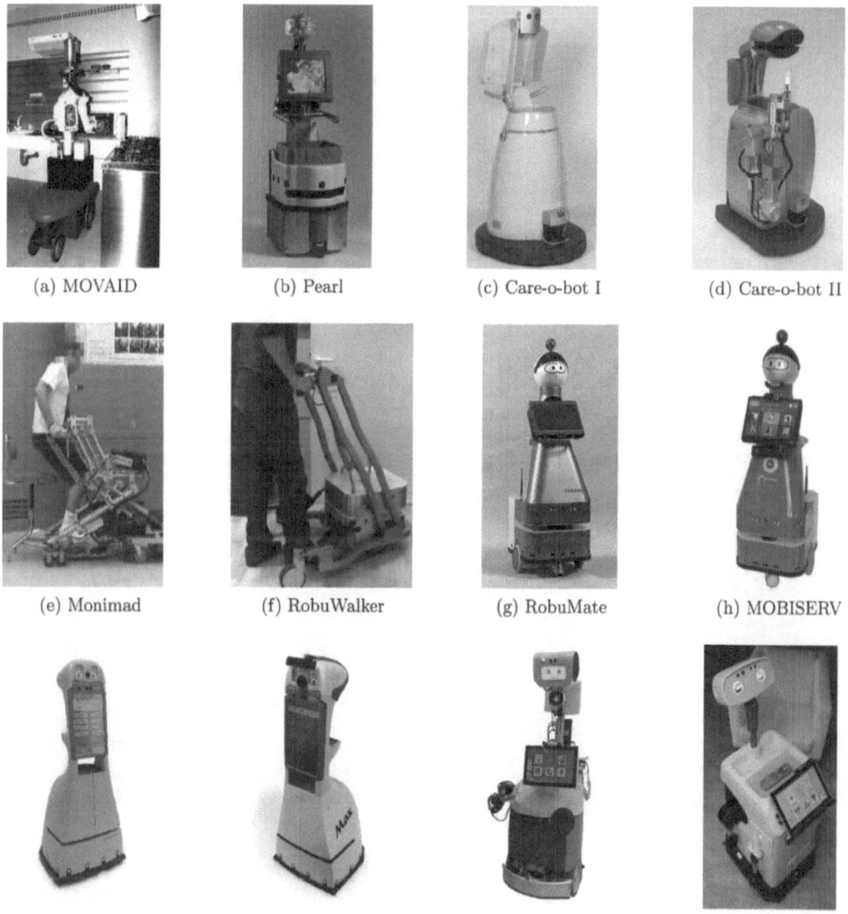

(a) MOVAID (b) Pearl (c) Care-o-bot I (d) Care-o-bot II

(e) Monimad (f) RobuWalker (g) RobuMate (h) MOBISERV

(i) Hector (j) Max (k) Hobbit PT1 (l) Hobbit PT2

Figure 7.5 (a-l) Different types of robots available of elderly persons [25].

but some several potential solutions and interventions can help improve their quality of life and well-being.

7.5 CASE STUDIES

EPFL's SoftHand Pro [26]: Researchers at École Polytechnique Fédérale de Lausanne(EPFL) developed a soft robotic hand called SoftHand Pro shown in Figure 7.6, which is designed to be sensitive and adaptable. Such technology can assist elderly individuals in performing daily tasks like grasping objects or handling delicate items, enhancing their independence.

Robo-Mate Project [28]: The Robo-Mate project, funded by the European Commission, focuses on developing soft exoskeletons to assist workers in handling heavy loads safely. Figure 7.7 describes the robo-mate

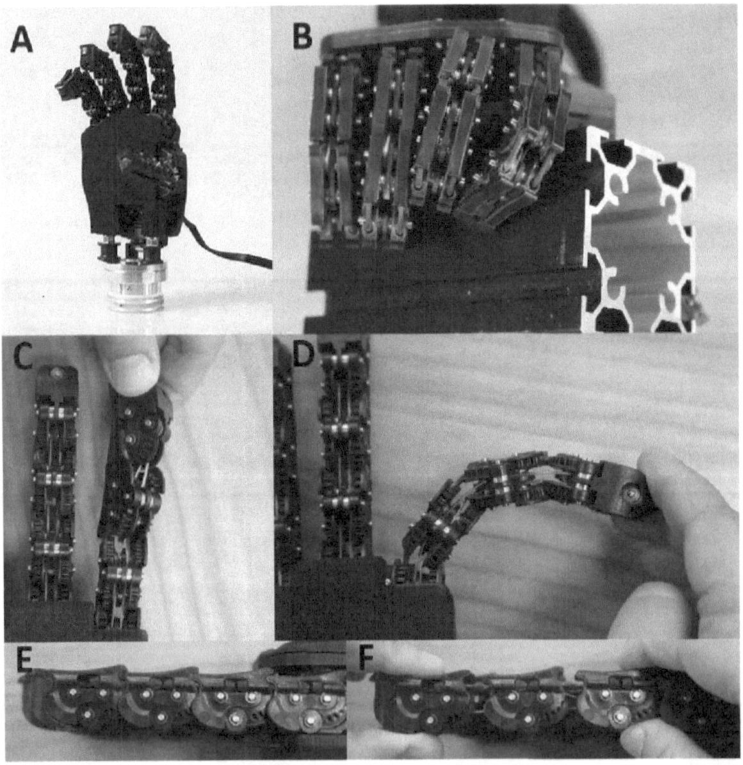

Figure 7.6 The SoftHand Pro (SHP) is displayed with a wrist interface. The SHP is seen gripping a large square tube, showcasing the benefits of its flexible joint design. The bottom two rows illustrate the twisting (C), bending (D), and disarticulating (E, F) capabilities of the SHP [27].

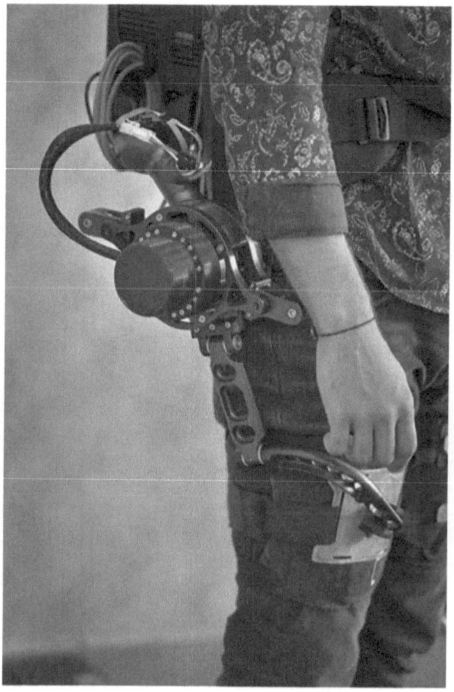

Figure 7.7 Active trunk which reduces the exoskeleton loading [29].

installed person leg. While not exclusively for elderly care, the technology could be adapted to provide support for elderly individuals with mobility issues, enabling them to move more comfortably and reducing the risk of injury.

RIBA (Robot for Interactive Body Assistance) [30]: RIBA was developed through a collaboration between RIKEN (a Japanese research institute) and Tokai Rubber Industries. The project aimed to create a robot that could alleviate some of the physical strain on caregivers while providing a safe and comfortable experience for patients. It features a soft, cushion-like body that can gently lift people from beds or wheelchairs. RIBA is a notable soft robotic system developed primarily for assisting elderly and disabled individuals in care settings. Figure 7.8 shows the RIBA with parts. RIBA is designed with a soft, cushion-like body covered in a flexible material resembling a soft robotic suit. Its appearance is non-threatening and comfortable, resembling a large cushion or pillow with robotic capabilities.

The main purpose of RIBA is to provide physical assistance with lifting and moving individuals who require support due to age-related frailty or physical disabilities. It is particularly useful in environments such as nursing homes or hospitals where caregivers may need assistance with tasks like

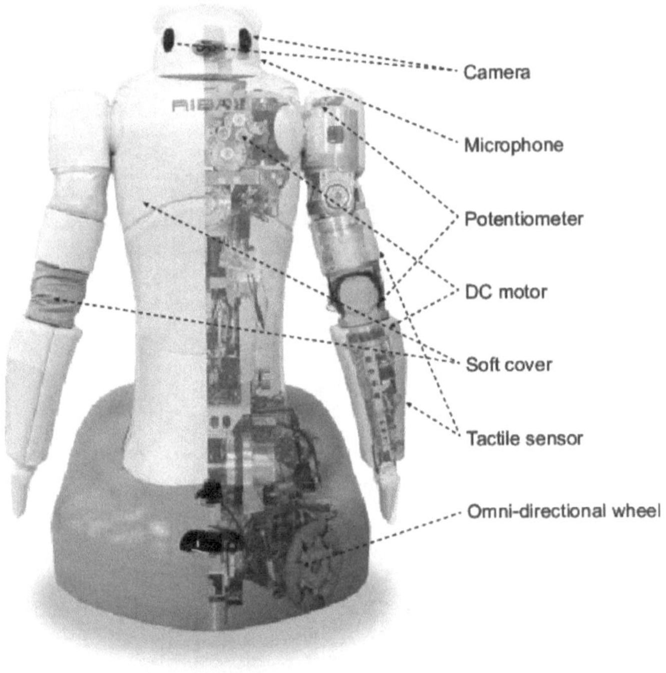

Figure 7.8 RIBA-nursing robot [30].

transferring patients from beds to wheelchairs or assisting in toileting. RIBA operates using pneumatic actuators embedded within its soft body. These actuators enable controlled and gentle movements, ensuring that lifting and positioning are done smoothly without causing discomfort or injury to the person being assisted.

By employing soft robotics technology, RIBA offers several benefits over traditional rigid robots or manual lifting methods. It reduces the risk of injury to both caregivers and patients, enhances the comfort of the lifting process, and promotes a sense of security and dignity for elderly individuals needing assistance. RIBA represents a significant advancement in assistive robotics for elderly care. Its success has spurred further research into soft robotics applications for healthcare, focusing on improving autonomy, safety, and quality of life for elderly and disabled populations. RIBA exemplifies how soft robotics can be applied effectively to address specific challenges in eldercare, providing practical solutions that enhance caregiving practices and improve the overall well-being of elderly individuals.

Exo-Glove Poly [31, 32]: Glove Poly is an innovative soft robotic glove designed to assist with hand movements and enhance grip strength, particularly beneficial for elderly individuals or those with hand

> disabilities. Exo-Glove Poly is constructed using soft, flexible materials that mimic the natural movement and flexibility of the human hand. It features a lightweight and ergonomic design, intended to be comfortable for extended use. The primary function of Exo-Glove Poly is to augment the user's hand strength and dexterity. The front view of the Exo-Glove Poly arm is shown in Figure 7.9. It incorporates soft robotic actuators and sensors that detect the wearer's movements and provide assistive force to support gripping and holding objects.

The dotted lines show the areas of tendons and Bowden cables that are on the opposite side of the hand. (a) The black arrows point out the pressure put on the TA support by the Bowden cables, and the red arrows point out the pressure spread on the TA support by the hand. (b) As the tendon approaches the joint, the pressure on the joint is higher than the pressure at the point of attachment [33].

It is designed for various applications where enhanced hand strength and precision are beneficial, such as in rehabilitation settings, activities of daily living (ADLs) for elderly persons, or industrial tasks requiring repetitive

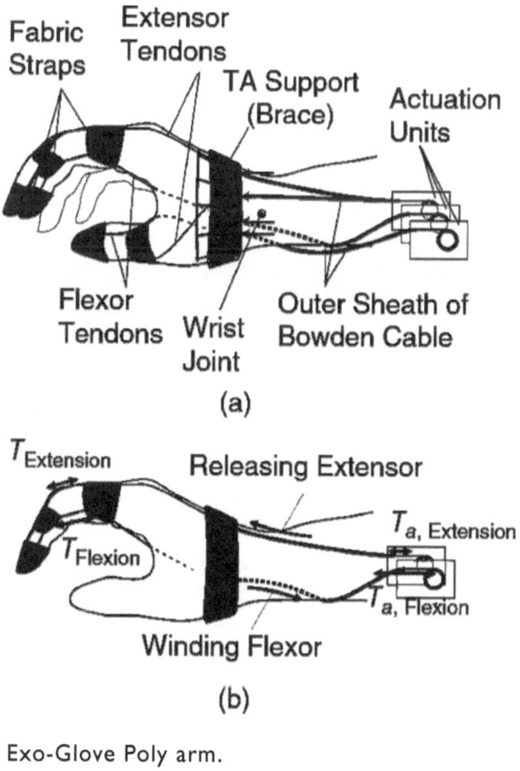

Figure 7.9 (a-b) Exo-Glove Poly arm.

gripping. Exo-Glove Poly was developed by ExoAtlet, a company specializing in wearable robotics. The glove has undergone iterative development to optimize its performance, usability, and comfort for users. Exo-Glove Poly offers several advantages over traditional rigid exoskeletons or prosthetic devices. It provides natural hand movements, reduces muscle fatigue, and assists users in performing tasks independently that may otherwise be challenging due to age-related weakness or disabilities.

The development of Exo-Glove Poly represents ongoing advancements in wearable robotics and assistive technologies. Future iterations will focus on enhancing the glove's capabilities, integrating more intuitive control systems, and expanding its applicability across different user demographics and industries. Exo-Glove Poly demonstrates how soft robotics can improve the quality of life for elderly individuals by restoring or augmenting hand function, promoting independence, and supporting activities that contribute to daily living and overall well-being.

PneuChair [34, 35]: PneuChair is an innovative soft robotic wheelchair developed by researchers at the Singapore-MIT Alliance for Research and Technology (SMART) and the National University of Singapore (NUS). Developed by researchers at Singapore's Nanyang Technological University. PneuChair is designed with soft robotics technology, using pneumatic (air-powered) actuators instead of traditional motors and rigid components. This design choice makes the wheelchair lightweight, flexible, and more energy-efficient compared to conventional wheelchairs.

The wheelchair's pneumatic actuators allow it to maneuver smoothly and navigate various terrains with greater agility. This includes handling slopes, uneven surfaces, and tight spaces more effectively, enhancing mobility and independence for users.

The soft materials used in its construction provide a more comfortable seating experience, reducing pressure points and improving overall comfort for long-term use. Its flexible design and pneumatic actuators enable precise control and smoother rides, enhancing user maneuverability and reducing physical strain on caregivers. The lightweight nature and improved maneuverability make PneuChair particularly suitable for indoor and outdoor use, including in environments with limited accessibility. PneuChair was developed as part of ongoing research efforts to explore the application of soft robotics in mobility devices. The project aims to improve the quality of life for wheelchair users by addressing common challenges associated with conventional wheelchairs.

The development of PneuChair highlights the potential of soft robotics to revolutionize mobility solutions for individuals with disabilities, including elderly persons who may benefit from enhanced comfort, maneuverability, and accessibility. Researchers continue to refine and optimize PneuChair, exploring additional functionalities and potential adaptations to further enhance its performance and suitability for a wider range of users and environments.

EPFL Soft Robot [36, 37]: MobiChair: Developed by EPFL and INRIA researchers, MobiChair is a soft wheelchair that adapts its shape to the user's body, providing customized support and comfort. It uses soft robotics technology to improve mobility and reduce pressure sores.

MobiChair is designed with a focus on adaptability and comfort using soft robotics principles. It features a flexible and modular structure that can adjust to the user's body shape and movements, providing a customized seating experience. The wheelchair incorporates soft actuators and materials that allow for dynamic adjustments in response to the user's weight distribution and posture. This enhances comfort and reduces the risk of pressure sores often associated with traditional wheelchair seating. MobiChair is equipped with advanced control systems that optimize its performance across various surfaces and environments. It offers improved stability and maneuverability, making it easier for users, including elderly individuals, to navigate both indoor and outdoor spaces. The development of MobiChair reflects ongoing research efforts in the field of soft robotics and assistive technology. Researchers aim to enhance mobility and independence for wheelchair users by addressing ergonomic challenges and improving overall user experience.

Its soft and adaptable design provides ergonomic support and reduces discomfort during prolonged use. Enhanced maneuverability and stability make it suitable for diverse settings, promoting greater independence and accessibility for users. By integrating soft robotics technology, MobiChair represents a forward-thinking approach to improving the quality of life for individuals with mobility impairments. Researchers continue to refine MobiChair's design and functionality, exploring opportunities to integrate more advanced sensing and control capabilities. Future developments may focus on enhancing user interface features and expanding its application in healthcare and personal mobility.

Automated Toilet Assistance Robot (ATARO)[38, 39]: Developed by researchers at Stanford University, ATARO is a soft robotic device designed to assist elderly individuals with toileting tasks. It can autonomously help with sitting down, standing up, and maintaining balance. While prosthetics typically serve individuals of all ages, advancements in soft robotics have led to more natural and comfortable prosthetic limbs. For elderly persons requiring prosthetic assistance, soft robotics can offer improved functionality and ease of use compared to traditional rigid prosthetics.

ATARO is an innovative soft robotic device designed to assist elderly and disabled individuals with toileting tasks. Developed by researchers at Stanford University, ATARO aims to enhance independence and improve the quality of life for users who may have difficulty using traditional toilets independently. ATARO features a soft and adaptable structure that integrates with existing toilet facilities. Its design includes soft robotic arms and sensors that facilitate safe and effective assistance during toileting activities. The primary function of ATARO is to assist users with tasks such as sitting down, standing up, and maintaining balance while using the toilet. It utilizes soft actuators and responsive control systems to provide gentle support tailored to the user's needs.

ATARO is designed to interact intuitively with users, adapting its assistance based on real-time feedback and user preferences. This approach aims to enhance comfort and promote user dignity during the toileting process. It enables elderly and disabled individuals to perform toileting tasks more independently, reducing reliance on caregivers for assistance. Soft robotics technology ensures gentle and secure assistance, minimizing the risk of injury or discomfort during use. By improving access to essential toileting facilities, ATARO enhances overall accessibility and supports greater autonomy for users.

ATARO represents a significant advancement in the application of soft robotics for healthcare and assistive technology. Its development is part of ongoing research efforts to address challenges faced by individuals with mobility impairments. Researchers are exploring potential enhancements and adaptations for ATARO, including improvements in user interface design, integration with smart home technologies, and scalability for broader healthcare applications.

Robear [40, 41]: Developed by RIKEN and Sumitomo Riko Company Limited, Robear is a gentle nursing care robot designed to provide assistance with lifting and carrying elderly individuals. It has a soft, bear-like appearance and is equipped with sensors for safe interaction.

Harvard's Soft Robotics Toolkit [42]: Harvard University's Wyss Institute developed a Soft Robotics Toolkit that provides resources for creating soft robotic devices. This toolkit enables researchers and developers to design custom soft robots tailored for specific applications in elder care, such as wearable devices for assistance with mobility or rehabilitation.

Gentle Robotic Companions: Research into robotic companionship for elderly individuals includes projects like PARO [43], a therapeutic robot seal developed by AIST in Japan. While not strictly soft robotics, it demonstrates the potential for soft materials in creating comforting and non-threatening robotic companions that can alleviate loneliness and provide mental stimulation. These examples highlight the potential of soft robotics in improving the quality of life for elderly individuals through enhanced mobility, assistance with daily tasks, and companionship. While comprehensive case studies specifically on autonomous applications in elder care may be limited, ongoing research and development in the field continue to explore and expand these possibilities.

7.6 CONCLUSIONS

Soft robotics offers a promising solution for enhancing the safety and comfort of elderly individuals during caregiving tasks. The use of compliant materials and gentle actuators reduces the risk of injury and discomfort compared to traditional rigid robotics. Applications such as soft robotic exoskeletons, prosthetics, and assistive devices contribute significantly to improving the quality of life for elderly persons. These technologies promote independence by augmenting mobility and aiding in ADLs.

Soft robotics allows for personalized and adaptable solutions tailored to the unique needs and capabilities of elderly individuals. This customization supports better integration into daily routines and addresses specific challenges related to aging and mobility limitations. Beyond physical assistance, soft robotic companions and social robots provide psychological benefits by reducing loneliness and promoting social interaction. These robots can engage with users in meaningful ways, enhancing cognitive stimulation and emotional well-being. Despite advancements, challenges remain in areas such as cost-effectiveness, robustness, and user acceptance. Future research should focus on addressing these challenges to facilitate broader adoption and integration of soft robotics in elder care settings. Ethical implications, including privacy concerns and the impact on human dignity, should be carefully considered and addressed in the development and deployment of soft robotics for elderly care. Soft robotics has the potential to alleviate the physical and emotional burden on caregivers by providing reliable assistance and support in caregiving tasks.

REFERENCES

[1] Cohen, J. E. (2001, November). World population in 2050: assessing the projections. In *Conference Series-Federal Reserve Bank of Boston*(Vol. 46, pp. 83–113). Federal Reserve Bank of Boston; 1998.

[2] Trancoso, R., Syktus, J., Allan, R. P., Croke, J., Hoegh-Guldberg, O., & Chadwick, R. (2024). Significantly wetter or drier future conditions for one to two thirds of the world's population. *Nature Communications*, 15(1), 483.

[3] Agarwal, A., Lubet, A., Mitgang, E., Mohanty, S., & Bloom, D. E. (2020). *Population Aging in India: Facts, Issues, and Options* (pp. 289–311). Springer Singapore.

[4] Vimarlund, V., Borycki, E. M., Kushniruk, A. W., & Avenberg, K. (2021). Ambient assisted living: Identifying new challenges and needs for digital technologies and service innovation. *Yearbook of Medical Informatics*, 30(01), 141–149.

[5] Yang, Y., Wu, Y., Li, C., Yang, X., & Chen, W. (2020). Flexible actuators for soft robotics. *Advanced Intelligent Systems*, 2(1), 1900077.

[6] Sharkey, A. (2014). Robots and human dignity: a consideration of the effects of robot care on the dignity of older people. *Ethics and Information Technology*, 16, 63–75.

[7] Kim, D., Kim, S. H., Kim, T., Kang, B. B., Lee, M., Park, W., ... & Jo, S. (2021). Review of machine learning methods in soft robotics. *PLoS One*, 16(2), e0246102.
[8] Woodbridge, R., Sullivan, M. P., Harding, E., Crutch, S., Gilhooly, K. J., Gilhooly, M. L. M., ... & Wilson, L. (2018). Use of the physical environment to support everyday activities for people with dementia: A systematic review. *Dementia*, 17(5), 533–572.
[9] Weiss, R. (1975). *Loneliness: The Experience of Emotional and Social Isolation.* MIT Press.
[10] Dessin, C. L. (1999). Financial abuse of the elderly. *Idaho L. Rev.*, 36, 203.
[11] Choi, N. G., & Mayer, J. (2000). Elder abuse, neglect, and exploitation: Risk factors and prevention strategies. *Journal of Gerontological Social Work*, 33(2), 5–25.
[12] https://www.iastoppers.com/articles/mains-article-indias-elderly-population
[13] Ingber, D. E. (2011). The Wyss institute at Harvard university. *IEEE Pulse*, 2(4), 43–46.
[14] https://www.azorobotics.com/News.aspx?newsID=14472
[15] Jumphoo, T., Uthansakul, M., Duangmanee, P., Khan, N., & Uthansakul, P. (2021). Soft robotic glove controlling using brainwave detection for continuous rehabilitation at home. *Computers, Materials & Continua*, 66(1), 961–976.
[16] van Veggel, S., Wiertlewski, M., Doubrovski, E. L., Kooijman, A., Shahabi, E., Mazzolai, B., & Scharff, R. B. (2024). Classification and evaluation of octopus-inspired suction cups for soft continuum robots. *Advanced Science*, 2400806, https://doi.org/10.1002/advs.202400806
[17] Perez Vidal, A. F., Rumbo Morales, J. Y., Ortiz Torres, G., Sorcia Vazquez, F. D. J., Cruz Rojas, A., Brizuela Mendoza, J. A., & Rodriguez Cerda, J. C. (2021, July). Soft exoskeletons: Development, requirements, and challenges of the last decade. In *Actuators* (Vol. 10, No. 7, p. 166). Basel, Switzerland; MDPI.
[18] Chen, B. L., & Lin, Y. P. (2022). Robot-assisted posterior endoscopic cervical decompression. In *Technical Advances in Minimally Invasive Spine Surgery: Navigation, Robotics, Endoscopy, Augmented and Virtual Reality* (pp. 327–337). Singapore: Springer Nature Singapore.
[19] https://www.istockphoto.com/photos/robot-older-person
[20] Park, H. W., Rosenberg-Kima, R., Rosenberg, M., Gordon, G., & Breazeal, C. (2017, March). Growing growth mindset with a social robot peer. In *Proceedings of the 2017 ACM/IEEE International Conference on Human-Robot Interaction*(pp. 137–145).
[21] Strengers, Y., & Kennedy, J. (2021). *The Smart Wife: Why Siri, Alexa, and Other Smart Home Devices Need a Feminist Reboot.* MIT Press.
[22] Zhu, K., & Zhang, T. (2021). Deep reinforcement learning based mobile robot navigation: A review. *Tsinghua Science and Technology*, 26(5), 674–691.
[23] Bhandari, S., & Baral Sapkota, R. (2023). The role of social robots to support elderly people's mental health: a literature review, University in Lahti, Finland
[24] Pu, L., Moyle, W., Jones, C., & Todorovic, M. (2019). The effectiveness of social robots for older adults: a systematic review and meta-analysis of randomized controlled studies. *The Gerontologist*, 59(1), e37–e51.
[25] Bardaro, Gianluca, Antonini, Alessio,& Motta, Enrico. (2022). Robots for elderly care in the home: A landscape analysis and co-design toolkit. *International Journal of Social Robotics*.14. 10.1007/s12369-021-00816-3

[26] Fras, J., Althoefer, K., (2018). Bio-mimetic pneumatic soft prosthetic hand. UK-RAS Conference: 'Robots Working For & Among Us' Proceedings, 90-92. https://doi.org/10.31256/UKRAS17.29
[27] Godfrey, Sasha, Zhao, Kristin, Theuer, Amanda, Catalano, Manuel, Bianchi, Matteo, Breighner, Ryan, Bhaskaran, Divya, Lennon, Ryan, Grioli, Giorgio, Santello, Marco, Bicchi, Antonio, & Andrews, Karen. (2018). The SoftHand Pro: Functional evaluation of a novel, flexible, and robust myoelectric prosthesis. *PLoS One*.13. e0205653. https://doi.org/10.1371/journal.pone.0205653
[28] van der Vorm, J., Nugent, R., & O'Sullivan, L. (2015). Safety and risk management in designing for the lifecycle of an exoskeleton: a novel process developed in the robo-mate project. *Procedia Manufacturing*, 3, 1410–1417.
[29] https://www.robo-mate.eu/active-trunk.html
[30] Ding, Ming, Ikeura, Ryojun, Mori, Yukim Mukai, Toshiharu, & Shigeyuki, Hosoe. (2014). Lift-up motion generation of nursing-care assistant robot based on human muscle force and body softness estimation. *IEEE/ASME International Conference on Advanced Intelligent Mechatronics, AIM*. 1302–1307. https://doi.org/10.1109/AIM.2014.6878262
[31] Kang, B. B., Choi, H., Lee, H., & Cho, K. J. (2019). Exo-glove poly II: A polymer-based soft wearable robot for the hand with a tendon-driven actuation system. *Soft Robotics*, 6(2), 214–227.
[32] Yun, S. S., Kang, B. B., & Cho, K. J. (2017). Exo-glove PM: An easily customizable modularized pneumatic assistive glove. *IEEE Robotics and Automation Letters*, 2(3), 1725–1732.
[33] https://www.wevolver.com/specs/exo.glove
[34] Daveler, B. J. (2020). *Development and Evaluation of Pneumatic Powered Mobility Devices*. University of Pittsburgh.
[35] Daveler, B., Gebrosky, B., Grindle, G. G., & Cooper, R. A. (2018). Development of the pneuchair: Pneumatic-powered wheelchair. *Technology & Innovation*, 20(1–2), 11–19.
[36] Wang, L., Nurzaman, S. G., & Iida, F. (2017). Soft-material robotics. Foundations and Trends® in *Robotics*, 5(3), 191–259.
[37] https://actu.epfl.ch/news/robots-transform-into-furniture-at-epfl/
[38] Mishra, A. (2019). Intelligent human-aware decision making for semi-autonomous human rehabilitation assistance using modular robots (Master's thesis, University of Nebraska at Omaha).
[39] Park, S., Won, D.D., Lee, B. J. et al. A mountable toilet system for personalized health monitoring via the analysis of excreta. Nat Biomed Eng 4, 624–635 (2020). https://doi.org/10.1038/s41551-020-0534-9
[40] https://www.riken.jp/en/news_pubs/research_news/pr/2015/20150223_2/
[41] Bedaf, S., Huijnen, C., van den Heuvel, R., & de Witte, L. (2017). Robots supporting care for elderly people. In *Robotic Assistive Technologies* (pp. 309–332). CRC Press.
[42] Holland, D. P., Park, E. J., Polygerinos, P., Bennett, G. J., & Walsh, C. J. (2014). The soft robotics toolkit: Shared resources for research and design. *Soft Robotics*, 1(3), 224–230.
[43] Šabanović, S., Bennett, C. C., Chang, W. L., & Huber, L. (2013, June). PARO robot affects diverse interaction modalities in group sensory therapy for older adults with dementia. In *2013 IEEE 13th international conference on rehabilitation robotics (ICORR)* (pp. 1–6). IEEE.

Chapter 8

Comprehensive study on materials used in soft robotics for medical and healthcare industries

Perabathula Satish and Shaik Himam Saheb

8.1 INTRODUCTION

Soft robotics is a subfield of robotics that involves the use of flexible, pliable, and compliant materials to create robots with more flexibility. Unlike traditional rigid robots, soft robots can manipulate and interact with delicate or irregularly shaped objects, and can even change shape to fit through tight spaces. Some of the soft robots include soft grippers, inflatable robots for search and rescue applications, wearable robots for rehabilitation and assistance, soft exoskeletons for medical applications, and soft swarm robots for environmental monitoring. Soft robotic materials exhibit unique properties that enable their use in soft robotics. These properties include:

- Elasticity: The ability to stretch and deform without breaking
- Flexibility: The ability to bend and conform to complex shapes
- Compliance: The ability to absorb and distribute forces
- Biocompatibility: The ability to safely interact with humans and biological tissues
- Conductivity: The ability to transmit electrical signals

8.2 TYPES OF SOFT ROBOTIC MATERIALS

Soft robotic materials can be broadly classified into several categories:

- Elastomers: Flexible and stretchable materials, such as silicone and polyurethane
- Hydrogels: Water-absorbing materials that can alter shape in retort to humidity
- Shape Memory Polymers: Metals that can change shape in response to temperature changes
- Conductive Materials: Materials that can transmit electrical signals, such as conductive silicone and carbon nanotubes
- Biocompatible materials
- Advanced composites

DOI: 10.1201/9781003539612-8

8.2.1 Elastomers

Elastomer materials play an essential role in the field of soft robotics, offering intrinsic flexibility and adaptability that are crucial for creating advanced robotic systems. These materials exhibit unique mechanical properties that allow them to deform under stress and return to their original shape, which mimics biological systems. The significance of elastomers in soft robotics lies in their potential to perform complex movements and interactions in unstructured environments, akin to living organisms. Their use enhances the capabilities of robots to engage in safe and effective interactions with humans and their surroundings. Multiple types of elastomers are utilized in soft robotics, each with distinct properties tailored for specific applications. Thermosensitive elastomers, for example, offer variable mechanical properties that can be controlled through temperature changes. This characteristic allows for programmable responses to environmental stimuli, making them suitable for applications where adaptability is essential. Dielectric elastomers (DEs) are another prominent category, converting electrical energy into mechanical work, making them ideal for actuators and artificial muscles in soft robotic systems [1–4].

Thermosensitive elastomers are soft smart materials whose properties can be adjusted by varying their temperature. This capability arises from the incorporation of thermoplastic filler particles within a soft and elastic PDMS matrix. The thermoplastic fillers used include PCL, PA6, and PMMA powder, with melting temperatures ranging from 58°C to 215°C. DEs are a class of electro-mechanical transducers whose shapes change significantly in response to an electric voltage [5]. A typical DE consists of a thin polymer membrane coated on both sides with flexible electrodes, with a thickness that can vary from tens to hundreds of micrometers. When a voltage is functional to the actuator, it generates electrostatic pressure between the electrodes, causing the material to compress in the thickness direction. Because DEs are nearly incompressible, this compression leads to an expansion in the in-plane direction, as shown in Figure 8.1.

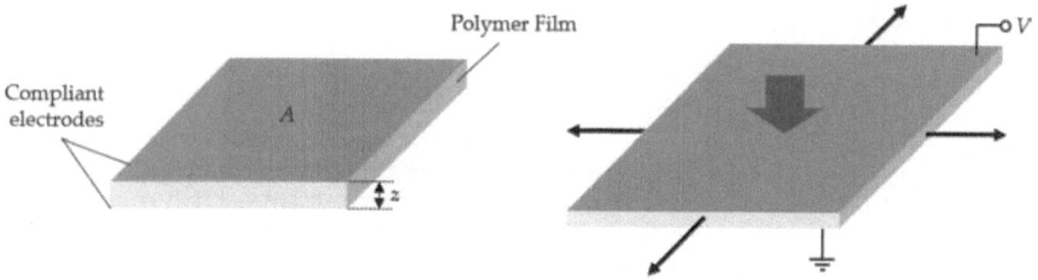

Figure 8.1 Operating principle of dielectric elastomers (DEs) through electrostatic forces.

A DE functions as a compliant variable capacitor that transforms electrical energy into mechanical energy. The capacitance CCC of the DE can be represented by the following equation:

$$C = \frac{\varepsilon_0 \varepsilon A}{z}$$

where ε represents the relative permittivity, ε_0 is the permittivity of free space, A is the area of the compliant electrode, and z denotes the thickness of the DE material. The electrical energy U stored in the DE with charge Q can be expressed as

$$U = \frac{0.5Q^2}{C} = \frac{0.5zQ^2}{\varepsilon_0 \varepsilon A}$$

As mentioned earlier, the DE material is essentially incompressible, which results in the constant volume equation

$$p = \varepsilon_0 \varepsilon E^2 = \varepsilon_0 \varepsilon \left(\frac{V}{z}\right)^2$$

Consequently, the electrostatic pressure p, known as Maxwell stress, acting across the two electrodes can be derived

$$S_z = -\frac{p}{Y} = -\frac{\varepsilon_0 \varepsilon E^2}{Y} = -\frac{\varepsilon_0 \varepsilon}{Y}\left(\frac{V}{z}\right)^2$$

where E is the electric field and V is the applied voltage. In the electrostatic pressure equation, it is assumed that the DE material exhibits uniform thickness and a consistent surface charge distribution. By applying free boundary conditions and assuming linear elasticity for small strains (less than 10%), the thickness strain S_z can be expressed as:

$$S_z = -\frac{p}{Y} = -\frac{\varepsilon_0 \varepsilon E^2}{Y} = -\frac{\varepsilon_0 \varepsilon}{Y}\left(\frac{V}{z}\right)^2$$

It is crucial to consider these variables to accurately determine the dynamic behavior of DEs. Generally, dielectric elastomer actuators (DEAs) are characterized by large strains (over 100%), high efficiency, significant energy density (exceeding 3.4 MJ/m^3), and rapid response times in the millisecond range. The performance of DEAs is primarily influenced by two main factors: the DE materials and the compliant electrodes.

The selection of DE materials is essential for optimizing the performance of DEAs. For enhanced effectiveness, acrylic elastomers provide significant advantages in achieving large strains. In contrast, silicone elastomers have lower dielectric constants, which require higher electric fields to generate comparable strains. However, due to their higher viscosity, acrylic elastomers may be less suitable for applications that operate at elevated frequencies, making silicone elastomers a better choice in those scenarios [6–9].

Compliant electrodes play a crucial role in enhancing the performance of DEAs, in addition to the selection of DE materials. These materials are cost-effective, highly conductive, and easy to apply; however, they may encounter stability issues over extended use. Additionally, ionic conductors are gaining attention as potential candidates for transparent compliant electrodes in DEAs, with reports suggesting that they exhibit lower resistance compared to other transparent electronic conductors like AgNWs or SWCNTs.

When comparing different elastomer materials used in soft robotics, it is crucial to consider their specific advantages and limitations. For example, while thermosensitive elastomers offer temperature-induced tunability, they may lack the robustness required for high-stress environments. On the other hand, DEs are particularly effective for applications requiring high actuation speed and efficiency but may struggle under mechanical loads without innovative design strategies. Thus, selecting the right elastomer depends largely on the intended application and the desired mechanical behavior's. The mechanical properties of elastomers are fundamental to their performance in soft robotics. Soft robotic systems often require materials with high stretchability and low stiffness, enabling them to effectively absorb shocks and impacts while maintaining mechanical stability [10, 11]. The ability to tune these properties dynamically is particularly advantageous, as it allows for fine control over the robot's movements and interactions with its environment. Consequently, understanding the relationship between the structural composition of elastomers and their mechanical behavior is essential for designing effective soft robotic systems. Recent advancements in elastomer formulations have led to the development of composite materials that combine elastomers with other substances, such as magnetic and conductive particles, which enhance their functional capabilities. For instance, magneto-sensitive elastomers can change their mechanical properties in response to external magnetic fields, allowing for precise control of robotic actions. Similarly, incorporating conductive materials into elastomers empowers the creation of smart actuators that monitor and respond to their operational environment, improving the functional quality of soft robots.

Elastomers are increasingly being integrated into various applications in soft robotics, such as grippers, soft actuators, and humanoid devices. Soft robotic grippers, which utilize elastomer materials, are often inspired by biological structures to improve dexterity and grasping capability. They can adapt their shapes to hold objects of different sizes and shapes, making them versatile tools for various industries, including construction, medicine, and manufacturing. Furthermore, elastomers enable the creation of soft actuators that can mimic the muscle movements found in biological organisms, allowing for smoother interactions in complex environments [12]. Despite the numerous advantages of elastomers in soft robotics, challenges remain in optimizing their performance and durability. Factors such as fatigue, environmental degradation, and limitations in the range of motion pose significant hurdles for practical applications. Future research is needed to develop more robust elastomer formulations that can sustain performance under varied conditions. Innovations in material science may lead to the discovery of new elastomer composites that exhibit enhanced properties, facilitating the design of next-generation soft robotic systems [13]. Functionalizing elastomers with additional materials further enhances their applicability in soft robotics. By incorporating elements such as carbon nanotubes or metal fibers, researchers have optimized elastomers for improved electrical conductivity or mechanical strength. This functionalization not only elevates the performance metrics of elastomeric materials but also expands their operational scope in soft robotic systems, allowing for more complex tasks that mimic intricate biological movements [14]. Real-world implementations of elastomer-based soft robots have demonstrated their effectiveness in a variety of scenarios. For instance, soft robots equipped with elastomer components have been deployed for minimally invasive surgeries, where their flexibility aids in navigating delicate anatomical structures without causing damage. Another notable application is in agriculture, where soft robots with elastomeric fingers can gently harvest fruits without bruising, showcasing the adaptability of these materials in specialized tasks.

8.2.2 Hydrogels

These are a class of materials characterized by their three-dimensional polymer networks that can hold substantial amounts of water. Their unique properties, including high flexibility, biocompatibility, and tunable mechanical characteristics, make them especially suitable for a variety of applications in soft robotics and healthcare. As the field of robotics integrates more closely with healthcare, hydrogels have emerged as critical components in the development of soft robotic systems designed for medical applications. Their ability to mimic biological tissues, facilitate fluid transport, and respond to environmental stimuli enhances their functionality in robotic platforms aimed at improving patient care and medical procedures. The mechanical and physical properties of hydrogels are significant for their applications in soft robotics. These materials are typically soft and pliable, exhibiting high elasticity and resilience under strain. Hydrogel materials can be engineered to possess specific tensile strengths, compressive strengths, and degrees of hydration, which are crucial for replicating the biomechanical behaviors of human tissues. The ability to finely tune these properties allows researchers to optimize hydrogels for specific tasks, such as soft manipulators, sensors, and actuators in medical devices [15–19].

One of the most critical aspects of using hydrogels in healthcare applications is their biocompatibility. Hydrogels can be formulated from various biocompatible materials, which minimizes the risk of adverse reactions when used in or on the human body. The hydrophilic nature of hydrogels also promotes cell adhesion and proliferation, which is vital for tissue engineering and regenerative medicine applications. The fabrication methods of hydrogels are varied and continue to evolve alongside technological advancements. Common techniques include chemical crosslinking, physical gelation, and 3D printing. 3D printing, in particular, has gained traction for fabricating hydrogels with complex geometries and customizable properties. This technique allows for the creation of intricate structures that can mimic the architecture of natural tissues, enhancing the functionality of soft robotic systems. Additionally, advances in photopolymerization and bio-ink development have opened new avenues for creating hydrogels with embedded biological factors, further improving their interaction with biological systems [20–22].

The integration of hydrogels into soft robotic systems has ushered in a new era of healthcare solutions. These soft robots are designed to perform delicate tasks, such as minimally invasive surgeries, patient monitoring, and rehabilitation therapies. For instance, soft robotic grippers made from hydrogels can handled, reducing the risk of damage during procedures. Similarly, hydrogel actuators can effectively simulate muscle contractions and movements, providing precise control in surgical applications. Hydrogel materials can be engineered to possess sensing capabilities essential for medical diagnostics and monitoring. For example, electrically conductive hydrogels can be used to develop soft sensors that detect pressure, strain, or temperature changes in physiological conditions. These sensors are invaluable in wearable health-monitoring devices, enabling real-time tracking of patient vitals without causing discomfort. Furthermore, by integrating functional nanomaterials, hydrogels can enhance their sensitivity and specificity, enabling accurate detection of biomarkers for disease diagnostics.

Hydrogels offer innovative solutions for controlled drug delivery applications, which are critical in managing diseases over prolonged periods. Soft robotic systems utilizing hydrogels have shown promise in rehabilitation therapies, providing tools for patients recovering from injuries or surgeries. These robots can assist in repetitive motion exercises, helping to facilitate muscle re-education and rehabilitation while minimizing strain on vulnerable tissues. The compliant nature of hydrogels allows these robotic systems to adapt to the movements of patients, creating a more natural and comfortable training environment. Research continues to explore how combining hydrogels with robotic technologies can lead to more effective rehabilitation solutions [23].

Despite their numerous advantages, several challenges persist in the use of hydrogels in soft robotics for healthcare. One of the main concerns is their mechanical robustness. While hydrogels are excellent for mimicking soft tissues, they can be sensitive to environmental conditions, leading to issues such as swelling, degradation, and loss of mechanical integrity under repeated stress. Researchers are actively seeking ways to enhance the mechanical properties of hydrogels, including the incorporation of reinforcing materials and the development of hybrid systems. The future of hydrogel materials in soft robotics and healthcare is brimming with potential. Emerging technologies such as 4D printing and bio printing are expected to revolutionize the way hydrogels are created, allowing for dynamic and responsive structures. Moreover, ongoing research into the combination of hydrogels with advanced materials such as liquid metals or conductive polymers may lead to more sophisticated and multifunctional devices, expanding their applications further into the realms of healthcare and beyond. Continued interdisciplinary collaboration between materials science, robotics, and healthcare disciplines will be paramount in overcoming existing challenges and harnessing the full capabilities of hydrogels in soft robotics.

1. Thermally responsive actuators (TRAs)
2. Chemically responsive actuators (CRAs)
3. Optically responsive actuators (ORAs)
4. Magnetically responsive actuators (MRAs)
5. Hydraulically responsive actuators (HRAs)
6. Electrically responsive actuators (ERAs)

8.3 TRA

Thermally responsive hydrogel actuators function by undergoing volumetric changes in reaction to fluctuations in ambient temperature. These actuators are designed to respond selectively to specific temperature ranges, resulting in significant deformations. Additionally, the ability to adjust the critical temperature increases their versatility for various applications. Thermally responsive hydrogel actuators can be divided into two categories: those with an LCST and those with a UCST. LCST and UCST actuators demonstrate opposite temperature responses. To enhance the performance of thermally responsive hydrogels, various strategies have been implemented, including improving agility, reducing hysteresis during the volume phase transition, and broadening their operational range. This fundamental property has prompted extensive research into controlling the actuation direction of hydrogels through methods such as geometric design, modulus gradients, and the use of passive layers. Biomolecule responsive hydrogels selectively react to specific input biomolecules; they enable independent control of multiple domains.

8.3.1 Optically responsive actuators

Optically responsive actuators are innovative devices that utilize light as a stimulus to induce movement or change in shape. These actuators are often made from smart materials, such as polymers or hydrogels, which undergo physical transformations when exposed to specific wavelengths of light. The mechanism typically involves photochemical or photothermal effects, allowing for precise control over their behavior. Applications of optically responsive actuators span various fields, including robotics, biomedical devices, and soft materials engineering. For instance, they can be used to create soft robotic components that mimic biological movements, or in drug delivery systems that release medication in response to light exposure.

One of the key advantages of these actuators is their remote activation capability, eliminating the need for physical connections or mechanical components. This feature enhances flexibility and scalability in design, paving the way for advanced applications in adaptive structures, sensors, and environmental monitoring. As research advances, the potential for integrating these actuators into everyday technologies continues to grow.

8.3.2 Magnetically responsive hydrogel

Magnetically responsive hydrogels are innovative materials that react to external magnetic fields, enabling controlled movement and deformation. Composed of a polymer network infused with magnetic nanoparticles, these hydrogels exhibit unique properties that allow them to change shape or volume in response to magnetic stimuli. This responsiveness can be finely tuned, making them ideal for applications in soft robotics, where they can function as actuators or sensors.

In addition to their use in robotics, magnetically responsive hydrogels are being explored in biomedical fields for drug delivery and tissue engineering. Their ability to release therapeutic agents in a targeted manner, triggered by magnetic fields, enhances the precision of treatments. Moreover, these hydrogels can adapt to their environment, providing potential solutions for dynamic and interactive systems. The versatility of magnetically responsive hydrogels makes them a promising avenue for advancements in various technological and medical applications. Given these benefits, hydraulically responsive hydrogel-based actuators are well-suited for applications that require stealthy operation.

8.3.3 Hydraulically responsive hydrogel

Hydraulically responsive hydrogels are advanced materials that change their volume and shape in response to hydraulic pressure or fluid dynamics. These hydrogels are typically composed of crosslinked polymers that can absorb significant amounts of water, allowing them to swell or shrink based on external stimuli. Their unique properties make them ideal for applications in soft robotics, where they can serve as actuators or sensors that respond dynamically to environmental changes. When subjected to pressure, these hydrogels can mimic muscle contractions, enabling precise movements. Additionally, they are being explored in biomedical applications, such as drug delivery systems and tissue engineering, due to their biocompatibility and ability to release therapeutic agents in a controlled manner. Overall, hydraulically responsive hydrogels hold great promise for innovative solutions across multiple fields.

8.4 SHAPE-MEMORY POLYMERS (SMPs)

SMPs are smart materials that can "remember" and revert to a predetermined shape when exposed to specific stimuli, such as heat or light. These polymers undergo a phase transition, allowing them to switch between a temporary and permanent shape. SMPs find applications in various fields, including medical devices, textiles, and aerospace, due to their flexibility and adaptability. Their ability to transform shape on command makes them particularly valuable for creating responsive systems and components in innovative designs.

In the healthcare sector, the use of SMPs has the potential to transform medical devices, surgical instruments, and therapeutic tools. Their flexibility, biocompatibility, and responsiveness offer innovative solutions to complex medical challenges. The origins of SMPs trace back to the development of heat-shrinkable tubing made from cross-linked polyethylene in the 1960s, but significant research interest did not emerge until the 1990s. Recently, SMPs have gained considerable attention for biomedical applications, including catheters, sutures, and cardiac valve repairs.

SMPs have found significant application in the development of surgical tools designed to operate within the human body. These tools can change shape to navigate complex anatomical structures, offering minimally invasive procedures that reduce recovery time and patient trauma. For example, shape memory stents can expand and contract to adapt to the unique geometries of blood vessels, thereby improving the effectiveness of treatment. The incorporation of SMPs in prosthetic devices allows for highly adaptable and customizable solutions that can conform to the residual limb's shape. This adaptability leads to improved comfort, better fitting, and increased functionality. Recent advancements have enabled the design of prosthetics that can change their stiffness and shape in response to physical activity, significantly enhancing user experience. Devices that utilize SMPs can be engineered to assist patients by evolving as their rehabilitation progresses. For instance, wearable support systems can be programmed to provide varying levels of support based on the patient's needs and recovery stages, thereby enhancing the rehabilitation process. Soft robotic systems equipped with

SMPs can be used for direct patient care, including tasks like lifting, support, and even basic mobility assistance. These systems are designed to interact safely and supportively, making them suitable for elderly care or for patients with limited mobility. Their gentle interaction minimizes the risk of harm, enhancing the overall patient experience.

8.4.1 PLA

Polylactic acid (PLA) is increasingly recognized in the field of soft robotics due to its biodegradable properties and straightforward processing. As a thermoplastic sourced from renewable materials, PLA presents significant environmental benefits compared to conventional substances. Its suitability for 3D printing enables quick prototyping and the creation of custom soft robotic components, allowing for complex designs that closely mimic biological movement. PLA is utilized to produce lightweight structures and actuators, striking a balance between durability and flexibility. Researchers are investigating ways to blend PLA with other materials, like elastomers, to improve its mechanical performance and responsiveness. Additionally, PLA's capacity to decompose over time makes it an excellent choice for biomedical applications where biocompatibility is crucial. Overall, the distinctive properties of PLA position it as a valuable material for developing sustainable and effective soft robotic systems, expanding the potential of these technologies across various sectors, including healthcare and environmental applications.

8.5 CONCLUSIONS

This comprehensive study highlights the critical role of materials in advancing soft robotics for medical and healthcare applications. Soft robotics, characterized by the use of flexible and compliant materials, offers unique advantages for interacting with delicate biological systems and performing complex tasks. A diverse range of materials, including elastomers, hydrogels, shape memory polymers, and biocompatible composites, can be tailored to meet specific functional requirements in healthcare applications. Each material type provides distinct benefits, such as elasticity, responsiveness, and safety. The use of biocompatible materials is essential for ensuring patient safety. Materials that minimize adverse immune responses and promote tissue integration are particularly valuable in medical devices and surgical tools.

Soft robotic materials enable devices to adapt to various shapes and sizes, enhancing their ability to perform tasks such as minimally invasive surgeries, rehabilitation, and patient monitoring. This adaptability improves patient outcomes and increases the efficacy of medical procedures. Incorporating conductive materials within soft robotics allows for real-time monitoring and control. This capability enhances the functionality of medical devices, facilitating precise responses to physiological changes. Despite significant progress, challenges remain, including the need for materials that can provide both strength and flexibility, as well as those capable of withstanding repeated use in dynamic environments. Ongoing research aims to address these challenges by developing innovative materials that enhance performance. The study emphasizes that the careful selection and development of materials are vital for the successful implementation of soft robotics in medical and healthcare settings. By leveraging the unique properties of these materials, the healthcare industry can enhance the effectiveness, safety, and adaptability of robotic systems, ultimately improving patient care and outcomes.

REFERENCES

[1] Hsiao, J. H., Chang, J. Y., & Cheng, C. M. (2019). Soft medical robotics: clinical and biomedical applications, challenges, and future directions. *Advanced Robotics*, 33(21), 1099–1111.

[2] Cianchetti, M., Laschi, C., Menciassi, A., & Dario, P. (2018). Biomedical applications of soft robotics. *Nature Reviews Materials*, 3(6), 143–153.

[3] Yang, Y., Wu, Y., Li, C., Yang, X., & Chen, W. (2020). Flexible actuators for soft robotics. *Advanced Intelligent Systems*, 2(1), 1900077.

[4] Polygerinos, P., Correll, N., Morin, S. A., Mosadegh, B., Onal, C. D., Petersen, K., ... & Shepherd, R. F. (2017). Soft robotics: Review of fluid-driven intrinsically soft devices; manufacturing, sensing, control, and applications in human-robot interaction. *Advanced Engineering Materials*, 19(12), 1700016.

[5] Majidi, C. (2019). Soft-matter engineering for soft robotics. *Advanced Materials Technologies*, 4(2), 1800477.

[6] Ashuri, T., Armani, A., Jalilzadeh Hamidi, R., Reasnor, T., Ahmadi, S., & Iqbal, K. (2020). Biomedical soft robots: current status and perspective. *Biomedical Engineering Letters*, 10, 369–385.

[7] Chen, S., Fan, S., Chan, H., Qiao, Z., Qi, J., Wu, Z., ... & Lim, C. T. (2024). Liquid metal functionalization innovations in wearables and soft robotics for smart healthcare applications. *Advanced Functional Materials*, 34(31), 2309989.

[8] El-Atab, N., Mishra, R. B., Al-Modaf, F., Joharji, L., Alsharif, A. A., Alamoudi, H.,& Hussain, M. M. (2020). Soft actuators for soft robotic applications: A review. *Advanced Intelligent Systems*, 2(10), 2000128.

[9] Hsiao, J. H., Chang, J. Y., & Cheng, C. M. (2019). Soft medical robotics: clinical and biomedical applications, challenges, and future directions. *Advanced Robotics*, 33(21), 1099–1111.

[10] Cianchetti, M., Laschi, C., Menciassi, A., & Dario, P. (2018). Biomedical applications of soft robotics. *Nature Reviews Materials*, 3(6), 143–153.

[11] Polygerinos, P., Correll, N., Morin, S. A., Mosadegh, B., Onal, C. D., Petersen, K., ... & Shepherd, R. F. (2017). Soft robotics: Review of fluid-driven intrinsically soft devices; manufacturing, sensing, control, and applications in human-robot interaction. *Advanced Engineering Materials*, 19(12), 1700016.

[12] Saheb, S. H., & Babu, G. S. (2020). Modeling and evaluation of performance characteristics of redundant parallel planar manipulator. In *Innovative Data Communication Technologies and Application: ICIDCA 2019* (pp. 229–236). Springer International Publishing.
[13] Ebrahimi, N., Bi, C., Cappelleri, D. J., Ciuti, G., Conn, A. T., Faivre, D., ... & Jafari, A. (2021). Magnetic actuation methods in bio/soft robotics. *Advanced Functional Materials*, 31(11), 2005137.
[14] Islam, M. A., Talukder, L., Al, M. F., Sarker, S. K., Muyeen, S. M., Das, P., ... & Abhi, S. H. (2023). A review on self-healing featured soft robotics. *Frontiers in Robotics and AI*, 10, 1202584.
[15] Zhu, J., Lyu, L., Xu, Y., Liang, H., Zhang, X., Ding, H., & Wu, Z. (2021). Intelligent soft surgical robots for next-generation minimally invasive surgery. *Advanced Intelligent Systems*, 3(5), 2100011.
[16] Chandrashekhar, A., Himam Saheb, S., & Pavan Kishore, M. L. (2021). Investigation of the static and dynamic path planning of mobile and aerial robots. *Computer Networks and Inventive Communication Technologies: Proceedings of Third ICCNCT* 2020, 1033–1044.
[17] Qu, J., Li, Z., Fan, Q., Cui, H., & Liu, Y. (2024). *Introduction to Advanced Soft Robotics*. Bentham Science Publishers.
[18] Gariya, N., Kumar, S., Shaikh, A., Prasad, B., & Nautiyal, H. (2024). A Review on Soft Pneumatic Actuators with Integrated or Embedded Soft Sensors. *Sensors and Actuators A: Physical*, 372, 1 July 2024, 115364.
[19] Ambaye, G., Boldsaikhan, E., & Krishnan, K. (2024). Soft Robot Design, Manufacturing, and Operation Challenges: A Review. *Journal of Manufacturing and Materials Processing*, 8(2), 79.
[20] Gong, S., Lu, Y., Yin, J., Levin, A., & Cheng, W. (2024). Materials-driven soft wearable bioelectronics for connected healthcare. *Chemical Reviews*, 124(2), 455–553.
[21] Tan, Y. J., Susanto, G. J., Anwar Ali, H. P., & Tee, B. C. (2021). Progress and roadmap for intelligent self-healing materials in autonomous robotics. *Advanced Materials*, 33(19), 2002800.
[22] Farooq, A. S., & Zhang, P. (2022). A comprehensive review on the prospects of next-generation wearable electronics for individualized health monitoring, assistive robotics, and communication. *Sensors and Actuators A: Physical*, 344, 113715.
[23] Budati, T. & Khang, A. (2024). Detection of Drowsiness in Drivers Using TensorFlow Framework. In *Medical Robotics and AI-Assisted Diagnostics for a High-Tech Healthcare Industry* (pp. 123–143). IGI Global.

Chapter 9

Data-driven soft robotics

P Sree Lakshmi and P Rohini

9.1 INTRODUCTION TO SOFT ROBOTICS

The field of soft robotics is developing and rapidly evolving field within robotics that focuses on the creation of robots made from materials that are extremely malleable and flexible. These materials often replicate the physical properties of living organisms, which allow for safer and more adaptable interactions with complex environments and humans [1, 2]. Traditional rigid robots, although powerful and precise, often lack the flexibility and adaptability required for many real-world applications. In contrast, gentle robots are designed to be more resilient, versatile, and able to perform tasks that require a significant level of compliance and versatility.

The concept of soft robotics is inspired by the natural world, where many organisms exhibit extraordinary flexibility and adaptability. For example, octopuses, starfish, and worms can contort their bodies to move through tight spaces, grasp irregular objects, and perform complex movements with ease. This biological inspiration has led researchers to explore new materials and design principles that enable robots to achieve similar capabilities.

The development of soft robotics is driven by several key factors. First, the requirement for capable robots to safely interact with individuals from a variety of settings, such as healthcare, elder care, and domestic environments, has become increasingly important. Traditional rigid robots pose safety risks due to their hard surfaces and high levels of force, making them unsuitable for direct physical interaction with humans. Soft robots, on the other hand, can absorb impacts and conform to the shapes of objects and human bodies, reducing the risk of injury. Second, the versatility of soft robots allows them to execute activities that are challenging for inflexible robots. For instance, soft robots can handle delicate objects without causing damage, navigate through unstructured and dynamic environments, and adapt their shape and stiffness to different tasks. This makes them ideal for applications in domains that includes industrial automation, medical equipment, environmental monitoring, and exploration.

Soft robotics is a field that comprises a wide range of materials and fabrication techniques. Commonly used materials include elastomers, hydrogels,

DOI: 10.1201/9781003539612-9

and shape-memory alloys (SMAs). Elastomers, such as silicone rubber, are highly stretchable and can return to their original shape after deformation. Hydrogels, which are capable of absorbing large amounts of water, can shape-shift in reaction to environmental stimuli. Shape-memory metals, like nickel–titanium (NiTi) alloys, can revert to a predetermined shape when heated. Manufacturing methods for soft robots include molding, 3D printing, and soft lithography. Molding involves pouring elastomeric materials into molds to create specific shapes. 3D Complex structures can be created by printing layer by layer, enabling the integration of multiple materials and components. Soft lithography involves patterning soft materials at the micro- and nanoscale, allowing for the creation of detailed structures and devices.

A critical Integrating soft robotics is one of its aspects of data-driven approaches. Data-driven methodologies are vital in enhancing capabilities and performance of soft robots. By collecting data from sensors and using advanced modeling and simulation techniques, researchers can develop sophisticated control systems that enable soft robots to adapt and react to their surroundings in real-time.

Data collection in soft robotics involves the use of various sensors, including pressure sensors, stretch sensors, and temperature sensors. Pressure sensors measure the force and pressure distribution on the surface of the robot, providing feedback for tasks such as gripping and manipulation. Stretch sensors monitor the robot's structure and behavior, allowing for precise control of its shape and motion. Temperature sensors detect changes in environmental temperature and the robot's own temperature, which is particularly useful for applications involving thermal actuation.

Data-driven modeling and simulation methods, like machine learning models and finite-element analysis (FEA), are employed to forecast and control the behavior of soft robots. FEA allows researchers to simulate how soft materials deform under various forces, helping to improve the robot's design. Machine learning models can predict and control the behavior of soft robots by learning from large datasets collected from sensors and simulations. Control systems for soft robots can be divided into traditional and data-driven methods. Traditional methodologies like model predictive control (MPC) and proportional–integral–derivative (PID) control provide a foundation for managing the basic movements and functions of soft robots. Data-driven methods, such as reinforcement learning (RL) and neural networks, offer significant advantages by enabling soft robots that can adapt to new tasks, learn from experience, and handle complex and nonlinear dynamics.

The applications of data-driven soft robotics are vast and varied. In the medical field, soft robots can be used for minimally invasive surgery (MIS), rehabilitation devices, and assistive technologies for patients with mobility impairments. In industrial settings, soft robots can perform tasks such as delicate object handling, adaptive manufacturing, and automated inspection.

Environmental and exploration applications include search and rescue operations, underwater exploration, and monitoring of hazardous environments.

Despite the significant advancements in soft robotics, several challenges remain. Technical challenges include finding materials that combine flexibility with strength, integrating sensors without compromising the softness of the robot, and developing more efficient and adaptive control algorithms. Ethical and societal implications, such as ensuring the safety of human–robot interactions and developing appropriate regulations, also need to be addressed.

9.2 FUNDAMENTALS OF SOFT ROBOTICS

9.2.1 Materials used in soft robotics

The choice of materials is a critical factor in the development of soft robots, as these materials must have features that allow for flexibility, deformability, and resilience. The primary materials used in soft robotics include elastomers, hydrogels, and SMAs.

9.2.1.1 Elastomers

Elastomers, also referred to as viscoelasticity, are polymers that display both viscosity and flexibility [20]. These materials are highly stretchable and can revert to their original state when altered. Silicone rubber is a common elastomer due to its exceptional physical characteristics, it can be used in soft robotics, biocompatibility, and ease of molding [3, 4]. Other types of elastomers include polyurethane and natural rubber. The use of elastomers allows soft robots to perform tasks that require significant bending, stretching, and compressing, such as gripping delicate objects or navigating through narrow spaces. Silicone elastomers, in particular, are favored for their thermal stability, chemical resistance, and ability to form tight seals. They can be tailored to specific applications by adjusting their hardness, elasticity, and transparency. This versatility makes elastomers an ideal choice for creating soft robotic components that need to endure repeated cycles of deformation without losing their mechanical integrity. Figure 9.1 shows the structure of elastomer material used in soft robotics [27].

9.2.1.2 Hydrogels

Hydrogels are networks of polymer chains that can hold and absorb enormous amounts of water, making them soft and flexible. These materials can undergo significant volume changes in response to outside factors which includes pH, temperature, and light [5]. Hydrogels are used in soft robotics for applications that require shape-changing capabilities.

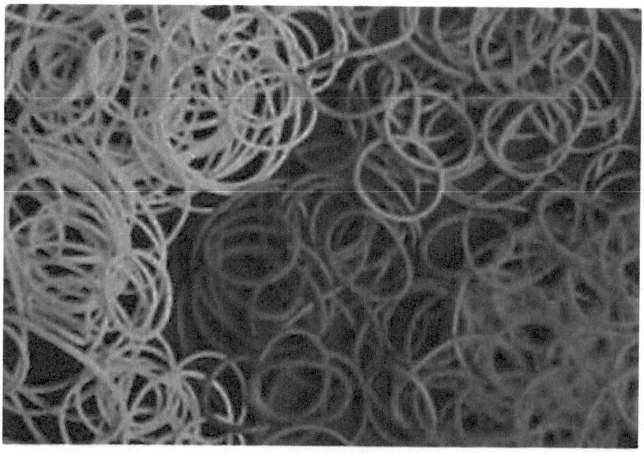

Figure 9.1 Elastomers.

For example, hydrogels can be engineered to alter their size in reaction to temperature changes, allowing for the creation of actuators that mimic muscle movements.

The biocompatibility of hydrogels makes them particularly useful in medical uses, including tissue engineering and medication delivery systems. Hydrogels can be designed to degrade in response to specific biological conditions, providing controlled release of therapeutic agents. In soft robotics, hydrogels are used to create soft actuators [19] and sensors that can operate in wet environments, such as inside the human body or underwater.

9.2.1.3 Shape-memory alloys (SMAs)

SMAs are materials that can revert back to a predetermined shape when heated above a certain temperature. NiTi alloys are the most frequently used SMAs in soft robotics. These materials are particularly useful for creating actuators that can produce significant movement with relatively small changes in temperature. SMAs exhibit unique features like super elasticity and the capacity to remember and revert to their original shape after deformation [6].

The application of SMAs in soft robotics involves embedding these materials into the structure of the robot, where they act as muscles or tendons. When an electrical current is applied, the SMA heats up and contracts, causing the soft robot to move. This property makes SMAs ideal for creating soft robots that require precise and controllable movements, such as robotic arms or surgical tools [28].

9.2.2 Design and fabrication techniques

A paradigm change in the domain of robotics is represented by soft robotics, which focuses on creating robots from incredibly flexible and pliable

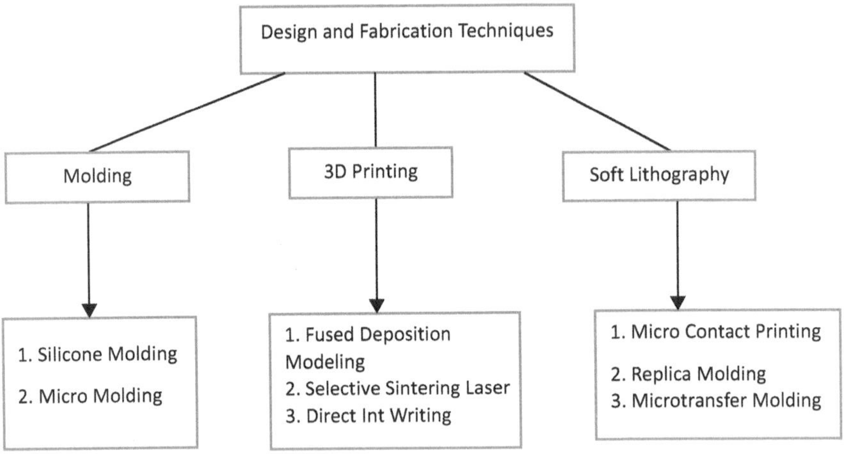

Figure 9.2 Design and fabrication techniques.

materials that resemble the mechanical properties of biological organisms [16]. Achieving these characteristics requires careful consideration of materials and precise control over fabrication techniques. This section explores the key methods employed in designing and fabricating soft robots: molding, 3D printing, and soft lithography. Figure 9.2 shows the different methods used in design and fabrication techniques.

9.2.2.1 Molding

Molding is a foundational technique in soft robotics, widely used due to its capacity for generating complex patterns and integrate functional components within soft structures. The procedure initiates with the development of a master mold, typically made from materials like silicone or epoxy, which serves as a template for producing multiple copies of the desired soft robotic component [4, 7].

9.2.2.2 Types of molding techniques

1. **Silicone Molding:** Silicone rubber is a preferred material for molding due to its elasticity, durability, and biocompatibility. The molding process involves preparing a liquid silicone elastomer mixed with a curing agent, which is then poured into the mold cavity. Curing can be achieved through heat, UV light, or chemical reactions, depending on the material requirements and desired properties of the final product.
2. **Micromolding:** For microscale soft robotic components, micromolding techniques are employed. These techniques utilize microstructured molds fabricated using photolithography or CNC micromachining.

Micromolding allows for the production of miniature soft robots with precise features, such as microactuators and microsensors, essential for applications in biomedicine and microfluidics.

9.2.2.3 Integration of functional elements

One of the significant advantages of molding in soft robotics is its ability to integrate sensors, actuators, and other functional elements directly into the structure of the robot. For instance, soft grippers designed for delicate object handling can incorporate embedded pneumatic channels for actuation and tactile sensors for feedback. This integration enhances the robot's ability to interact with its environment intelligently and perform complex tasks autonomously [8].

9.2.2.4 Applications

Molding techniques are applied across various soft robotic applications, including medical devices, wearable robotics, and soft manipulators for industrial automation. The ability to customize the mechanical properties and surface textures of soft robots through molding enables their deployment in diverse environments where interaction with humans or delicate objects is required.

9.2.3 3D printing

3D printing, or additive production, has revolutionized the fabrication of soft robots By allowing the creation of complex, customized geometries layer by layer [8, 9]. This technique offers unparalleled design flexibility, allowing researchers to incorporate multiple materials with varying stiffness and functionality within a single print.

9.2.3.1 Types of 3D-printing techniques

1. **Fused Deposition Modeling (FDM)**: FDM is commonly used for printing soft robots using thermoplastic elastomers. The process involves extruding molten material via a hot nozzle and onto a construction platform, where it solidifies layer by layer. FDM allows for the creation of large-scale soft robotic structures with relatively simple geometries.
2. **Selective Laser Sintering (SLS)**: In SLS, a laser is used to sintering materials that are powdered such as nylon or elastomers, into solid layers based on a 3D CAD model. This technique enables the fabrication of robust, high-resolution soft robotic components suitable for applications requiring mechanical strength and durability.
3. **Direct-Ink Writing (DIW)**: DIW is a precise 3D printing method that extrudes highly viscous materials, including hydrogels and conductive

using a tiny nozzle to apply inks to form complex structures with controlled rheological properties. DIW is ideal for printing soft actuators, sensors, and microfluidic devices with complex internal architectures.

9.2.3.2 *Multimaterial printing*

Advances in multimaterial 3D printing technologies have expanded the capabilities of soft robotics [18]. Researchers can now fabricate soft robots with hybrid structures incorporating both rigid and compliant materials. For example, a soft robotic hand can feature articulated fingers with embedded sensors and actuators tailored for dexterous manipulation tasks [6].

9.2.3.3 *Customization and prototyping*

The ability to rapidly prototype and customize soft robots through 3D printing accelerates innovation in the field. Design iterations can be quickly tested and refined, leading to the development of optimized robotic systems for specific applications in healthcare, agriculture, and beyond.

9.2.3.4 *Soft lithography*

Soft lithography encompasses a suite of techniques for patterning soft materials at micro- and nanoscales, essential for creating intricate features and functionalities in soft robots [10]. These techniques enable the fabrication of microfluidic channels, microvalves, and sensors critical for precise control and manipulation tasks.

9.2.3.5 *Techniques in soft lithography*

1. **Microcontact Printing:** Microcontact printing involves using a patterned elastomeric stamp to transfer molecules or materials onto a substrate with high precision. This technique is utilized in soft robotics to create microscale patterns for sensors and actuators integrated into the robot's structure.
2. **Replica Molding:** Replica molding uses a master mold to replicate microstructured surfaces onto soft substrates, enabling the mass production of soft robotic components with consistent microscale features. This technique is valuable for applications requiring uniformity and reproducibility in microfluidic devices and biomedical implants.
3. **Microtransfer Molding:** Microtransfer molding involves transferring predefined microstructured patterns from a mold onto a soft substrate using a stamping process. This technique is instrumental in fabricating soft robots with intricate geometries and functionalities, such as biomimetic structures and soft grippers for robotic manipulation tasks [13].

9.2.3.6 *Soft robotics applications*

Soft lithography techniques facilitate the development of miniaturized soft robots capable of performing tasks at small scales, such as micro assembly, drug delivery, and biomedical diagnostics [17, 21]. The integration of microfluidic channels and valves enables precise control over fluid flow and chemical reactions within soft robotic systems, expanding their utility in biotechnology and environmental monitoring.

9.3 THE ROLE OF DATA IN SOFT ROBOTICS

Data-driven approaches are fundamentally transforming the area of soft robotics through improved precision, adaptability, and overall capabilities of these robots. By leveraging vast amounts of data, researchers and engineers can develop more sophisticated models and control systems, enabling soft robots to perform complex tasks with high levels of efficiency and accuracy. This section delves into the critical role of data in soft robotics, focusing on data collection through sensors and the application of Data-driven simulation and modeling techniques.

9.3.1 Data collection and sensors

The integration of various sensors is essential for soft robots to interact effectively with their environment. These sensors provide real-time data that are essential for keeping an eye on and managing the robot's motions. and functions. The primary types of sensors used in soft robotics include stretch sensors, pressure sensors, and temperature sensors.

9.3.1.1 *Pressure sensors*

Pressure sensors are critical for measuring the force and pressure distribution [11] on the surface of a soft robot. These sensors are particularly important for applications that involve gripping or manipulating objects, as they provide feedback on the amount of force being applied. For instance, in a soft robotic gripper, pressure sensors can help ensure that delicate objects are handled with the appropriate amount of force to avoid damage. The data collected from pressure sensors can also be used to adjust the grip strength in real-time, enhancing the robot's ability to adapt to different objects and tasks.

Pressure sensors typically work by converting physical pressure into an electrical signal, which can then be analyzed by the robot's control system. Advanced pressure sensors can detect even slight variations in force, providing precise feedback that is crucial for delicate and nuanced tasks.

9.3.1.2 *Stretch sensors*

Stretch sensors monitor the deformation and movement of soft robotic components. These sensors are essential for understanding how the robot's structure changes in response to external forces and movements. By providing data on the extent and direction of deformation, stretch sensors enable more accurate control of the robot's shape and movements [12].

Stretch sensors are often made from conductive elastomers or other flexible materials that change their electrical properties in response to stretching. This change can be measured and translated into data that reflects the degree of deformation. This information is vital for applications where precise movement and flexibility are required, such as in medical devices or adaptive manufacturing processes.

9.3.1.3 *Temperature sensors*

Temperature sensors detect changes in environmental temperature and the robot's internal temperature [13]. These sensors are particularly useful in applications where thermal effects play a significant role, such as in SMAs used for actuation. SMAs rely on temperature changes to trigger movement, making temperature sensors critical for their control.

Temperature sensors can also help monitor the robot's thermal environment, ensuring that the materials and components do not overheat and become damaged. For example, in a soft robot used for underwater exploration, temperature sensors can provide data on the surrounding water temperature, which can affect the robot's performance and durability.

By integrating these sensors, soft robots can collect comprehensive data about their interactions with the environment. This data is then used to inform control systems and enable real-time adjustments, enhancing the robot's performance and adaptability.

9.3.2 Data-driven modeling and simulation

Data-driven modeling and simulation techniques are essential for interpreting and predicting the behavior of soft robots. These techniques allow researchers to create accurate models that can simulate how soft materials and structures respond to various forces and conditions [14]. Two primary methods used in this context are Machine learning and FEA learning models.

9.3.2.1 *Finite-element analysis (FEA)*

A type of computing called FEA is used to predict how materials and structures will deform under different forces and conditions. In FEA is used in soft robotics to model the properties of soft materials like hydrogels and elastomers, providing insights into their mechanical properties and performance.

FEA involves dividing the robot's partition into a limited quantity of little, discrete elements. Each element is analyzed separately to determine how it will respond to specific forces. By combining the results of these individual analyses, researchers can create a comprehensive model that predicts the overall behavior of the robot [15].

FEA is particularly useful for optimizing the design of soft robots. By simulating various scenarios and conditions, researchers can identify potential weaknesses and areas for improvement. This iterative process helps in developing more robust and efficient soft robots capable of challenging tasks with greater precision and reliability.

9.3.2.2 Machine learning models

Machine learning models leverage large datasets to anticipate and manage the behaviors of soft robots. These models can learn from data collected by sensors and simulations, identifying patterns and making predictions about the robot's performance. Examples of these types of machine learning techniques are RL and neural networks, are increasingly being used to enhance the control systems of soft robots.

Neural networks are one type of machine learning algorithm that may be trained to recognize complex patterns in data and forecast the behaviors and interactions of the robot. For example, a neural network can learn to predict how a soft robot will deform in response to different forces, allowing for more accurate and adaptive control.

RL is another powerful machine learning technique used in soft robotics. In RL, the robot learns to perform tasks through committing mistakes and receiving feedback in either the way of rewards or penalties. This approach allows soft robots to develop optimal strategies for performing specific tasks, such as navigating through complex environments or manipulating objects with varying shapes and sizes.

The combination of FEA and machine learning models provides a comprehensive approach to data-driven simulations and modeling in soft robotics. FEA offers detailed insights into the mechanical behavior of soft materials, while machine learning models provide adaptive and predictive capabilities that enhance the robot's control systems. Together, these techniques enable the development of more sophisticated and competent soft robots with the capacity to complete a variety of jobs with a high degree of precision and efficiency.

9.4 SOFT ROBOTICS CONTROL SYSTEMS

The control systems used in soft robotics are pivotal to their functionality, enabling these robots to perform complex tasks with precision and adaptability. Control systems in soft robotics can be broadly classified into traditional control methods and data-driven control methods. Each approach has its unique strengths and is employed according to the specific needs of the application.

9.4.1 Traditional control methods

Traditional control methods have been adapted from rigid robotics to meet the unique challenges posed by soft robotics. These methods establish a framework for the effective control of soft robots, ensuring stability and accuracy in their movements.

9.4.1.1 PID control: Proportional–integral–derivative

PID control is among the most popular control methods in both rigid and soft robotics [11]. Three distinct components make up this method: derivative, integral, and proportional controls, which work together to reduce the variation between the intended position and the actual position of the robot.

- **Proportional Control** (P): The portion of proportionate control responds to the current error, providing a correction that is proportional to the error magnitude. This rapidly lowers the inaccuracy but might not eliminate it entirely.
- **Holistic Control** (I): The holistic control component responds to the cumulative error over time, helping to clear any residual stable-state error that the proportional control alone cannot address.
- **Differential Control** (D): The differential control component reacts to the rate at which the error is changing, providing a damping effect that helps prevent overshoot and oscillations.

In soft robotics, PID control is adapted to account for the flexible and often nonlinear soft material behavior. For example, when controlling the deformation of a soft robotic arm, the PID controller must handle the continuous and complex changes in shape and resistance. To provide responsive and steady control, the PID parameters need to be carefully modified.

9.4.1.2 Model predictive control (MPC)

A more sophisticated control approach termed MPC makes use of a model of the robot's dynamics to forecast future states and maximize control actions [10]. The optimal set of control inputs for MPC entails solving an optimization problem at each control step to minimize a cost function over a future time horizon.

MPC is very suitable for soft robotics due to its ability to handle multi-variable control problems and constraints. It can predict the behavior of soft robots with complex dynamics and optimize their movements to achieve desired outcomes while respecting physical limitations.

For example, a flexible robotic grasp, MPC can be used to predict the deformation of the gripper's fingers as they interact with an object. By optimizing the control inputs, MPC ensures that the gripper applies the right amount of force to securely grasp the object without causing damage. This predictive capability is necessary for tasks that require high precision and adaptability, such as handling fragile items or performing delicate manipulations.

9.4.2 Data-based control techniques

Data-based control techniques represent a transformative approach in soft robotics, harnessing machine learning and artificial intelligence to develop adaptive and intelligent control strategies. These methods empower soft robots that use experiences to learn, optimize their performance, and autonomously adjust to dynamic environments and tasks.

9.4.2.1 Reinforcement learning (RL)

When agents interact with their environment and receive feedback in the form of rewards or penalties based on their behaviors, RL stands out as a potent machine learning model. In the realm of soft robotics, RL enables robots to autonomously explore and learn effective strategies to accomplish tasks through trial and error [15].

9.4.2.2 Mechanism and implementation

In RL-based control for soft robots, the robot is equipped with sensors that continuously monitor its state and the outcomes of its actions. For instance, a soft robotic gripper tasked with object manipulation would use tactile and proximity sensors to gather data about the object's shape, size, and position. The RL agent then explores various gripping strategies, learning which actions yield the best outcomes in terms of securely grasping and manipulating objects.

9.4.2.3 Learning and adaptation

Through iterative interactions with the environment, the soft robot refines its decision-making process. By optimizing the policy that dictates its actions based on cumulative rewards, the robot gradually improves its performance. For example, a soft robotic arm deployed in a manufacturing setting could learn to pick and place items more efficiently over time by adapting its movements to varying shapes and weights of objects.

9.4.2.4 Applications and advancements

RL holds promise across various applications in soft robotics, including autonomous navigation, object manipulation, and adaptive locomotion. For instance, in the development of soft robotic prosthetics, RL enables personalized learning of gait patterns and fine motor control tailored to individual users' needs and capabilities (Kober et al., 2013).

9.4.2.5 Neural networks

Neural networks are a cornerstone of artificial intelligence, capable of learning complex patterns and relationships from data. In the context of soft robotics, neural networks play a pivotal role in developing sophisticated control systems that can interpret sensory inputs and generate precise motor commands [14].

9.4.2.6 Architecture and functionality

A typical neural network comprises artificial neurons with interconnected layers that process input data and generate output signals. In soft robotics, these networks are trained using datasets that link sensory information—such as proprioceptive feedback from joint angles, tactile information from pressure sensors, or visual data from cameras—to desired robotic actions.

9.4.2.7 Training and optimization

Training neural networks involves presenting them with labeled datasets to learn the mapping between inputs and outputs. For instance, a neural network controlling a soft robotic gripper might be trained on a dataset of different object shapes and textures paired with optimal grasping forces and positions. Through iterative training, the network adjusts its internal parameters to improve accuracy and reduce prediction errors in controlling the gripper's movements.

9.4.2.8 Versatility and adaptability

Neural networks excel in tasks requiring real-time decision-making and adaptation to changing conditions. They can learn to handle uncertainties and variations in the environment, enabling soft robots to perform complex gentle robots to carry out complex maneuvers precisely and reliability. For example, in soft robotic exoskeletons used for rehabilitation, neural networks facilitate intuitive control of joint movements based on the user's intended actions and physiological responses [14].

9.5 ARCHITECTURES REPRESENTING DATA-DRIVEN SOFT ROBOTICS

Soft robotics, characterized by robots made from highly flexible and deformable materials, is increasingly leveraging data-driven approaches to enhance their capabilities across various applications. Data-driven architectures in soft robotics encompass several key frameworks and methodologies that integrate sensing, control, modeling, learning, adaptation, and deployment strategies. These architectures are crucial for optimizing robot performance, adapting to dynamic environments, and advancing the field towards more autonomous and intelligent systems. Figure 9.3 shows the different types of architectures representing data-driven soft robotics

9.5.1 Sensor-actuator architecture

The foundation of data-driven soft robotics lies in the integration of sensor-actuator architectures. Soft robots possess a variety of sensors that capture current data from their surroundings and internal states. These sensors include pressure sensors, stretch sensors, temperature sensors, and more, each providing critical information about the way the robot engages with its surroundings. The data collected from these sensors is processed and analyzed to inform decision-making processes within the robot's control system.

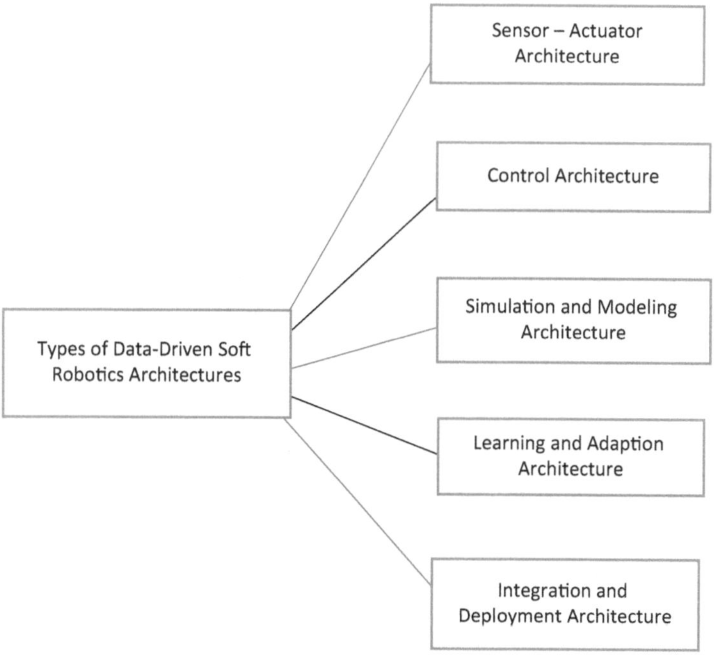

Figure 9.3 Types of data-driven soft robotics architectures.

The actuation mechanisms in soft robots are designed to respond to the data gathered by sensors. Actuators, which can be pneumatic, hydraulic, or based on SMAs, among others, translate control signals into physical movements and deformations. Data-driven sensor-actuator architectures enable soft robots to dynamically adjust their behavior based on sensory inputs, facilitating tasks such as adaptive grasping, locomotion on varied terrains, and interaction with delicate objects in industrial settings.

9.5.2 Control architecture

Control architectures in data-driven soft robotics encompass both traditional and advanced control methodologies. Conventional control techniques like MPC and PID control are adapted to suit the unique characteristics of soft materials and compliant structures. These methods rely on mathematical models that incorporate data inputs from sensors to regulate the robot's movements and interactions with its environment.

In data-driven control methods employ machine learning algorithms and RL techniques to optimize performance and adaptability. Machine learning models, trained on extensive datasets, enable soft robots to acquire knowledge from experience and improve their decision-making processes over time. RL algorithms allow robots to autonomously discover optimal behaviors through trial and error, enhancing their ability to navigate complex environments and perform tasks with greater efficiency.

9.5.3 Simulation and modeling architecture

Data-driven soft robotics heavily relies on accurate simulation and modeling architectures to predict and optimize robot behavior. FEA [22] is commonly used to simulate how soft materials deform under different forces and conditions. These simulations help in designing robots with optimal structural integrity and performance characteristics. Machine learning-based models, such as neural networks, are employed to predict complex interactions between the robot and its environment, enabling real-time adjustments and optimizations based on incoming data.

Moreover, data-driven modeling architectures facilitate the creation of digital twins—virtual replicas of physical robots that simulate their behavior under various scenarios. Digital twins are instrumental in testing and validating control strategies, refining algorithms, and predicting long-term performance without the need for extensive physical prototyping.

9.5.4 Adaptation and learning architecture

Adaptation and learning architectures empower soft robots to autonomously enhance their output and adjust to changing environments. Supervised and unsupervised learning algorithms analyze data collected from sensors to identify patterns, correlations, and anomalies. These algorithms enable robots to recognize objects, predict outcomes, and optimize their actions based on past experiences.

Furthermore, RL architectures enable soft robots to figure out the most effective behaviors through communication with the environment. By rewarding desirable actions and penalizing undesirable ones, RL algorithms facilitate adaptive learning and continuous improvement. Adaptive soft robots can adjust their strategies in real-time, making them appropriate for dynamic works such as exploration, rescue and search missions, collaborative interactions with humans.

9.5.5 Integration and deployment architecture

Integrating and deploying data-driven soft robotics involves designing robust architectures that encompass hardware, software, and data processing capabilities. Modular design principles are employed to facilitate the seamless integration of new sensors, actuators, and control algorithms into existing robotic systems. This modularity enhances flexibility, scalability, and interoperability, allowing soft robots to evolve with technological advancements and application requirements.

Moreover, deployment architectures ensure that data-driven soft robots operate effectively in diverse environments, from industrial production lines to unstructured outdoor settings. Real-time data processing capabilities enable robots to respond swiftly to environmental changes and unforeseen obstacles, optimizing efficiency and safety during operation.

9.6 APPLICATIONS OF DATA-DRIVEN SOFT ROBOTICS

Soft robotics, enhanced by data-driven approaches, has marked the beginning of a new versatility and adaptability in various fields. The underlying section explores the transformative applications of data-driven soft robotics across medical, industrial, and environmental domains, highlighting how these robots are revolutionizing traditional practices and expanding the scope of what is achievable.

9.6.1 Medical applications

Soft robotics holds tremendous promise in the field of medicine, where the ability to interact gently with biological tissues and adapt to complex anatomical structures is crucial.

9.6.1.1 Soft robotic exoskeletons

Among the most promising purposes for soft robotics in medicine is in the growth of soft robotic exoskeletons. These wearable devices can assist patients with mobility impairments by providing support and enhancing their ability to perform daily activities [12]. Unlike traditional exoskeletons, which are often rigid and cumbersome, soft robotic exoskeletons are made from flexible materials that mimic the natural movements of human muscles and joints.

Data-driven approaches perform a significant part in optimizing the design and control of flexible robotic exoskeletons. By collecting data from sensors embedded in the exoskeleton and analyzing the biomechanics of the wearer, researchers can tailor the exoskeleton's movements to suit individual needs. Machine learning algorithms can be employed to adapt the exoskeleton's assistance levels based on real-time feedback, ensuring optimal support and comfort for the user.

For instance, a soft robotic exoskeleton designed for patients with spinal cord injuries can adjust its gait assistance based on the wearer's walking patterns and muscle activity. This adaptive capability not only improves mobility but also promotes rehabilitation by encouraging natural movement patterns.

9.6.1.2 Minimally invasive surgery

Soft robots are also making significant strides regarding MIS, where precise and delicate maneuvers are required within confined spaces of the human body.

In MIS, soft robots equipped with miniature cameras and surgical instruments can navigate through complex anatomical structures with greater precision and minimal trauma to surrounding tissues [13]. These robots can perform intricate procedures such as biopsies, tumor removals, and even suturing with unprecedented dexterity and accuracy.

Data-driven control systems enable soft surgical robots to interpret real-time imaging data and adjust their movements accordingly. By integrating machine learning models, these robots can learn from past surgeries and optimize their surgical techniques for better patient outcomes. For example, a soft robotic surgical assistant can learn to identify and avoid critical structures based on preoperative imaging, reducing the risk of complications during surgery.

9.6.2 Industrial applications

In industrial settings, soft robotics is transforming manufacturing processes by offering new possibilities for automation and flexibility.

9.6.2.1 Soft grippers

Traditional rigid grippers used in manufacturing often struggle with handling delicate and irregularly shaped objects without causing damage [10].

Soft grippers, on the other hand, are designed from compliant materials that are able to take on the form of objects and exert gentle yet firm grasping forces.

Data-driven soft grippers are equipped with sensors that provide feedback on the texture, size, and shape of objects being manipulated. This sensory data allows the gripper to adjust its grasp in real-time, ensuring a secure hold without compromising the integrity of the object. Machine learning algorithms enable the gripper to adapt its gripping strategy based on the characteristics of different entities, reducing product damage and enhancing efficiency.

For example, in electronics assembly, soft grippers can delicately handle sensitive components such as microchips and circuit boards without causing deformation or breakage. By leveraging data-driven control methods, these grippers can optimize their grasp force and finger positions to accommodate variations in component sizes and shapes, improving manufacturing throughput and product quality.

9.6.2.2 *Adaptive manufacturing*

Soft robots are also revolutionizing adaptive manufacturing processes, where the potential for manipulation and assembling entities of varying sizes and shapes is essential [9].

In adaptive manufacturing, data-driven soft robots can autonomously reconfigure their movements and tooling to accommodate changes in production requirements. By analyzing real-time data from sensors and integrating predictive models, these robots can optimize their manufacturing processes for efficiency and precision. The application of machine learning strategies allows adaptive robots to get insights from production data and adjust their operations to minimize downtime and optimize resource utilization.

For instance, in automotive manufacturing, soft robotic arms equipped with vision systems can precisely assemble vehicle components with varying geometries. These robots can adapt their movements based on data collected from sensors that monitor part dimensions and alignment, ensuring accurate assembly and minimizing manufacturing errors.

9.6.3 Environmental and exploration applications

Beyond medicine and industry, data-driven soft robotics is opening up new frontiers in environmental monitoring, exploration, and disaster response.

9.6.3.1 *Search and recovery*

Soft robots are ideally suited for search and recovery operations in challenging and hazardous environments where conventional robots may struggle to navigate [7].

Equipped with sensors for detecting heat signatures, sounds, and structural weaknesses, data-driven soft robots can traverse rubble and debris to locate and rescue individuals trapped in collapsed buildings or disaster zones. These robots can autonomously analyze environmental data to identify optimal paths and strategies for reaching survivors quickly and safely.

Machine learning algorithms enable search and rescue robots to adapt their search patterns based on evolving environmental conditions and sensory inputs. For example, a soft robot deployed in a disaster scenario can learn to prioritize areas with the highest likelihood of survivor presence based on real-time data from seismic sensors and thermal imaging cameras.

9.6.3.2 Ocean exploration

Soft robots are also proving invaluable for exploring underwater environments where delicate ecosystems and marine life must be preserved [9].

Data-driven soft robotic vehicles can navigate through coral reefs and underwater caves with minimal disturbance, collecting scientific data and samples for marine biologists and environmental researchers. These robots are equipped with sensors that monitor water quality, temperature, and marine biodiversity, providing valuable insights into ecosystem health and climate change impacts.

Neural networks and machine learning models enable underwater soft robots to analyze complex sensory data and make autonomous decisions about navigation and data collection. For instance, a soft robotic fish inspired by biological locomotion can adjust its swimming patterns based on underwater currents and environmental conditions, maximizing energy efficiency and mission endurance.

9.7 CHALLENGES AND FUTURE DIRECTIONS

Soft robotics has grown into a more prominent area with transformative potential across various applications. However, like any burgeoning technology, it encounters multiple technical, ethical, and research difficulties that need to be addressed to unlock its full capabilities and ensure responsible deployment.

9.7.1 Technical challenges

Soft robots present unique technical challenges primarily related to materials [23] and sensor integration, crucial for their functionality and performance in diverse applications.

9.7.1.1 Material limitations

In soft robotics, a significant challenge is finding materials that strike a balance between flexibility and strength [6, 8]. Conventional inflexible robots are typically made from materials like hard plastics and metals, which provide structural integrity but lack the flexibility required for soft robots to imitate natural movements and engage in safe human interaction [18].

On the other hand, soft robots are fabricated from elastomers, hydrogels, and other soft materials that can deform and bend without losing functionality. However, these materials often struggle to maintain strength and durability over extended periods or under varying environmental conditions. For instance, while silicone rubber offers excellent stretchability, it may lack the robustness needed for rigorous applications like industrial manipulation or outdoor exploration [24].

Addressing this challenge requires advancements in material science and engineering. Researchers are exploring new composite materials and hybrid structures that combine the flexibility of soft materials with the strength of traditional rigid materials. For example, incorporating carbon nanotubes into elastomers can enhance their mechanical properties without compromising their softness, thereby expanding the operational capabilities of soft robots.

Moreover, additive manufacturing methods like 3D printing are enabling the fabrication of complex soft robotic structures with tailored material properties. By precisely controlling the composition and microstructure of materials, researchers can overcome existing limitations and pave the way for more resilient and versatile soft robots.

9.7.1.2 Sensor integration

Another critical challenge in soft robotics is the incorporation of sensors without compromising the softness and compliance of the robot's [13]. Sensors play a significant role in enabling soft robots to understand and respond to their surroundings, facilitating tasks such as navigation, object detection, and interaction with humans.

However, embedding sensors into soft materials poses critical challenges due to the material's deformable nature and the need to maintain sensor functionality under mechanical strain and environmental factors. Traditional sensors designed for rigid robots may not be suitable for soft robotics applications, as they can impede the robot's flexibility or become damaged during operation.

To overcome these challenges, researchers are developing innovative sensor technologies specifically tailored for soft robots. For example, stretchable and conformable sensors based on flexible electronics can seamlessly integrate into soft materials, allowing robots to detect pressure, strain, and temperature changes without sacrificing compliance.

Furthermore, advancements in wireless communication and various strategies for collecting energy enable robots to tackle autonomously while maintaining continuous sensor data transmission. This capability is especially advantageous in applications such as disaster response and environmental monitoring, where real-time data collection is critical for decision-making.

9.7.2 Ethical and societal implications

Beyond technical challenges, the deployment of soft robotics rises significant social and ethical issues that need to be properly considered in order to guarantee responsible and safe use.

9.7.2.1 *Safety concerns*

One of the key challenges ethical concerns surrounding soft robotics is ensuring the safety of human–robot interactions. Unlike rigid robots, which are typically confined to controlled environments, soft robots are intended for close human interaction [12] in everyday settings such as homes, hospitals, and public spaces.

Ensuring the safety of soft robots involves mitigating risks associated with physical contact, potential malfunction, and unintended interactions. For instance, soft robotic exoskeletons used in rehabilitation must be equipped with fail-safe mechanisms [26] and ergonomic designs to prevent injury to patients during assisted movements.

Moreover, advances in sensor technology and artificial intelligence make possible soft robots to perceive and react to human presence and gestures, enhancing their ability to operate safely in dynamic environments. Reducing risks and fostering confidence in soft robotics technologies need putting strong safety procedures into place and carrying out thorough risk analyses.

9.7.2.2 *Regulatory issues*

The rapid growth of soft robotics also necessitates the establishment of regulatory frameworks to govern their use and ensure compliance with safety standards across different applications. Regulatory agencies face the challenge of adapting existing guidelines, which are mainly intended for rigid robots, to accommodate the distinct characteristics and capabilities of soft robots.

Developing comprehensive regulatory frameworks involves collaboration between researchers, industry stakeholders, and policymakers to address potential risks and ethical concerns effectively. For example, regulatory guidelines may stipulate safety certifications for soft robotic devices used in medical procedures or set operational limits for autonomous soft robots deployed in public spaces.

Regulating authorities can encourage innovation while preserving public health and safety by establishing clear norms and standards, thereby fostering responsible adoption of soft robotics in diverse societal contexts [14].

9.7.3 Future research directions

Looking ahead, the future of soft robotics hinges on overcoming current challenges and advancing research in key areas such as materials science, control algorithms, and human–robot interaction.

9.7.3.1 Advanced materials

The growth of advanced materials is essential to enhancing the performance and versatility of soft robots in demanding applications. Future research efforts are focused on engineering materials with superior mechanical properties, such as enhanced elasticity, durability, and biocompatibility [5, 10].

For instance, bioinspired materials inspired by natural organisms, such as muscles and tendons, offer promising avenues for creating soft robots that can mimic complex movements and adapt to changing environments. Integrating nanomaterials and smart polymers into soft robotic systems enables dynamic responsiveness and self-healing capabilities, further expanding their operational lifespan and functionality [25].

9.7.3.2 Improved control algorithms

Advancements in control algorithms are essential for enabling soft robots to achieve greater autonomy, adaptability, and efficiency in performing tasks across various domains. Researchers are exploring novel approaches, including machine learning, RL, and adaptive control strategies [11, 15], to enhance the cognitive capabilities and decision-making abilities of soft robots.

Machine learning algorithms help robots to learn from experience and optimize their behaviors based on real-time data inputs. For example, RL techniques allow robots to autonomously adapt their actions in reaction to changing task needs or external circumstances, leading to more robust and adaptive performance in complex scenarios.

Moreover, integrating predictive modeling and simulation techniques into control algorithms enables soft robots to anticipate future states and proactively adjust their operations to achieve desired outcomes. These predictive capabilities are particularly valuable in applications such as predictive maintenance in industrial settings or real-time navigation in unpredictable environments.

9.7.3.3 Human–robot interaction

Enhancing the ways in which soft robots interact with humans [12] is another crucial research direction for advancing the field. Human–robot interaction encompasses aspects such as user interface design, intuitive control mechanisms, and social acceptance of robotic technologies in everyday life.

Designing soft robots with natural and intuitive interfaces promotes seamless collaboration between humans and robots, enabling users to interact with robots effectively and comfortably. For example, soft robotic prostheses equipped with intuitive control interfaces allow users to perform dexterous tasks with ease, enhancing their quality of life and independence.

Furthermore, incorporating principles from psychology and social sciences into robot design facilitates the development of robots with social awareness and empathy that can recognize, comprehend, and react to human intentions and feelings. These advancements promote trust and acceptance of soft robotics technologies in diverse societal contexts, from healthcare and rehabilitation to education and entertainment.

Finally, addressing the technical, moral, and research challenges outlined within this segment is essential for realizing the full potential of soft robotics and ensuring its responsible integration into society. By fostering interdisciplinary collaboration and innovation, researchers and stakeholders can drive forward the development of soft robots that are not only advanced in functionality but also safe, ethical, and socially beneficial.

9.8 CONCLUSION

Data-driven methodologies are spearheading a transformative era in soft robotics, facilitating the development of highly advanced and adaptable systems. Through the integration of state-of-the-art materials that offer superior flexibility and resilience, alongside cutting-edge sensor technologies for real-time data acquisition, soft robots are achieving unprecedented levels of functionality and performance. These innovations are not only enhancing the efficiency and precision of tasks traditionally performed by rigid robots but also opening up new frontiers in fields such as healthcare and industrial automation. With the aid of sophisticated algorithms rooted in machine learning and artificial intelligence, soft robots can autonomously learn and optimize their behaviors based on extensive datasets, thereby overcoming challenges and operating more effectively in dynamic and unpredictable environments. This synergy of materials, sensors, and algorithms promises to revolutionize various sectors by offering safer, more adaptable, and more responsive robotic solutions.

REFERENCES

[1] Kim, S., Laschi, C., & Trimmer, B. (2013). Soft robotics: A bioinspired evolution in robotics. *Trends in Biotechnology*, *31*(5), 287–294. https://doi.org/10.1016/j.tibtech.2013.03.002

[2] Rus, D., & Tolley, M. T. (2015). Design, fabrication and control of soft robots. *Nature*, *521*(7553), 467–475. https://doi.org/10.1038/nature14543

[3] Majidi, C. (2014). Soft robotics: A perspective—current trends and prospects for the future. *Soft Robotics*, *1*(1), 5–11. https://doi.org/10.1089/soro.2013.0001

[4] Ilievski, F., Mazzeo, A. D., Shepherd, R. F., Chen, X., & Whitesides, G. M. (2011). Soft robotics for chemists. *Angewandte Chemie International Edition*, *50*(8), 1890–1895. https://doi.org/10.1002/anie.201006464

[5] Whitesides, G. M. (2018). Soft robotics. *Angewandte Chemie International Edition*, *57*(16), 4258–4273. https://doi.org/10.1002/anie.201800907

[6] Truby, R. L., & Lewis, J. A. (2016). Printing soft matter in three dimensions. *Nature*, *540*(7633), 371–378. https://doi.org/10.1038/nature21003
[7] Gong, Z., Wang, T., Zhang, C., Qian, L., Su, H., & Tolley, M. T. (2021). An origami-inspired electromechanical soft robot for locomotion and object manipulation. *Soft Robotics*, *8*(1), 25–36. https://doi.org/10.1089/soro.2019.0133
[8] Laschi, C., Cianchetti, M., Mazzolai, B., Margheri, L., Follador, M., & Dario, P. (2012). Soft robot arm inspired by the octopus. *Advanced Robotics*, *26*(7), 709–727. https://doi.org/10.1163/156855312X626343
[9] Katzschmann, R. K., DelPreto, J., MacCurdy, R., & Rus, D. (2018). Exploration of underwater life with an acoustically controlled soft robotic fish. *Science Robotics*, *3*(16), eaar3449. https://doi.org/10.1126/scirobotics.aar3449
[10] Yang, Y., Chen, B., Wang, Q., Allen, S., Wu, X., Li, G., & Zhao, J. (2020). Bioinspired robotic fingers based on pneumatic actuator and 3D printing of smart material with self-healing and sensing capabilities. *Scientific Reports*, *10*(1), 1–11. https://doi.org/10.1038/s41598-020-60355-9
[11] Marchese, A. D., Katzschmann, R. K., & Rus, D. (2015). A recipe for soft fluidic elastomer robots. *Soft Robotics*, *2*(1), 7–25. https://doi.org/10.1089/soro.2014.0022
[12] Hughes, J., Culha, U., Giardina, F., Guenther, F., Rosendo, A., & Iida, F. (2016). Soft manipulators and grippers: A review. *Frontiers in Robotics and AI*, *3*, 69. https://doi.org/10.3389/frobt.2016.00069
[13] Polygerinos, P., Correll, N., Morin, S. A., Mosadegh, B., Onal, C. D., Petersen, K., ... & Walsh, C. J. (2017). Soft robotics: Review of fluid-driven intrinsically soft devices; manufacturing, sensing, control, and applications in human-robot interaction. *Advanced Engineering Materials*, *19*(12), 1700016. https://doi.org/10.1002/adem.201700016
[14] Liu, Y., Sun, L., Xu, W., Gu, G., & Liu, H. (2020). Design and control of a soft robotic glove for hand rehabilitation. *IEEE Robotics and Automation Letters*, *5*(3), 2613–2620. https://doi.org/10.1109/LRA.2020.2976825
[15] Rich, S. I., Wood, R. J., & Majidi, C. (2018). Untethered soft robotics. *Nature Electronics*, *1*(2), 102–112. https://doi.org/10.1038/s41928-018-0024-1
[16] Marchese, A. D., Rus, D., & Palagi, S. (2016). Designing soft robots: A review. *Smart Materials and Structures*, *25*(9), 093001. https://doi.org/10.1088/0964–1726/25/9/093001
[17] Cianchetti, M., Laschi, C., Mazzolai, B., & Dario, P. (2018). Biomedical applications of soft robotics. *Nature Reviews Materials*, *3*(6), 143–153. https://doi.org/10.1038/s41578-018-0015-0
[18] Shepherd, R. F., Ilievski, F., Choi, W., Morin, S. A., Stokes, A. A., Mazzeo, A. D., ... & Whitesides, G. M. (2011). Multigait soft robot. *Proceedings of the National Academy of Sciences*, *108*(51), 20400–20403. https://doi.org/10.1073/pnas.1116564108
[19] Conn, A. T., Rossiter, J., & Walters, P. (2020). A review of soft actuator and sensor materials for soft robotics. *Soft Robotics*, *7*(4), 371–391. https://doi.org/10.1089/soro.2019.0136
[20] Martinez, R. V., Branch, J. L., Fish, C. R., Jin, L., Shepherd, R. F., Nunes, R. M., ... & Whitesides, G. M. (2013). Robotic tentacles with three-dimensional mobility based on flexible elastomers. *Advanced Materials*, *25*(2), 205–212. https://doi.org/10.1002/adma.201203102

[21] Yuan, W., Dong, X., Yang, H., Pan, S., Yang, C., Zhang, D., & Zhang, H. (2021). Soft robotics: Definitions, trends, and challenges in the construction of biomimetic machines. *Advanced Science*, *8*(8), 2004718. https://doi.org/10.1002/advs.202004718
[22] Thuruthel, T. G., Shintake, J., Maeda, S., & Floreano, D. (2019). Soft robotics: Academic insights and perspectives through bibliometric analysis. *Soft Robotics*, *6*(3), 272–289. https://doi.org/10.1089/soro.2018.0130
[23] Calisti, M., & Laschi, C. (2019). Bioinspired soft robotics: Material selection, actuation, and applications. *Innovative Superconductivity and Cryogenics*, *1*(1), 1–14. https://doi.org/10.1016/j.iscryd.2019.100003
[24] Tolley, M. T., Shepherd, R. F., Mosadegh, B., Galloway, K. C., Wehner, M., Karpelson, M., ... & Wood, R. J. (2014). A resilient, untethered soft robot. *Soft Robotics*, *1*(3), 213–223. https://doi.org/10.1089/soro.2014.0008
[25] Hines, L., Petersen, K., Lum, G. Z., & Sitti, M. (2017). Soft actuators for small-scale robotics. *Advanced Materials*, *29*(13), 1603483. https://doi.org/10.1002/adma.201603483
[26] Kober, J., Bagnell, J., & Peters, J. (2013). Reinforcement learning in robotics: A survey. *The International Journal of Robotics Research*, 32, 1238–1274. https://doi.org/10.1177/0278364913495721
[27] https://www.nature.com/articles/s41467-022-28015-2
[28] https://www.azom.com/article.aspx?ArticleID=17396

Chapter 10

Machine learning in soft robotics

Techniques and applications

Shaik Himam Saheb

10.1 INTRODUCTION

Soft robotics is a subfield of robotics that deals with robots constructed using compliant materials, often inspired by biological systems like octopus arms or elephant trunks. Unlike traditional rigid robots, soft robots can deform and adapt to their environment, making them suitable for tasks requiring delicate manipulation or interaction with humans [1]. Robotics has been a rapidly evolving field, driven by advancements in various domains, including materials science, control systems, and most notably machine learning (ML) [2]. The integration of ML techniques into soft robotics has opened up new possibilities, revolutionizing the way these systems are designed, controlled, and adapted to their environments [3, 4].

One of the key advantages of employing ML in soft robotics is the ability to handle the inherent complexity and uncertainty associated with these systems [5]. Soft robotic systems often operate in unstructured environments, where traditional control methods may struggle to adapt [6]. ML, on the other hand, allows for the development of more robust and adaptive control algorithms that can learn from data and continuously improve their performance [7]. Reinforcement learning, for instance, has been successfully applied to soft robotic control, where the robot learns an optimal policy through trial-and-error interactions with its environment [8, 9]. This approach is particularly well-suited for soft robotics, as it can handle the highly nonlinear and dynamic nature of these systems. Additionally, techniques like transfer learning and active learning can further enhance the learning capabilities of soft robotic systems, enabling them to adapt to new tasks and environments more efficiently [10].

ML, with its ability to model complex and nonlinear relationships, has proven to be a valuable tool in addressing the unique challenges posed by soft robotic systems, particularly in the domains of sensing and control [11]. Data-driven methods, such as supervised and reinforcement learning, have been successfully applied to soft robotic systems, enabling the encoding of dynamic behavior and the handling of hysteresis and nonstationary phenomena that can be challenging to model analytically [12].

DOI: 10.1201/9781003539612-10

The high structural compliance and maneuverability of soft robots, coupled with advances in manufacturing and the development of new actuators and functional materials, have further fueled the integration of ML techniques [13]. Figure 10.1 describes the human hand mimicking developed by TU/e soft robotics lab. This human hand is helpful for handicapped persons. These learning algorithms such as KNN, ANN, CNN, and RNN were applied for the signal processing of individual soft sensors, soft tactile array sensors, and soft stretch sensors [14]. Researchers have been exploring unconventional materials for robotic systems, focusing on soft materials like polymers for innovative sensory devices and actuators [15, 16].

The newly developed smart materials, sensors, and actuators were subsequently integrated into various types of soft micro-robots [17]. Additionally, the flexible body structures of animals were replicated in reconfigurable robots [18, 19].

Zhong and other researchers [21, 22] provide insights into the applications of ML in environmental science and engineering. While the study does not explicitly focus on soft robotics, the findings emphasize the growing importance of ML tools in addressing environmental challenges. The integration of soft robotics with ML in environmental monitoring and remediation represents a potential research area that warrants further exploration [23].

Raschka and others [24, 25] discuss the main developments and technology trends in data science, ML, and artificial intelligence (AI). The authors provide a comprehensive overview of the advancements in ML and data

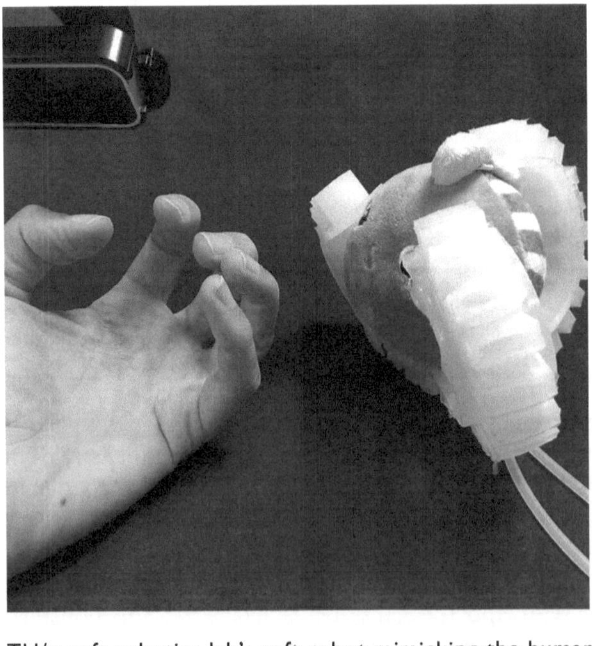

Figure 10.1 TU/e soft robotics lab's soft robot mimicking the human hand [20].

science, highlighting the increasing relevance of these fields in various domains [26]. Although the study does not specifically address soft robotics, it underscores the need to examine the intersection of ML and data science with soft robotics to unlock new opportunities and applications. Sarker [27] presented an overview of cybersecurity data science from an ML perspective. While the study does not directly focus on soft robotics, it underscores the critical role of ML in cybersecurity applications. This insight suggests the potential for leveraging ML techniques to enhance the security and robustness of soft robotic systems, thereby opening avenues for interdisciplinary research at the intersection of soft robotics, ML, and cybersecurity.

The integration of soft robotics with ML and data science presents a promising avenue for advancing the capabilities and applicability of soft robotic systems. By addressing the identified knowledge gaps and pursuing the suggested research directions, scholars and practitioners can unlock new opportunities and contribute to the advancement of this interdisciplinary field.

10.2 MACHINE LEARNING

ML is a subset of AI that involves the development of algorithms and statistical models that enable computers to learn from and make decisions based on data. Instead of being explicitly programmed to perform a specific task, ML systems use patterns and inference to perform tasks and improve their performance over time with experience. ML has emerged as an indispensable tool across various domains, revolutionizing how data-driven decisions are made and automation is achieved. This chapter explores why ML has become essential in contemporary applications, highlighting its transformative impact on industries, technology, and everyday life.

ML relies on large amounts of data, which can include numbers, images, text, or any other type of information. In today's interconnected world, the volume and complexity of data exceed human capacity to analyze and derive insights manually. ML algorithms offer a scalable solution to extract meaningful patterns, trends, and predictions from large datasets, driving informed decision-making and innovation. Various algorithms are used to process and analyze the data. Common types of ML algorithms include supervised learning, unsupervised learning, semi-supervised learning, and reinforcement learning. The ML model is trained using a portion of the data. During training, the algorithm adjusts its parameters to minimize errors and improve accuracy.

Evaluation and Testing is done after training, the model is evaluated and tested with new data to assess its performance and accuracy. Once trained and tested the data to the model can make predictions or decisions based on new, unseen data. Many ML systems are designed to continue learning and improving over time as they are exposed to more data. ML is used in a wide

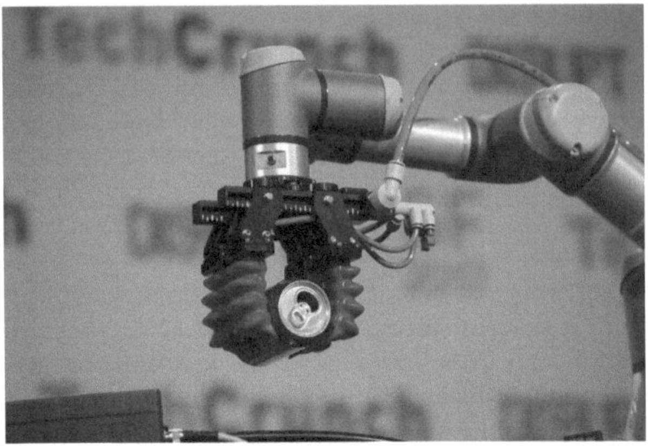

Figure 10.2 Soft robotic arm holding and lifting the Coke can.

range of applications, including image and speech recognition, natural language processing, recommendation systems, autonomous vehicles, soft robots and many other applications. These training and testing of data is useful to the robots to identify the type of object lifting and to hold the object properly to avoid damage to the object. Figure 10.2 demonstrates the serial robotic arm that holds and lifts the Coke can without spillover. The robot takes the decision based on the training the force is applied and this force is sufficient to hold the object and operate as per the requirement.

10.3 NECESSITY OF MACHINE LEARNING

ML algorithms process vast amounts of data to uncover hidden patterns and correlations, enabling businesses to make data-driven decisions with accuracy and speed, as data don't have proper insights the information and knowledge is assimilated from the data and its interpretation. With automation of repetitive tasks and optimizing processes, ML enhances efficiency, reduces operational costs, and improves overall productivity. Personalization and User Experience is improved with ML, which powers personalized recommendations, targeted marketing campaigns, and tailored user experiences, enhancing customer satisfaction and loyalty. ML tackles complex problems that are difficult to address using traditional algorithms, such as image recognition, natural language processing, and autonomous decision-making.

ML aids in medical industries in disease diagnosis, personalized medicine, drug discovery, and healthcare management systems, improving patient outcomes and operational efficiency. ML algorithms analyze financial data for fraud detection, risk assessment, algorithmic trading, and personalized financial advice, ensuring security and optimizing investments. ML powers autonomous vehicles, traffic management systems, predictive maintenance for fleets, and route optimization, transforming urban mobility and logistics. Even having these many advantages, the ML needs to ensure the integrity, quality, and privacy of data used in ML models to maintain trust and compliance with regulatory standards.

10.3.1 Unsupervised method

Unsupervised classification occurs when the training data is neither labeled nor classified. The primary goal of an unsupervised algorithm is to explore how a system can infer patterns and define the underlying structure from unlabeled data. In other words, you don't need to supervise the model. Instead, the model independently identifies and learns from the information.

10.3.2 Supervised method

Unsupervised classification occurs when the training data is neither labeled nor classified. The primary goal of an unsupervised algorithm is to explore how a system can infer patterns and define the underlying structure from unlabeled data. In other words, you don't need to supervise the model. Instead, the model independently identifies and learns from the information.

10.3.3 Semi-supervised method

The term "semi" in semi-supervised algorithms indicates that they fall between supervised and unsupervised algorithms. In this approach, both labeled (known) and unlabeled (unknown) data are used during the training process. Typically, a large amount of unlabeled data is combined with a smaller amount of labeled data. This method is often more accurate than purely supervised or unsupervised algorithms. Semi-supervised algorithms are particularly effective when acquiring labeled data requires significant expertise and resources, while obtaining unlabeled data is much less resource-intensive.

10.3.4 Reinforcement method

In this algorithm, the learning process involves taking actions and identifying errors through interactions with the surrounding environment. The main characteristic of a reinforcement algorithm is its trial-and-error search. To function effectively, it enables software agents and machines to autonomously choose the optimal behavior within a given context. For an agent to learn quickly, it must receive simple reward feedback for its actions. This feedback is known as the reinforcement signal.

ML is a leading trend because it enables the analysis of large volumes of data. Different ML techniques are shown in Figure 10.3. However,

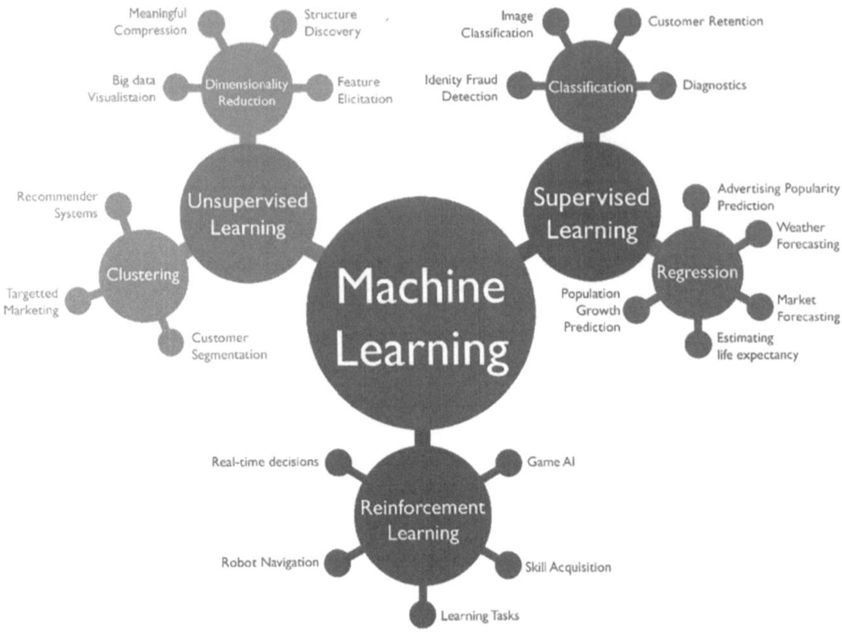

Figure 10.3 Machine learning types and its applications [28].

to achieve effective and fast results, it requires substantial time and resources. While it is highly effective on its own, integrating ML with cognitive technology and AI can streamline and enhance the overall process [29].

10.4 SOFT ROBOTICS

Soft robotics is a specialized field within robotics that focuses on designing and developing robots constructed from highly compliant materials, such as silicone, rubber, fabric, or flexible plastics. Soft robots are a subset of robotics that are characterized by their flexible and compliant structures, designed to mimic the properties of biological systems. Soft robotics have various advantages and disadvantages those are shown in Figure 10.4. These robots are fundamentally different from traditional rigid robots in that they emphasize flexibility, adaptability, and deformability, akin to natural organisms [30]. Flexibility and Deformability is a major advantage with soft robots which can change shape and deform to navigate through complex environments or manipulate delicate objects without causing damage. Their soft and compliant nature makes them inherently safer to interact with humans and delicate surroundings compared to rigid robots, reducing the risk of injury or damage [31].

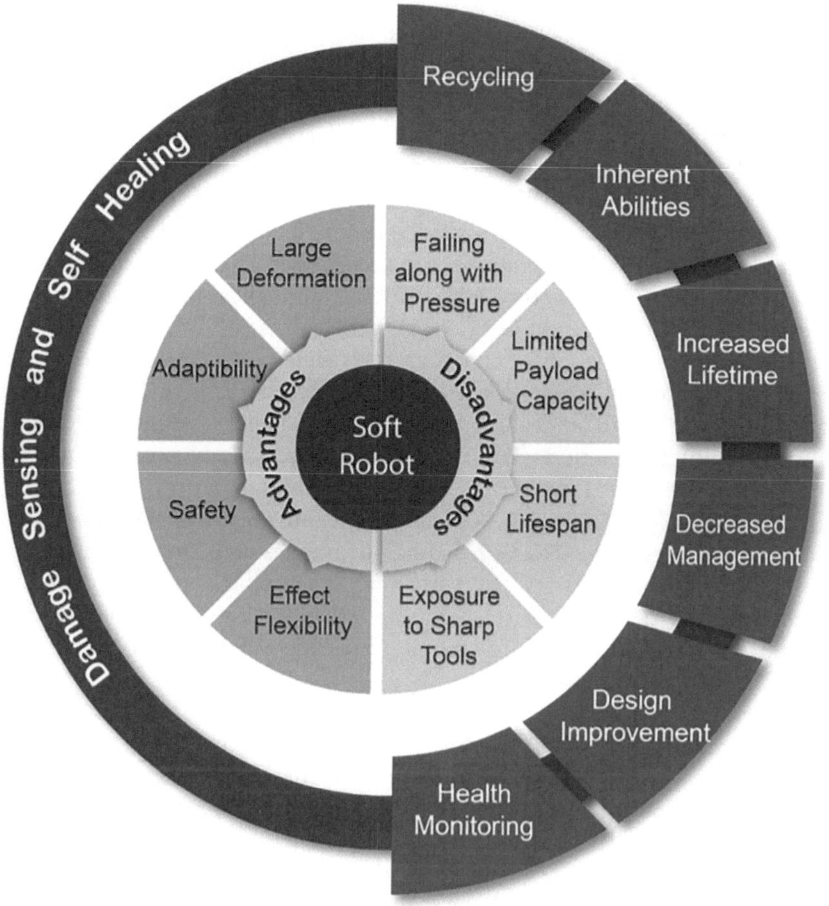

Figure 10.4 Soft robots' advantages and disadvantages [32].

Soft robots can perform a wide range of tasks that are challenging for traditional robots, such as gripping irregularly shaped objects, squeezing through tight spaces, or conforming to various surfaces. Many soft robotic designs draw inspiration from biological systems, such as muscles, tentacles, or octopus arms, to mimic natural movements and functionalities. Soft robots are used in minimally invasive surgeries, rehabilitation therapies, prosthetics, and assistive devices due to their gentle interaction with human tissues.

They are deployed in disaster scenarios to navigate through rubble or confined spaces where rigid robots cannot access, aiding in search and rescue operations. Soft robots assist in tasks like harvesting delicate fruits, monitoring crops, and performing precision agriculture tasks in variable environments. They are utilized in underwater exploration, surveillance missions, and space exploration due to their ability to withstand harsh conditions and navigate complex terrains.

Soft robots are made from materials such as silicone, rubber, and other elastomers [33], which allow them to bend, stretch, and twist. This flexibility enables them to navigate through complex environments and interact safely with humans and delicate objects. Due to their soft and deformable nature, soft robots can adapt to a wide range of shapes and surfaces. This adaptability makes them suitable for applications in search and rescue, where they can maneuver through rubble, or in medical procedures, where they can conform to the shape of organs and tissues.

Soft robots are inherently safer than their rigid counterparts when interacting with humans. Their soft materials reduce the risk of injury during collisions, making them ideal for use in collaborative environments, such as human–robot interaction (HRI) and healthcare. Many soft robots are inspired by biological organisms, such as octopuses, worms, and human muscles. This biomimicry allows them to replicate the movements and functionalities of these organisms, providing advantages in locomotion, manipulation, and sensing. robots often use unconventional actuation methods, such as pneumatic (air pressure), hydraulic (fluid pressure), or shape-memory alloys. These actuators require complex control systems to achieve precise movements and responses.

Soft robots can integrate various sensors within their structures, such as pressure, strain, and tactile sensors. These sensors allow the robots to perceive and respond to their environment in a manner similar to biological systems. The materials used in soft robots are typically lightweight, which can be advantageous for applications requiring mobility and dexterity. This lightweight nature also contributes to their energy efficiency. Soft robotic systems can be designed at various scales, from micro-scale robots for minimally invasive surgery to larger robots for industrial and environmental applications [34]. Soft robots can be manufactured using techniques like 3D printing, casting, and molding. These methods allow for rapid prototyping and customization, making it easier to develop robots tailored to specific tasks. There are different types of rapid prototyping techniques are useful for variety of applications. The material of rapid prototyping decides the outcome for example the metal 3D-printing prints high-strength metal parts compared to FDM [35] printer where the plastic components are printed. Figure 10.5 depicts the various 3D-printing materials used for soft robotics applications.

Despite their advantages, soft robots face challenges such as limited force generation, complex control algorithms, and durability issues under repeated use or extreme conditions. Soft robots are a rapidly evolving field with the potential to revolutionize many industries by providing safe, adaptable, and efficient solutions to complex problems.

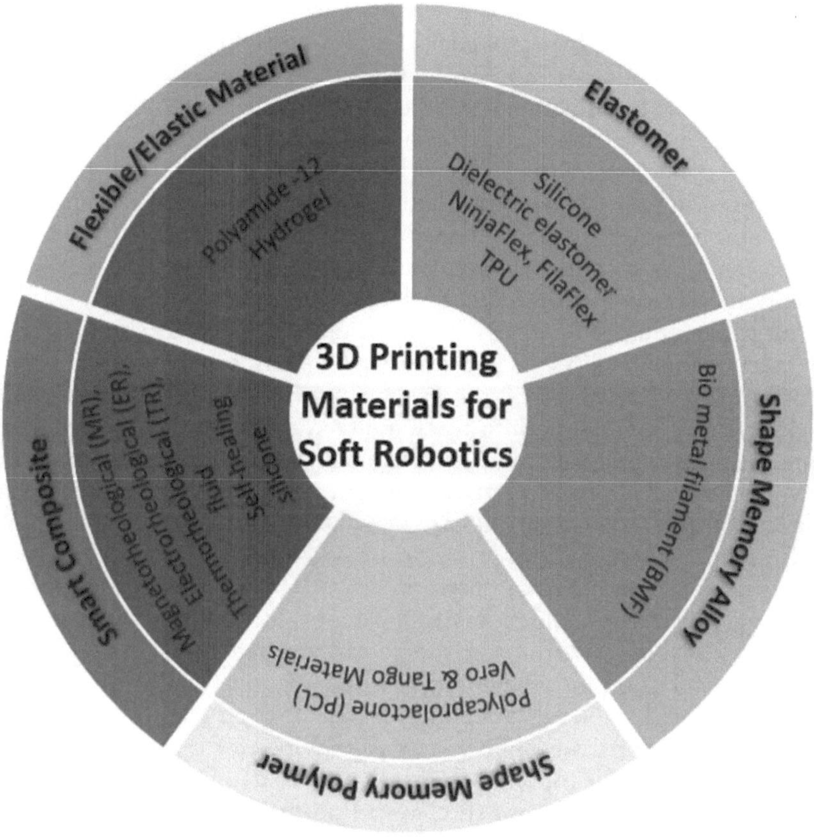

Figure 10.5 Different materials used for soft robotics.

10.5 COLLABORATION OF SOFT ROBOTICS WITH MACHINE LEARNING

The collaboration of soft robotics with ML represents a significant advancement that enhances the capabilities and functionalities of soft robotic systems.

ML algorithms can analyze sensory data from soft robotic sensors (such as pressure sensors and stretch sensors) to interpret the robot's interaction with its environment. This enables the robot to understand and respond to external stimuli more effectively. ML can be used to train soft robots to recognize and classify objects they encounter, allowing them to adapt their behaviors based on the objects' properties. ML enables soft robots to adapt their movements and behaviors based on feedback from the environment. This adaptive control helps them navigate complex terrains, manipulate objects more precisely, and perform tasks with greater efficiency.

Soft robots can utilize reinforcement learning algorithms to learn optimal strategies for achieving specific goals. For example, they can learn to grasp objects of varying shapes and sizes using different gripping techniques based on trial-and-error interactions. ML models can predict potential failures or degradation in soft robotic components based on historical data and environmental conditions. This capability helps in scheduling proactive maintenance, reducing downtime, and extending the lifespan of the robots. ML algorithms optimize the performance of soft robotic systems by adjusting parameters such as actuator movements, control strategies, and energy consumption based on real-time data feedback.

Soft robots equipped with ML can autonomously navigate complex environments, avoiding obstacles and adapting their paths in real-time based on sensor inputs. ML enables soft robots to make decisions autonomously, such as determining the best path to reach a target, adjusting their behaviors in response to changing conditions, or deciding when to initiate specific tasks.

ML-enhanced soft robots can assist in minimally invasive surgeries, rehabilitation therapies, and patient care by adapting to the patient's anatomy and responding dynamically to surgical environments. In agriculture, soft robots equipped with ML can perform delicate tasks such as fruit picking, handling fragile crops, and monitoring plant health based on real-time sensor data [36]. ML-powered soft robots can navigate disaster sites, locate survivors, and assist in rescue operations by adapting their movements to navigate through debris and confined spaces. The integration of ML with soft robotics continues to unlock new possibilities for creating intelligent, adaptive, and versatile robotic systems. As both fields advance, collaborative research and innovation are expected to lead to further breakthroughs in robotics applications across various industries and domains.

10.6 NOTABLE EXAMPLES OF SOFT ROBOTICS

Octobot [37]: Developed by researchers at Harvard University, Octobot is a completely soft robot inspired by octopuses which is shown in Figure 10.6. It is powered by a microfluidic soft circuit that controls its movements.

The Octobot is the first completely autonomous soft robot, manufactured with the combination of embedded 3D printing, modeling, and soft lithography. Inspired by actual octopuses, the Octobot is composed entirely of flexible parts. Its fuel flow is regulated by a microfluidic logic circuit, which is fueled by a chemical reaction. This logic circuit controls the fuel flow on its own, much like a circuit board. Soft robots of a new generation are made possible by the Octobot. Companies like Soft Robotics Inc. have developed soft grippers that can handle a variety of objects with different shapes, sizes, and textures. These grippers are used in industries such as food processing and packaging.

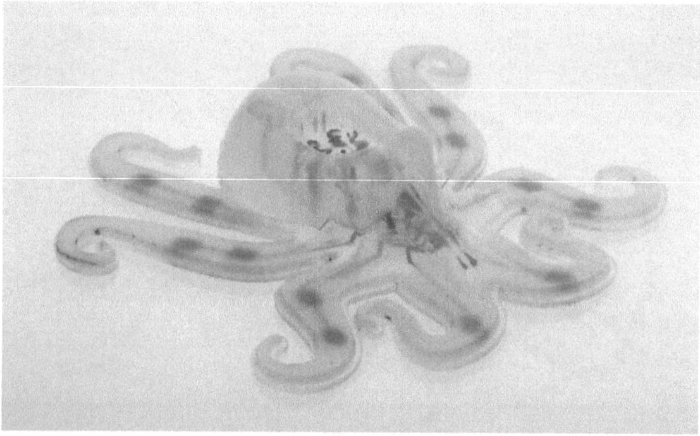

Figure 10.6 Octopus autonomous soft robot.

RoboBee [38]: is developed at Harvard, RoboBee is a small, insect-inspired robot with flexible wings. It is designed for tasks such as environmental monitoring and crop pollination. Researchers at the Wyss Institute are creating artificial systems called RoboBees, which are inspired by the biology of bees and have the potential to play a wide range of functions in agriculture and disaster assistance. A RoboBee is roughly half the size of a paper clip, weighs less than tenth of an ounce, and uses materials for its "artificial muscles"—which contract when electricity is applied—to fly. Certain RoboBee versions can now fly and swim underwater, as well as "perch" on surfaces by using static electricity thanks to additional improvements.

Developing autonomous micro-aerial vehicles that can fly alone and in large groups, as well as exhibit coordinated behavior, was the driving force behind the creation of the RoboBee. Consequently, the Body, Brain, and Colony constitute the three primary components of the RoboBee evolution. The Versatile Crawling Microrobot is bio mimic robot developed by RoboBee as shown in Figure 10.7 [39]. Building autonomous robotic insects with the aid of a small, seamlessly integrated power source is the goal of body development; creating "smart" sensors and control electronics that resemble a bee's eyes and antennae and are capable of sensing and reacting to their surroundings dynamically is the goal of brain development; and coordinating the actions of numerous independent robots to function as a cohesive unit is the main goal of the colony.

Soft Exosuits also autonomous soft robots developed by teams, one at Harvard's Wyss Institute, soft exosuits are wearable robots that assist with human movement [40]. They are designed to help people with mobility impairments or to enhance the performance of soldiers and athletes.

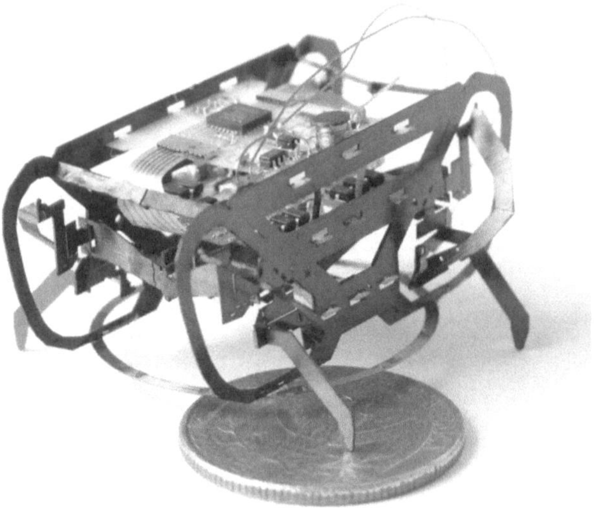

Figure 10.7 HAMR: versatile crawling microrobot.

Pneumatic Network (PneuNet) Actuators are a type of soft actuator that uses air pressure to create movement. They are used in various soft robotic applications, including grippers and manipulators [41]. Soft Robotic Fish Developed by MIT, this robot mimics the movements of a real fish using flexible silicone. It is used for underwater exploration and research [42]. Vincent Systems' Soft Robotic Prosthetic Hand is prosthetic hand uses soft robotics technology to provide a more natural and flexible range of motion for amputees [43]. Robot Sleeve is developed by CSAIL at MIT, this soft robotic sleeve can be placed around a heart to help it beat, potentially providing a new treatment option for heart failure patients [44].

Soft Caterpillar Robot [45] Developed by researchers at Seoul National University, this robot mimics the movements of a caterpillar and can navigate through narrow and complex environments. These examples highlight the versatility and potential of soft robotics across various fields, including medical, industrial, and environmental applications.

Soft Robotics Toolkit developed at Harvard University is an open-source platform that combines ML with soft robotics to provide tools and resources for designing, fabricating, modeling, and controlling soft robots [46]. Researchers use ML algorithms to optimize the design and functionality of these robots. Self-healing Soft Robots are developed by researchers at the University of California, San Diego, have developed soft robots with self-healing capabilities using ML algorithms [47]. These robots can detect damage and autonomously initiate a self-repair process. Researchers at Harvard's Wyss Institute have integrated reinforcement learning algorithms into soft exoskeletons [48]. These algorithms enable the exoskeletons to learn and adapt to the user's movements, providing personalized assistance and improving walking efficiency. Soft robotic worms developed by Seoul National University use ML algorithms to enhance their navigation capabilities [49]. These algorithms enable the robots to learn and adapt to complex environments, making them useful for search and rescue missions. ML algorithms are used to process data from integrated soft sensors in various soft robotic systems. These sensors provide real-time feedback on pressure, strain, and other parameters, allowing the robots to adapt their actions accordingly.

Data-driven design of soft robots are developed at institutions like ETH Zurich use ML to create data-driven models for designing soft robots [50]. These models help optimize the shape, material properties, and control strategies of the robots to achieve desired performance. Soft robot hands, such as those developed at the University of California, Berkeley, use deep learning algorithms to improve their dexterity and manipulation capabilities [51]. These algorithms enable the hands to learn from large datasets of grasping and manipulation tasks. Soft robotic skins embedded with tactile sensors use ML to interpret and respond to tactile stimuli. These systems can be used in applications like prosthetics, where the robot's ability to sense and adapt to touch is crucial.

10.7 CONCLUSIONS

Soft robotics benefits from the integration of ML techniques to enhance control, adaptability, and autonomy. ML enables soft robots to adapt to changing environments and tasks. This adaptability is crucial for applications in dynamic and unpredictable settings, such as medical robotics or search and rescue operations. Algorithms such as reinforcement learning, deep learning, and Bayesian methods (not limited to) are applied to optimize robot behavior and performance. The major problem to adopt the supervised and unsupervised ML is the preparation of dataset, as most of the soft robots are meant for specific applications. These robots generate task specific data which cannot be applied to other soft robots.

ML-based approaches are used for optimizing the design of soft robots, considering factors such as material selection, shape optimization, and energy efficiency. This contributes to the development of more efficient and effective robotic systems. The chapter also discusses the challenges such as the need for large-scale data collection, robustness in real-world applications, and ethical considerations. Advances in ML facilitate natural and intuitive HRI with soft robots. This includes recognizing and responding to human gestures, speech, and intentions, making them safer and more user-friendly. The field continues to evolve with ongoing research focusing on more sophisticated learning algorithms, bio-inspired designs, multimodal sensing, and collaborative robotics. Future directions may include integrating AI explainability into soft robotic systems and advancing towards fully autonomous and intelligent robotic assistants.

REFERENCES

[1] Yang, Y., Wu, Y., Li, C., Yang, X., & Chen, W. (2020). Flexible actuators for soft robotics. *Advanced Intelligent Systems*, 2(1), 1900077.

[2] Hippalgaonkar, K., Li, Q., Wang, X., Fisher III, J. W., Kirkpatrick, J., & Buonassisi, T. (2023). Knowledge-integrated machine learning for materials: lessons from gameplaying and robotics. *Nature Reviews Materials*, 8(4), 241–260.

[3] Chi, Y., Zhao, Y., Hong, Y., Li, Y., & Yin, J. (2024). A perspective on miniature soft robotics: Actuation, fabrication, control, and applications. *Advanced Intelligent Systems*, 6(2), 2300063.

[4] Xiong, J., Chen, J., & Lee, P. S. (2021). Functional fibers and fabrics for soft robotics, wearables, and human–robot interface. *Advanced Materials*, 33(19), 2002640.

[5] Johnson, C. C., Quackenbush, T., Sorensen, T., Wingate, D., & Killpack, M. D. (2021). Using first principles for deep learning and model-based control of soft robots. *Frontiers in Robotics and AI*, 8, 654398.

[6] Pinskier, J., & Howard, D. (2022). From bioinspiration to computer generation: Developments in autonomous soft robot design. *Advanced Intelligent Systems*, 4(1), 2100086.

[7] Noye, S., Martinez, R. M., Carnieletto, L., De Carli, M., & Aguirre, A. C. (2022). A review of advanced ground source heat pump control: Artificial intelligence for autonomous and adaptive control. *Renewable and Sustainable Energy Reviews*, 153, 111685.

[8] Yao, J., Cao, Q., Ju, Y., Sun, Y., Liu, R., Han, X., & Li, L. (2023). Adaptive actuation of magnetic soft robots using deep reinforcement learning. *Advanced Intelligent Systems*, 5(2), 2200339.

[9] Schegg, P., Ménager, E., Khairallah, E., Marchal, D., Dequidt, J., Preux, P., & Duriez, C. (2023). SofaGym: An open platform for reinforcement learning based on soft robot simulations. *Soft Robotics*, 10(2), 410–430.

[10] Hua, J., Zeng, L., Li, G., & Ju, Z. (2021). Learning for a robot: Deep reinforcement learning, imitation learning, transfer learning. *Sensors*, 21(4), 1278.

[11] Chin, K., Hellebrekers, T., & Majidi, C. (2020). Machine learning for soft robotic sensing and control. *Advanced Intelligent Systems*, 2(6), 1900171.

[12] Fuhg, J. N., Padmanabha, G. A., Bouklas, N., Bahmani, B., Sun, W., Vlassis, N. N., ... & De Lorenzis, L. (2024). A review on data-driven constitutive laws for solids. arXiv preprint arXiv:2405.03658.

[13] Pal, A., Restrepo, V., Goswami, D., & Martinez, R. V. (2021). Exploiting mechanical instabilities in soft robotics: Control, sensing, and actuation. *Advanced Materials*, 33(19), 2006939.

[14] Chandrashekhar, A., Saheb, S., & Pavan Kishore, M. L. (2021). Investigation of the static and dynamic path planning of mobile and aerial robots. *Computer Networks and Inventive Communication Technologies: Proceedings of Third ICCNCT* 2020, 1033–1044.

[15] Walker, J., Zidek, T., Harbel, C., Yoon, S., Strickland, F. S., Kumar, S., & Shin, M. (2020, January). Soft robotics: A review of recent developments of pneumatic soft actuators. In *Actuators* (Vol. 9, No. 1, p. 3). MDPI.
[16] Regis, J. E., Renteria, A., Hall, S. E., Hassan, M. S., Marquez, C., & Lin, Y. (2021). Recent trends and innovation in additive manufacturing of soft functional materials. *Materials*, 14(16), 4521.
[17] Lin, Z., Jiang, T., & Shang, J. (2022). The emerging technology of biohybrid micro-robots: a review. *Bio-Design and Manufacturing*, 5, 107–132.
[18] Martella, D., Nocentini, S., Parmeggiani, C., & Wiersma, D. S. (2020). Photonic artificial muscles: from micro robots to tissue engineering. *Faraday Discussions*, 223, 216–232.
[19] Ahmed, F., Waqas, M., Jawed, B., Soomro, A. M., Kumar, S., Hina, A., ... & Choi, K. H. (2022). Decade of bio-inspired soft robots: A review. *Smart Materials and Structures*, 31(7), 073002.
[20] Da Cunha, M. P., Debije, M. G., & Schenning, A. P. (2020). Bioinspired light-driven soft robots based on liquid crystal polymers. *Chemical Society Reviews*, 49(18), 6568–6578.
[21] Liu, X., Lu, D., Zhang, A., Liu, Q., & Jiang, G. (2022). Data-driven machine learning in environmental pollution: gains and problems. *Environmental Science & Technology*, 56(4), 2124–2133.
[22] Zhong, S., Zhang, K., Bagheri, M., Burken, J. G., Gu, A., Li, B., ... & Zhang, H. (2021). Machine learning: new ideas and tools in environmental science and engineering. *Environmental Science & Technology*, 55(19), 12741–12754.
[23] Hegde, C., Su, J., Tan, J. M. R., He, K., Chen, X., & Magdassi, S. (2023). Sensing in soft robotics. *ACS Nano*, 17(16), 15277–15307.
[24] Raschka, S., Patterson, J., & Nolet, C. (2020). Machine learning in python: Main developments and technology trends in data science, machine learning, and artificial intelligence. *Information*, 11(4), 193.
[25] Kumar, P. R., Bikash, S., Rout, L., & Sutar, S. (n.d.), Python-based machine learning: Key advancements and technological trends in data science, machine learning, and AI.
[26] Sarker, I. H. (2021). Deep learning: a comprehensive overview on techniques, taxonomy, applications and research directions. *SN Computer Science*, 2(6), 420.
[27] Sarker, I. H., Kayes, A. S. M., Badsha, S., Alqahtani, H., Watters, P., & Ng, A. (2020). Cybersecurity data science: an overview from machine learning perspective. *Journal of Big Data*, 7, 1–29.
[28] Shekhar, A. C., & Shahab, S. (2021). Analysis of Geneva mechanism using dwell symmetrical coupler curve mechanism. *Materials Today: Proceedings*, *39*, 1402–1406.
[29] Kumar, Y., Kaur, K., & Singh, G. (2020, January). Machine learning aspects and its applications towards different research areas. In *2020 International conference on computation, automation and knowledge management (ICCAKM)* (pp. 150–156). IEEE.
[30] Fang, J., Zhuang, Y., Liu, K., Chen, Z., Liu, Z., Kong, T., ... & Qi, C. (2022). A shift from efficiency to adaptability: recent progress in biomimetic interactive soft robotics in wet environments. *Advanced Science*, 9(8), 2104347.
[31] Mazzolai, B., Mondini, A., Del Dottore, E., Margheri, L., Carpi, F., Suzumori, K., & Lendlein, A. (2022). Roadmap on soft robotics: multifunctionality,

adaptability and growth without borders. *Multifunctional Materials*, 5(3), 032001.

[32] Islam, M. A., Talukder, L., Al, M. F., Sarker, S. K., Muyeen, S. M., Das, P., … & Abhi, S. H. (2023). A review on self-healing featured soft robotics. *Frontiers in Robotics and AI*, 10, 1202584.

[33] Gariya, N., & Kumar, P. (2021). A review on soft materials utilized for the manufacturing of soft robots. *Materials Today: Proceedings*, 46, 11177–11181.

[34] Ghanbarzadeh-Dagheyan, A., Jalili, N., & Ahmadian, M. T. (2021). A holistic survey on mechatronic Systems in Micro/Nano scale with challenges and applications. *Journal of Micro-Bio Robotics*, 17(1), 1–22.

[35] Frohn-Sörensen, P., Geueke, M., Tuli, T. B., Kuhnhen, C., Manns, M., & Engel, B. (2021). 3D printed prototyping tools for flexible sheet metal drawing. *The International Journal of Advanced Manufacturing Technology*, 115(7), 2623–2637.

[36] Hegde, C., Su, J., Tan, J. M. R., He, K., Chen, X., & Magdassi, S. (2023). Sensing in soft robotics. *ACS Nano*, 17(16), 15277–15307.

[37] Zhao, W., Zhang, Y., & Wang, N. (2021). Soft robotics: Research, challenges, and prospects. *Journal of Robotics and Mechatronics*, 33(1), 45–68.

[38] Finio, B. M. (2012). *Roll, Pitch and Yaw Torque Control for a Robotic Bee* (Doctoral dissertation, Harvard University).

[39] De Rivaz, S. D., Goldberg, B., Doshi, N., Jayaram, K., Zhou, J., & Wood, R. J. (2018). Inverted and vertical climbing of a quadrupedal microrobot using electroadhesion. *Science Robotics*, 3(25), eaau3038.

[40] Campbell, S. (2018). The robotics revolution will be soft: soft robotics proliferate-along with their sources of inspiration. *IEEE pulse*, 9(3), 19–24.

[41] Yu, M., Liu, W., Zhao, J., Hou, Y., Hong, X., & Zhang, H. (2022). Modeling and analysis of a composite structure-based soft pneumatic actuators for soft-robotic gripper. *Sensors*, 22(13), 4851.

[42] Katzschmann, R. K., DelPreto, J., MacCurdy, R., & Rus, D. (2018). Exploration of underwater life with an acoustically controlled soft robotic fish. *Science Robotics*, 3(16), eaar3449.

[43] Capsi-Morales, P., Piazza, C., Catalano, M. G., Grioli, G., Schiavon, L., Fiaschi, E., & Bicchi, A. (2021). Comparison between rigid and soft poly-articulated prosthetic hands in non-expert myo-electric users shows advantages of soft robotics. *Scientific Reports*, 11(1), 23952.

[44] Davenport, R. D. (2005). Robotics. *Smart Technology for Aging, Disability, and Independence: The State of the Science*, 67–109.

[45] Lin, H. T., Leisk, G. G., & Trimmer, B. (2011). GoQBot: a caterpillar-inspired soft-bodied rolling robot. *Bioinspiration & biomimetics*, 6(2), 026007.

[46] Glick, P. E. (2021). *Soft Robots for Operation on Unknown Surfaces in Extreme Environments*. University of California, San Diego.

[47] Subad, R. A. S. I., Cross, L. B., & Park, K. (2021). Soft robotic hands and tactile sensors for underwater robotics. *Applied Mechanics*, 2(2), 356–382.

[48] Chandrashekhar, A. S., & Pavan Kishore, M. L. (2021). Investigation of the static and dynamic path planning of mobile and aerial robots. *Computer Networks and Inventive Communication Technologies: Proceedings of Third ICCNCT 2020*, 1033–1044.

[49] Baud, R., Manzoori, A. R., Ijspeert, A., & Bouri, M. (2021). Review of control strategies for lower-limb exoskeletons to assist gait. *Journal of NeuroEngineering and Rehabilitation*, 18, 1–34.
[50] Sapai, S., Loo, J. Y., Ding, Z. Y., Tan, C. P., Baskaran, V. M., & Nurzaman, S. G. (2023). A deep learning framework for soft robots with synthetic data. *Soft robotics*, 10(6), 1224–1240.
[51] Wang, J., & Chortos, A. (2022). Control strategies for soft robot systems. *Advanced Intelligent Systems*, 4(5), 2100165.

Chapter 11

3D and 4D printing

Revolutionizing soft robotics

S Gopinath and A Ranjith Raj

11.1 INTRODUCTION

The field of soft robotics, inspired by the flexibility and adaptability found in biological systems, has made significant strides in recent years. This progress is primarily driven by the advent of 3D- and 4D-printing technologies, which have transformed the way these innovative robotic systems are designed and fabricated. Unlike conventional rigid robots, soft robots have the distinct ability to deform, adapt to their surroundings, and safely interact with humans and delicate objects, leading to numerous applications in areas ranging from healthcare to manufacturing.

Although the potential for soft robotics is vast, its development presents unique challenges related to material selection, design complexity, and fabrication methods. Traditional manufacturing techniques often fail to overcome these challenges, slowing the progress of creating more advanced soft robotic systems.

3D printing, commonly referred to as additive manufacturing, has gained prominence as a groundbreaking solution. This technology allows for the precise, layer-by-layer construction of complex 3D structures, enabling the integration of materials with different properties in a single object. This is crucial for forming the complex and varied structures seen in soft robots (Wang et al., 2017). Ongoing advancements in 3D printing, such as greater precision, speed, and material versatility, have reinforced its role as a key technology in the research and development of soft robotics.

Expanding on 3D printing, 4D printing introduces the dimension of time, allowing structures to alter their shape or properties over time in response to external factors like temperature, moisture, or light (Tibbits, 2014). This dynamic feature is perfectly suited to the adaptive qualities of soft robots, enabling the creation of autonomous systems capable of real-time environmental responses.

This chapter explores the transformative influence of 3D and 4D printing in soft robotics. It provides a thorough overview of the historical evolution of these technologies, their core principles and techniques, and their

DOI: 10.1201/9781003539612-11

wide-ranging applications. In addition, the chapter examines the current challenges and limitations, recent advancements, and future research directions in this rapidly advancing field.

11.2 HISTORICAL DEVELOPMENT

The rise of 3D printing, also known as additive manufacturing, has significantly transformed the robotics sector, particularly soft robotics. This chapter outlines the historical development of 3D and 4D printing, emphasizing their game-changing influence on the design and production of soft robotic systems.

The origins of 3D printing date back to the early 1980s. Hideo Kodama's pioneering work in 1981, although not patented, set the stage for rapid prototyping using photopolymers (Kodama, 1981). Charles Hull's 1984 patent for stereolithography (SLA), a method that uses ultraviolet light to cure layers of photopolymer resin, marked a critical breakthrough, leading to the commercialization of 3D printing by his company, 3D Systems.

Significant advancements in 3D printing technologies occurred during the 1990s, marked by the development of Fused Deposition Modeling (FDM) and Selective Laser Sintering (SLS). These innovations expanded the variety of printable materials and made it possible to create more intricate structures, including some of the earliest soft robotic components.

In 2006, the release of the first commercially available SLS printer represented a major turning point, making 3D printing more accessible across industries and research domains, thereby driving innovation in robotics. By 2019, improvements in precision, material compatibility, and repeatability cemented 3D printing as a reliable manufacturing process for industrial applications.

While 3D printing primarily focused on static objects, researchers soon explored dynamic functionality, leading to the advent of 4D printing. In 2013, Skylar Tibbits introduced the concept of 4D printing, defining it as 3D printing with the added element of time (Tibbits, 2014). 4D-printed objects can alter their shape or properties when exposed to external stimuli like temperature, moisture, or light.

This capability is ideal for soft robotics, which aims to create flexible, adaptive robots capable of safe environmental interactions. 4D printing enables the development of dynamic structures that autonomously respond to stimuli, mirroring the adaptability of living organisms.

Since its introduction, 4D printing has seen rapid growth in materials and techniques. Researchers have developed smart materials such as shape-memory polymers (SMPs), hydrogels, and responsive composites, unlocking new possibilities for creating soft robotic systems with exceptional abilities.

The evolution of 3D and 4D printing has had a profound impact on soft robotics. These additive manufacturing methods allow researchers to design complex, customizable robotic structures with properties resembling biological systems. The precise integration of functional materials and responsive elements has allowed for the development of soft robots capable of performing complex tasks, adapting to their surroundings, and even self-repairing.

As these technologies advance, they are expanding the potential of soft robotics. From medical devices that navigate the human body to industrial robots with unprecedented dexterity, 3D- and 4D-printed soft robots are charting new frontiers in robotics and automation.

11.2.1 Principles and techniques

The foundation of 3D and 4D printing in soft robotics is based on the core ideas of additive manufacturing, combined with advanced material science and intelligent design strategies. These methods enable the production of intricate, varied structures with characteristics customized for specific robotic uses.

11.3 3D PRINTING IN SOFT ROBOTICS

3D printing has become crucial for soft robotics, as it allows for the creation of complex, flexible forms that emulate the adaptability of biological systems. Below are the primary 3D printing methods used in soft robotics, each with distinct advantages and limitations.

1. **FDM:** Initially intended for rigid plastics, FDM has advanced to use flexible filaments for soft robotics. This method involves extruding heated thermoplastic through a nozzle, building up layers to form the desired structure. While FDM is cost-effective and easy to access, it has limitations in resolution and material options.
2. **SLA and Digital Light Processing (DLP):** These techniques use light to harden liquid photopolymer resins, offering high precision and the ability to create intricate, flexible structures. By carefully controlling the curing process, researchers can produce objects with varying degrees of elasticity.
3. **SLS:** Although primarily for rigid materials, SLS can be adapted for elastomeric powders, allowing for flexible designs. However, material limitations and higher costs make SLS less common in soft robotics.
4. **Direct Ink Writing (DIW):** DIW is a highly adaptable method, capable of handling diverse materials such as hydrogels, silicones, and even biological inks. This technique involves extruding viscous ink to create complex, multi-material structures with specific properties.

11.4 ADVANCEMENTS EXPANDING CAPABILITIES

Researchers are continually pushing 3D printing boundaries for soft robotics through innovative approaches.

- **UltiCast:** Developed at Delft University of Technology, this method combines 3D printing with silicone casting. A printed shell serves as a mold for crafting intricate soft robotic structures with complex internal features (Wallin et al., 2018).
- **Omnidirectional Printing:** Jennifer A. Lewis's group at Harvard University has pioneered omnidirectional printing, allowing for the creation of soft materials, including liquids, which are polymerized into stable forms, enabling highly deformable soft robots (Lewis, 2015).

  These innovations show the ongoing evolution of 3D printing technologies, constantly expanding the possibilities for soft robotics. As research advances, more sophisticated materials and methods will further enhance these systems' capabilities.

11.5 4D PRINTING IN SOFT ROBOTICS

4D printing advances the potential of 3D printing by introducing the element of time, enabling the creation of structures that can change shape, adapt, and even function autonomously. This is achieved by incorporating smart materials that respond to external stimuli, adding a "fourth dimension" to the process.

Key principles of 4D printing in soft robotics are as follows

1. **Shape-Memory Effect:** Materials like SMPs and shape-memory alloys (SMAs) can be programmed to remember and revert to a specific shape when triggered by heat or light, allowing soft robots to change form.
2. **Swelling and Deswelling:** Hydrogels, capable of absorbing and releasing water, are used to create actuators that expand and contract, enabling soft robots to move, grip, or pump fluids.
3. **Anisotropic Thermal Expansion:** Different materials expand and contract at varying rates when heated. By strategically designing the structure, components can be made to bend or twist predictably in response to temperature changes.
4. **Magnetic Responsiveness:** By embedding magnetic particles in materials, soft robots can be manipulated remotely using magnetic fields, offering precise control and navigation.

11.5.1 Multimaterial printing: A blend of functions

One of the most exciting developments in 4D printing is multimaterial printing, where various materials are printed together to create robots with heterogeneous structures. For example, a soft gripper may have a flexible outer layer for adaptability and a more rigid core for strength.

11.5.2 Microstructures: Nanoscale engineering

High-resolution printing methods now allow for the creation of microstructures within soft robotics components. These can enhance mechanical properties, create unique responsive behaviors, or act as tiny sensors or actuators.

Though still in its early stages, the potential of 4D printing in soft robotics is vast. Continued exploration of new materials, techniques, and designs will lead to the development of more advanced soft robots capable of navigating complex environments, interacting with delicate objects, and performing tasks that traditional robots cannot.

Applications: The integration of 3D and 4D printing with soft robotics is unlocking vast new opportunities, revolutionizing sectors ranging from healthcare to industrial manufacturing. These flexible, adaptable, and environmentally responsive robots are reshaping how we tackle complex tasks and interact with the world.

Healthcare Transformation: The medical field is undergoing significant change due to the advent of 3D- and 4D-printed soft robots. Their adaptability, biocompatibility, and ability to navigate delicate anatomical structures make them ideal for numerous Healthcare applications

- **Minimally Invasive Surgery:** Picture robotic tools capable of traversing the body with the precision of a surgeon's hand, causing minimal tissue damage. Soft robotic tentacles created via 3D printing are in development for this, promising less invasive operations and quicker recovery times (Cianchetti et al., 2014).
- **Customized Implants:** With 4D printing, implants can grow or adapt with the patient. Bioresorbable, 3D-printed tracheal splints, for example, expand as children grow, eliminating the need for repeat surgeries (Morrison et al., 2015).
- **Targeted Drug Delivery:** Microscopic soft robots printed in 3D can serve as delivery systems, navigating blood vessels and releasing medication directly to diseased cells, revolutionizing treatments for cancer and other illnesses (Li et al., 2020).
- **Regenerative Medicine:** 4D-printed scaffolds simulate the natural cellular environment, guiding tissue growth and repair, offering tremendous promise for healing damaged tissues and advancing regenerative medicine (Gao et al., 2016).

Industry Transformation: Beyond healthcare, 3D- and 4D-printed soft robotics are transforming various industries

- **Adaptive Grippers:** Imagine grippers that can gently handle delicate items such as electronics or fresh produce. Soft grippers, 3D printed for use in assembly lines, provide a safer, more efficient alternative to traditional rigid grippers (Hao et al., 2017).
- **Inspection and Maintenance:** In fields like aerospace and oil and gas, accessing tight spaces can be challenging. Soft robots, with their flexibility, are proving invaluable for inspecting and maintaining complex structures, reducing downtime and improving safety.
- **Collaborative Robotics:** Safety is paramount in environments where humans and robots work together. Soft exoskeletons and assistive devices, produced using 3D printing, enhance human capabilities while reducing the risk of injury, advancing human–robot collaboration.

Environmental Exploration and Disaster Response: The adaptability of 3D- and 4D-printed soft robots makes them ideal for operating in dynamic and challenging environments

- **Underwater Exploration:** Soft robots inspired by marine life, printed using 3D techniques, can navigate coral reefs and the ocean's depths without disturbing ecosystems. These bio-inspired robots can adapt to varying water pressures and change shape to interact with their surroundings (Cianchetti et al., 2015).
- **Disaster Response:** In disaster situations, time is critical. 4D-printed robots can change shape to move through debris or tight spaces, aiding search-and-rescue operations and delivering essential supplies or information in disaster zones (Wang et al., 2017).
- **Sustainable Agriculture:** The gentle nature of 3D-printed soft robots makes them perfect for handling delicate crops. These robots can carefully harvest fruits and vegetables without damaging them, as well as apply pesticides or fertilizers precisely, minimizing environmental harm (Hughes et al., 2016).

Wearable Technology: 3D and 4D printing are transforming wearable technology, creating soft, personalized, and highly responsive devices that seamlessly integrate with the human body

- **Personalized Assistance:** Custom-fit exoskeletons and orthotic devices, produced through 3D printing, offer mobility support tailored to individuals' specific needs, providing comfort and functionality for people with disabilities (Yap et al., 2016).
- **Adaptive Clothing:** Imagine clothing that changes in response to temperature, humidity, or even the wearer's emotions. 4D printing enables the creation of smart textiles that adjust to various stimuli, offering a blend of comfort, protection, and style (Guo et al., 2017).

- **Health Monitoring:** Wearable sensors created using 3D printing can conform to the body, providing continuous and comfortable health monitoring, opening new avenues for personalized healthcare and early disease detection (Gao et al., 2016). As 3D and 4D printing continue to evolve, their applications in soft robotics will likely grow, further transforming industries, enhancing human lives, and enabling unprecedented exploration and technological integration.

11.6 CHALLENGES AND CONSTRAINTS

Despite the remarkable progress in 3D and 4D printing for soft robotics, several hurdles remain. Overcoming these barriers is essential for broader adoption and commercial use.

1. **Material Constraint:** While 3D and 4D printing have reshaped soft robotics, challenges remain to maximize their potential. Addressing these is vital for wider application.
   - **Material Science in Soft Robotics:** Soft robotics heavily relies on advanced materials. Balancing flexibility, strength, and responsiveness is an ongoing challenge.
   - **Pursuit of Optimal Materials:** Imagine materials that combine extreme flexibility and durability for real-world applications. Researchers are tirelessly seeking new materials with ideal properties (Wang et al., 2017).
   - **Combining Different Materials:** Creating soft robots often requires integrating multiple materials with different characteristics. Achieving seamless integration and ensuring strong interfaces is a key challenge (Truby & Lewis, 2016).
   - **Safety Considerations:** In medical applications, biocompatibility is crucial. Researchers are focusing on developing materials that are safe and functional for internal use (Morrison et al., 2015).
2. **Fabrication Challenges:** Beyond materials, fabricating soft robots presents unique difficulties
   - **Resolution Constraints:** Achieving the high resolution required to print complex microstructures, especially with soft materials, remains difficult (Trimmer et al., 2015).
   - **Support Structures:** Very soft materials often need support structures during printing. Removing these without damaging the product is challenging (Wallin et al., 2018).
   - **Scaling for Mass Production:** Scaling up production of soft robots while maintaining accuracy and cost-effectiveness is essential for broad usage (Hao et al., 2017).

3. **Integrating Sensors and Actuators:** Building fully functional soft robots demands seamless integration of sensors, actuators, and control systems
   - **Embedding Electronics:** Incorporating rigid electronics into flexible, soft bodies without impairing function is complex. Research is exploring flexible electronics capable of bending with soft robots (Rus & Tolley, 2015).
   - **Sensitivity of Sensors:** Soft robots' flexibility can reduce sensor accuracy. Developing reliable sensing methods for such deformable robots is crucial (Wang et al., 2018).
   - **Efficiency of Actuators:** Current soft actuators often lack the force and speed of rigid ones. Improving power density and efficiency remains an area of focus (Polygerinos et al., 2017).
4. **Control and Modeling:** The nonlinear, flexible nature of soft robots introduces control and modeling issues
   - **Complex Dynamics:** Soft robots exhibit complex, unpredictable dynamics due to constant deformation, complicating accurate modeling and control algorithm development (Cianchetti & Laschi, 2014).
   - **Real-Time Control:** Controlling soft robots with multiple degrees of freedom in real-time is challenging due to their dynamics and current technology limits (Thuruthel et al., 2018).
   - **Simulation Shortcomings:** A lack of advanced simulation tools capable of modeling soft robots hinders design and performance prediction (Hiller & Lipson, 2014).
5. **Durability and Longevity:** Ensuring the long-term use and durability of 3D- and 4D-printed soft robots is crucial for their viability
   - **Material Durability:** Soft robotic materials, especially 4D-responsive ones, can degrade over time. Research is focusing on improving their long-term stability (Ge et al., 2016).
   - **Resistance to Fatigue:** Soft robots undergo large, repeated movements, risking material fatigue. Creating materials that endure extended use is vital (Rus & Tolley, 2015).
   - **Environmental Durability:** Soft robots need to withstand environmental factors such as temperature, moisture, and chemicals, especially for harsh applications (Cianchetti et al., 2015).
6. **Sustainability and Environmental Concerns:** As technology advances, reducing the environmental impact of soft robotics becomes critical
   - **Material Recycling:** Soft robotic materials, particularly composites, pose recycling challenges. Developing eco-friendly, recyclable materials is essential (Gao et al., 2016).
   - **Energy Usage:** Both the printing process and the robots themselves need to become more energy efficient to support sustainable growth (Wang et al., 2017).

   - **Life Cycle Assessment:** Conducting life cycle assessments of soft robots helps understand and reduce their environmental footprint from creation to disposal (Faludi et al., 2015).
7. **Cost and Accessibility:** While 3D and 4D printing has become more accessible, cost-related barriers persist
   - **Equipment Costs:** High-resolution 3D printers for complex soft robotics are expensive, limiting access for smaller businesses and researchers (Trimmer et al., 2015).
   - **Material Expenses:** Specialized materials, particularly in 4D printing, are costly, hampering large-scale applications (Ge et al., 2016).
   - **Skill Demands:** Designing and producing soft robots requires expertise across disciplines, which can be a major barrier for many potential users (Rus & Tolley, 2015).

11.7 RECENT PROGRESS AND FUTURE PROSPECTS

Despite ongoing challenges, there have been major breakthroughs in 3D- and 4D-printed soft robotics in recent years. These innovations, along with continued research, are shaping the future of this dynamic field.

Material Advances: New materials tailored for 3D and 4D printing are essential for soft robotics progression.

1. **Multiscale Heterogeneous Polymer Composites:** Researchers have developed composites with elastic modulus four orders of magnitude higher than current 4D-printed materials, alongside tunable electrical conductivity. These advancements address scalability and load-bearing issues in 4D structures (Ge et al., 2016).
2. **Biocompatible and Biodegradable Materials:** The development of biocompatible compounds, like the soybean oil–epoxidized acrylate by Dr. Lijie Grace Zhang's team, opens new possibilities for soft robots in healthcare, combining functionality with eco-friendliness (Zhang et al., 2019).
3. **Self-Healing Materials:** Innovations in self-repairing polymers extend the lifespan of soft robots by allowing autonomous damage.
4. **Stimuli-Responsive Materials:** Materials responsive to stimuli such as light and magnetic fields enable the creation of adaptable 4D-printed structures (Zerin et al., 2020).

11.8 FABRICATION IMPROVEMENTS

Advancements in fabrication techniques are overcoming traditional 3D printing limitations

1. **High-Resolution Printing:** Two-photon polymerization allows for the production of soft robots with microscale details, facilitating the development of miniaturized structures (Kawata et al., 2001).
2. **Rapid Liquid Printing:** MIT researchers introduced this method for quickly creating large objects with materials like rubber, solving scalability issues (Hajash et al., 2017).
3. **Embedded 3D Printing:** This technique allows the direct integration of sensors and actuators within soft structures during the printing process, simplifying complex systems (Muth et al., 2014).
4. **4D Bioprinting:** Bioprinting advancements enable the creation of tissue constructs that change over time, with implications for regenerative medicine (Gao et al., 2016).

Control and Sensing: Alongside material and fabrication innovations, significant progress has been made in control and sensing technologies

1. **Machine Learning for Control:** Traditional control methods struggle with soft robotics' non-linear dynamics. Machine learning algorithms can learn and adapt, enhancing control precision (Thuruthel et al., 2018).
2. **Soft Sensors:** New developments in flexible electronics enable the seamless integration of soft sensors, improving accuracy in measuring deformation, pressure, and temperature (Wang et al., 2018).
3. **Closed-Loop 4D Printing:** Combining 4D printing with machine learning, this method enables robots to adjust shape and function in real-time based on environmental cues, opening doors to adaptive robotic systems (Kempaiah & Nie, 2014).

Future Trends: Several promising trends could dramatically expand the impact of 3D- and 4D-printed soft robotics across various sectors

1. **Bio-Inspired Design:** Nature offers inspiration for efficient, adaptable systems. Biomimetic research could yield robots with enhanced locomotion and sensory abilities (Laschi et al., 2016).
2. **Multifunctional Soft Robots:** Future designs may combine sensing, actuation, and energy harvesting in a single structure, allowing more versatile, autonomous robots (Wallin et al., 2018).
3. **Swarm Robotics:** The ability to quickly fabricate customized soft robots could lead to coordinated swarms for complex tasks like environmental monitoring or search and rescue (Rubenstein et al., 2014).
4. **Environmental Applications:** As robots grow more durable and adaptable, their potential in environmental monitoring, pollution cleanup, and conservation will expand (Laschi & Cianchetti, 2014).
5. **Human–Robot Interaction:** Advances in soft robotics are leading to safer human–robot interactions, especially in healthcare, rehabilitation, and collaborative industrial settings (Rus & Tolley, 2015).

6. **Space Exploration:** Lightweight, adaptable, and self-repairing soft robots are ideal for tasks like planetary exploration and habitat construction in space missions (Rossiter et al., 2017).

11.9 CONCLUSIONS

The fusion of 3D and 4D printing with soft robotics has revolutionized robotic design and functionality, paving the way for a new era of possibilities. These additive manufacturing technologies have facilitated the creation of flexible, adaptive, and responsive robotic systems, capable of interacting safely with both humans and sensitive environments. Minimally invasive medical devices that navigate the intricacies of the human body to industrial robots with unmatched dexterity, 3D- and 4D-printed soft robots are redefining the limits of robotics and automation.

The evolution from early 3D printing to the sophisticated 4D-printed soft robots we see today has been driven by technological advancements and interdisciplinary collaboration. Researchers have tackled challenges in materials science, fabrication methods, and control systems to create complex, multifunctional structures with precise properties. This progress has unlocked new opportunities for innovation across a variety of industries.

Despite these achievements, several challenges remain. Continued research is needed to develop materials that combine flexibility, strength, and responsiveness. Enhancing the resolution and speed of printing processes, integrating sensors and actuators seamlessly, and advancing control algorithms are all critical to further development. Further, addressing sustainability, cost-effectiveness, and scalability will be key for widespread adoption of these technologies.

Even with these obstacles, the future of 3D- and 4D-printed soft robotics is promising. Ongoing research in bio-inspired designs, multifunctional materials, and advanced control systems is likely to produce robots with greater adaptability and functionality. The potential applications extend well beyond current uses, impacting areas such as healthcare, environmental monitoring, space exploration, and advanced manufacturing.

3D- and 4D-printed soft robotics will play an increasingly significant role in shaping how we interact with technology and the environment. The ability to create robots that adapt, learn, and respond to their surroundings—much like biological organisms—opens exciting possibilities for solving complex challenges across various fields.

3D and 4D printing are set to transform the world of soft robotics, by creating new possibilities for innovation and progress. These technologies allow for flexible, multifunctional, and affordable robotic systems that can easily adapt to various real-time problems. They promise to bring about significant changes, offering practical solutions and opening up exciting new opportunities.

REFERENCES

Cianchetti, M., Laschi, C., Menciassi, A., & Dario, P. (2014). Biomedical applications of soft robotics. *Nature Reviews Materials*, 3(6), 143–153.

Cianchetti, M., Calisti, M., Margheri, L., Kuba, M., & Laschi, C. (2015). Bioinspired locomotion and grasping in water: the soft eight-arm OCTOPUS robot. *Bioinspiration & Biomimetics*, 10(3), 035003.

Faludi, J., Bayley, C., Bhogal, S., & Iribarne, M. (2015). Comparing environmental impacts of additive manufacturing vs traditional machining via life-cycle assessment. *Rapid Prototyping Journal*, 21(1), 14–33.

Gao, B., Yang, Q., Zhao, X., Jin, G., Ma, Y., & Xu, F. (2016). 4D Bioprinting for Biomedical Applications. *Trends in Biotechnology*, 34(9), 746–756.

Ge, Q., Sakhaei, A. H., Lee, H., Dunn, C. K., Fang, N. X., & Dunn, M. L. (2016). Multimaterial 4D Printing with Tailorable Shape Memory Polymers. *Scientific Reports*, 6, 31110.

Guo, S. Z., Qiu, K., Meng, F., Park, S. H., & McAlpine, M. C. (2017). 3D Printed Stretchable Tactile Sensors. *Advanced Materials*, 29(27), 1701218.

Hajash, K., Sparrman, B., Guberan, C., Laucks, J., & Tibbits, S. (2017). Large-Scale Rapid Liquid Printing. *3D Printing and Additive Manufacturing*, 4(3), 123–132.

Hao, Y., Wang, T., Ren, Z., Gong, Z., Wang, H., Yang, X., ... & Wen, L. (2017). Modeling and experiments of a soft robotic gripper in amphibious environments. *International Journal of Advanced Robotic Systems*, 14(3), 1729881417707148.

Hiller, J., & Lipson, H. (2014). Dynamic simulation of soft multimaterial 3D-printed objects. *Soft Robotics*, 1(1), 88–101.

Hughes, J., Culha, U., Giardina, F., Guenther, F., Rosendo, A., & Iida, F. (2016). Soft Manipulators and Grippers: A Review. *Frontiers in Robotics and AI*, 3, 69.

Kawata, S., Sun, H. B., Tanaka, T., & Takada, K. (2001). Finer features for functional microdevices. *Nature*, 412(6848), 697–698.

Kempaiah, R., & Nie, Z. (2014). From nature to synthetic systems: shape transformation in soft materials. *Journal of Materials Chemistry B*, 2(17), 2357–2368.

Kodama, H. (1981). Automatic method for fabricating a three-dimensional plastic model with photo-hardening polymer. *Review of Scientific Instruments*, 52(11), 1770–1773.

Laschi, C., Mazzolai, B., & Cianchetti, M. (2016). Soft robotics: Technologies and systems pushing the boundaries of robot abilities. *Science Robotics*, 1(1), eaah3690.

Laschi, C., & Cianchetti, M. (2014). Soft robotics: new perspectives for robot bodyware and control. *Frontiers in Bioengineering and Biotechnology*, 2, 3.

Lewis, J. A. (2015). Direct ink writing of 3D functional materials. *Advanced Functional Materials*, 25(29), 5840–5846.

Li, J., Wu, C., Chu, P. K., & Gelinsky, M. (2020). 3D printing of hydrogels: Rational design strategies and emerging biomedical applications. *Materials Science and Engineering: R: Reports*, 140, 100543.

Morrison, R. J., Hollister, S. J., Niedner, M. F., Mahani, M. G., Park, A. H., Mehta, D. K., ... & Green, G. E. (2015). Mitigation of tracheobronchomalacia with 3D-printed personalized medical devices in pediatric patients. *Science Translational Medicine*, 7(285), 285ra64–285ra64.

Muth, J. T., Vogt, D. M., Truby, R. L., Mengüç, Y., Kolesky, D. B., Wood, R. J., & Lewis, J. A. (2014). Embedded 3D printing of strain sensors within highly stretchable elastomers. *Advanced Materials*, 26(36), 6307–6312.

Polygerinos, P., Correll, N., Morin, S. A., Mosadegh, B., Onal, C. D., Petersen, K., ... & Shepherd, R. F. (2017). Soft robotics: Review of fluid-driven intrinsically soft devices; manufacturing, sensing, control, and applications in human-robot interaction. *Advanced Engineering Materials*, 19(12), 1700016.

Rossiter, J., Winfield, J., & Ieropoulos, I. (2017). Here today, gone tomorrow: biodegradable soft robots. *Electroactive Polymer Actuators and Devices (EAPAD) 2017*, 10163, 101630X.

Rubenstein, M., Cornejo, A., & Nagpal, R. (2014). Programmable self-assembly in a thousand-robot swarm. *Science*, 345(6198), 795–799.

Rus, D., & Tolley, M. T. (2015). Design, fabrication and control of soft robots. Nature, 521(7553), 467–475.

Thuruthel, T. G., Shih, B., Laschi, C., & Tolley, M. T. (2018). Soft robot perception using embedded soft sensors and recurrent neural networks. *Science Robotics*, 3(24), eaau3098.

Tibbits, S. (2014). 4D printing: multi-material shape change. *Architectural Design*, 84(1), 116–121.

Trimmer, B. A., Lin, H. T., Baryshyan, A., Leisk, G. G., & Kaplan, D. L. (2015). Towards a biomorphic soft robot: design constraints and solutions. In *The 4th IEEE RAS/EMBS International Conference on Biomedical Robotics and Biomechatronics* (pp. 599–605). IEEE.

Truby, R. L., & Lewis, J. A. (2016). Printing soft matter in three dimensions. *Nature*, 540(7633), 371–378.

Wallin, T. J., Pikul, J., & Shepherd, R. F. (2018). 3D printing of soft robotic systems. *Nature Reviews Materials*, 3(6), 84–100.

Wang, W., Yao, L., Cheng, C. Y., Zhang, T., Atsumi, H., Wang, L., ... & Yao, L. (2017). Harnessing the hygroscopic and biofluorescent behaviors of genetically tractable microbial cells to design biohybrid wearables. *Science Advances*, 3(5), e1601984.

Wang, T., Ge, L., & Gu, G. (2018). Programmable design of soft pneu-net actuators with oblique chambers can generate coupled bending and twisting motions. *Sensors and Actuators A: Physical*, 271, 131–138.

Yap, H. K., Ng, H. Y., & Yeow, C. H. (2016). High-force soft printable pneumatics for soft robotic applications. *Soft Robotics*, 3(3), 144–158.

Zerin, I., Sabouri, A., Ohiri, K. A., Jaradat, S., Ren, L., & Zadeh, M. H. (2020). 4D Printed Tunable Mechanical Metamaterials with Shape Memory Operations. *ACS Applied Materials & Interfaces*, 12(37), 41986–41995.

Zhang, B., Kowsari, K., Serjouei, A., Dunn, M. L., & Ge, Q. (2019). Reprocessable thermosets for sustainable three-dimensional printing. *Nature Communications*, 9(1), 1–7.

Chapter 12

Designing bio-inspired soft robotics for medical applications

Vinay K M and M Prasanna Kumar

12.1 INTRODUCTION

Biological systems seldom consist of rigid mechanical components; instead, they predominantly employ flexible, soft, and elastic materials to thrive in intricate, unstructured environments. This is in contrast to robotic systems, which are typically made of hard materials like steel and aluminum. For instance, the body of animals is made up of flexible muscles and tendons, soft skin with hairs, and a variety of shaky organs. Figure 12.1 shows the human hand and the fabricated hand combinedly shaking hands. Because control designs reflect variations in underlying material qualities, they are also highly distinct from one another. Traditional robotic systems frequently

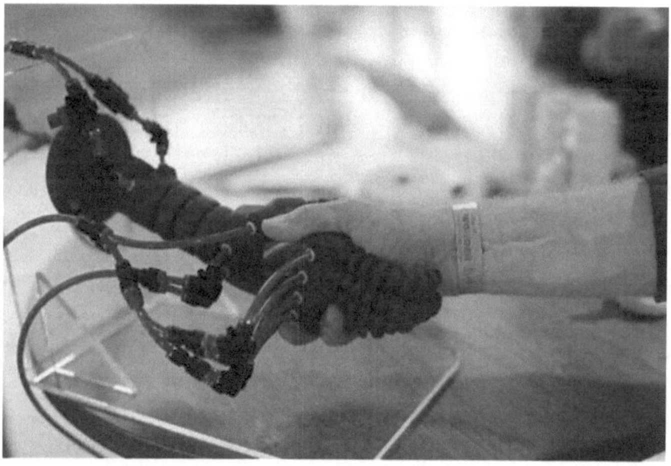

Figure 12.1 Shake hands with a 3D-printed robot.

(source: https://all3dp.com/soft-robotics-shake-hands-with-3d-printed-robot-hand/).

DOI: 10.1201/9781003539612-12

depend on pre-established motion patterns, while biological systems dynamically modify their brain circuitry to adapt to significant changes in body forms [1].

12.2 SOFT ROBOTICS

Due to the significant differences between the components of natural autonomous and artificial systems, there is an increasing interest in the study of "softness" in the framework of embodied intelligence research, which has given rise to the field of soft robotics. There are a few unique study paths with similar motivations, despite the field's youth and lack of definition. For instance, several researchers have been looking into unusual materials for robotic systems. Soft materials, such as those based on polymers, are being looked at for potential new actuators and sensory devices [2, 3]. Following their development, the smart materials, sensors, and actuators were incorporated into a variety of microrobots [4]. Additionally, the robots that could reconfigure themselves mirrored the adaptable bodily systems of animals [5]. Over the past two decades, soft robotics has emerged as a novel and rapidly developing scientific topic that is gaining significant attention from both academic and industrial sectors [6]. An investigation of traditional hard robotics, the counterpart of soft robotics, becomes essential to comprehending the appeal of soft robotics. Hard robots are well known for their many attributes, including (a) high force, (b) accuracy, and (c) complex feedback systems made up of multiple sensors. However, they are also limited to operating in a predefined environment, (d) have discrete rigid links connecting to each other, meaning that their degrees of freedom (DoF) are finite, resulting in discrete topology, (e) very little human interaction, and (f) are very expensive due to hard materials and significant electronics. To address all of these problems, soft robotics was created [7]. Soft robots are characterized by their continuously malleable structure, which can encompass individual body segments or the entire robot in specific cases [8, 9]. This structure typically comprises elastomeric polymers, including silicones [10] and polyurethanes [11], among other materials. The soft body parts exhibit a relatively high number of DoF, leading to intriguing large-scale deformation modes [12]. Soft robotics represents a pioneering frontier in the field of robotics, propelled by the necessity for machines capable of adapting to complex environments and safely interacting with biological tissues. Drawing inspiration from the impressive abilities of living organisms, bio-inspired soft robots utilize materials and designs that emulate natural flexibility and resilience. This chapter explores the medical applications of such soft robots, highlighting their contributions to improving medical procedures and patient care.

12.3 CLASSIFICATION OF SOFT ROBOTS [13]

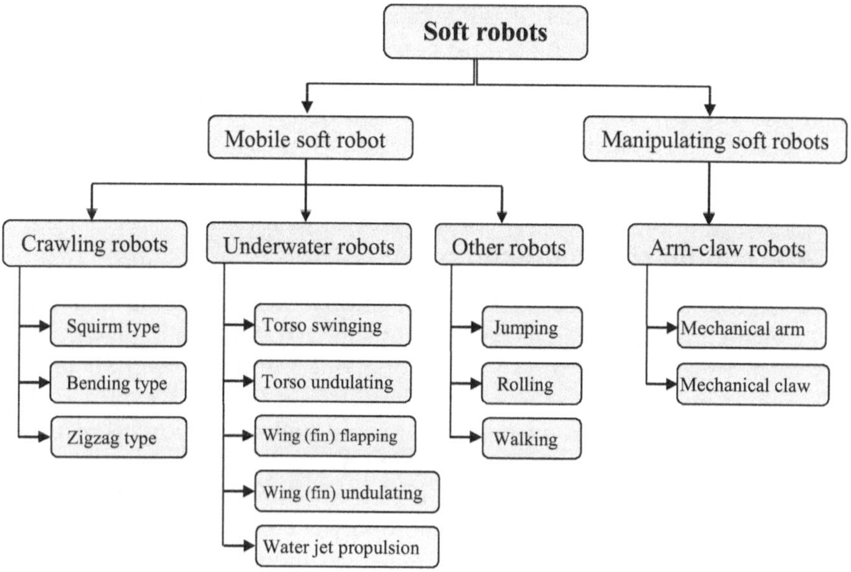

12.4 MANUFACTURING (3D PRINTING) TECHNOLOGY FOR ROBOTIC SOFT ACTUATOR

Three-dimensional (3D)-printed soft actuators are fascinating devices that combine the flexibility of soft materials with the precision and customization of 3D printing. These actuators are widely used in robotics, prosthetics, and various adaptive systems due to their ability to mimic the movement and flexibility of biological muscles.

12.4.1 Material selection

a. **Soft Polymers:** Common materials include silicones, urethanes, and thermoplastic elastomers. These materials are chosen for their flexibility, stretchability, and the capacity to regain their previous shape after being deformed.
b. **Composite Materials:** Sometimes, materials are combined to enhance performance, such as embedding fibers or particles to improve strength or add functionalities.

12.4.2 Design and modeling

a. **CAD Software:** Using computer-aided design (CAD) software, a comprehensive 3D model of the actuator is created at the start of the design phase. The design must consider the desired movement, force requirements, and integration with other components.
b. **Simulation:** Often, simulations are conducted to predict the actuator's performance, including its deformation behavior, stress distribution, and interaction with other parts.

12.4.3 Manufacturing techniques

a. **Stereolithography (SLA):** SLA is an additive manufacturing technique where liquid resin is cured by a light source to form solid plastic. It is sometimes referred to as vat photopolymerization or resin 3D printing, using a UV laser to solidify liquid resin into layers. SLA is the best method for producing intricate and high-resolution geometries. Figure 12.2 shows the schematic of SLA.
b. **Digital Light Processing (DLP):** DLP, a 3D printing technique, allows for the rapid production of photopolymer components. With one notable exception whereas SLA machines use a laser to trace a layer, DLP machines utilize a projected light source to cure the entire layer at once. Other than that, they are very similar to SLA machines. The component is built layer by layer. This printing technique is used to print tremendously intricate resin design items such as jewelry models, dental molds, toys, figurines, and other items with fine details. It cures the entire layer at once, which makes it significantly faster than SLA. Figure 12.3 shows the schematic of DLP.

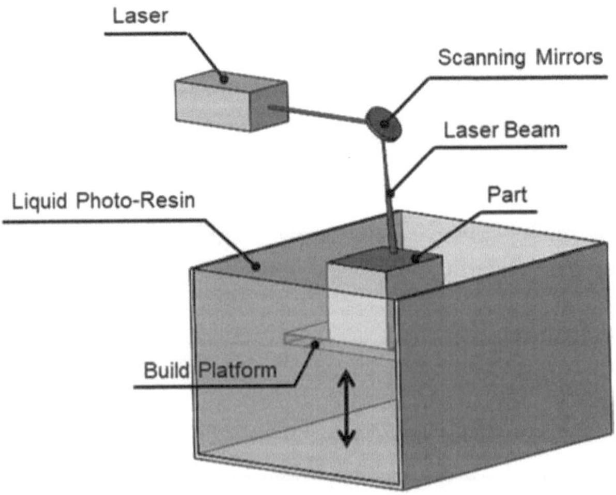

Figure 12.2 Schematic of stereolithography (SLA) [14].

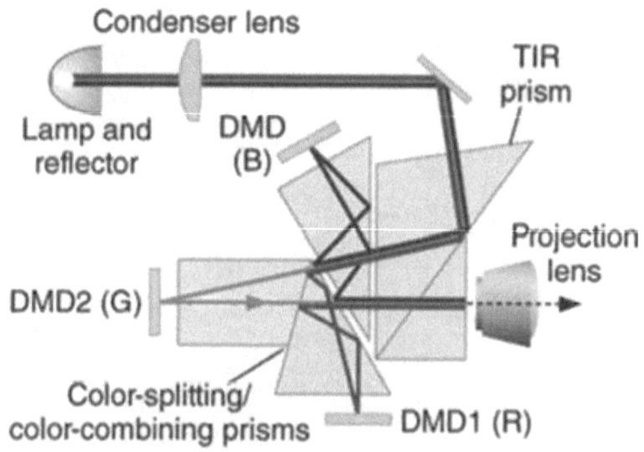

Figure 12.3 Digital light processing (DLP).

c. **Fused Deposition Modeling (FDM):** FDM is one of the most widely used 3D printing processes. To create a 3D model, it works by extruding thermoplastic material layer by layer. FDM is appreciated for its versatility, cost-effectiveness, and ease of use, making it one of the most accessible 3D printing technologies for a variety of users [15].
d. **Inkjet Printing:** It's a 3D printing technology, often referred to as "Inkjet 3D Printing" or "Inkjet-Based Additive Manufacturing," is a method that uses inkjet printing technology to build up 3D objects layer by layer. This approach involves selectively depositing droplets of material to create the final structure; with the help of this technology, we can print multiple materials in a single layer, allowing for complex structures and material gradients.
e. **Direct Ink Writing (DIW):** DIW is a 3D printing technique that involves the extrusion of a material, often referred to as "ink," to build up a 3D object. Unlike other 3D printing methods that use molten plastic or cured resin, DIW uses a range of materials, together with ceramics, polymers, and even biological substances, which are dispensed through a nozzle or a similar extrusion system, as shown in Figure 12.4. DIW supports complicated geometries and functional integration and may be printed on a variety of soft materials.

12.4.4 Postprocessing

Postprocessing is an essential part of 3D printing that involves finishing and refining the printed object to achieve the desired quality, appearance, and functionality. Here are presented some common postprocessing techniques used in 3D printing

a. **Curing:** Many soft actuators need extra curing processes; they can range from only employing light (UV nail salons, natural sunshine, DIY UV cure boxes, etc.) to using both light and heat, as shown in

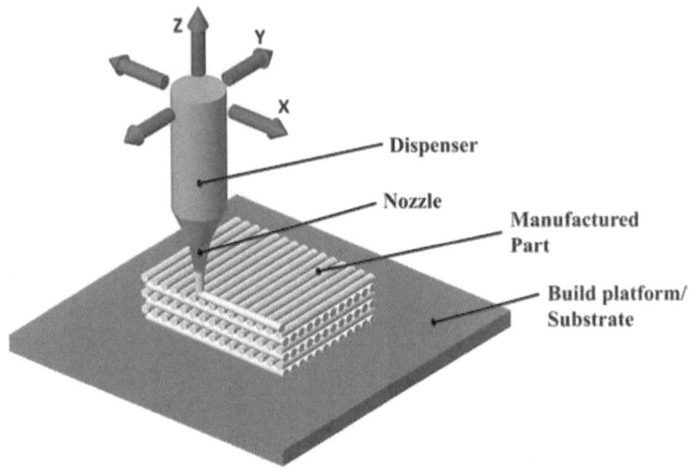

Figure 12.4 Direct ink writing (DIW).

Figure 12.5. Increases in material qualities that are not possible to accomplish with light alone are produced by heat, which speeds up the process and permits even more thorough bond formation.

b. **Support Removal:** If you have any angles in your model that are more than 45 degrees, you will need to activate the "support structure" feature. A support structure provides a secure foundation from which overhanging sections can be constructed safely, much like scaffolding does on a building. The software generates the support structure automatically if the checkbox is checked. When the print is finished, the lattice-like structure may usually be snapped off easily, but occasionally, sandpaper or nail clippers are needed to remove any leftover material, as shown in Figure 12.6(a). This is where dual-extruder 3D printers are useful since they can create support structure with a separate dissolvable filament, like HIPS (high-impact polystyrene), which

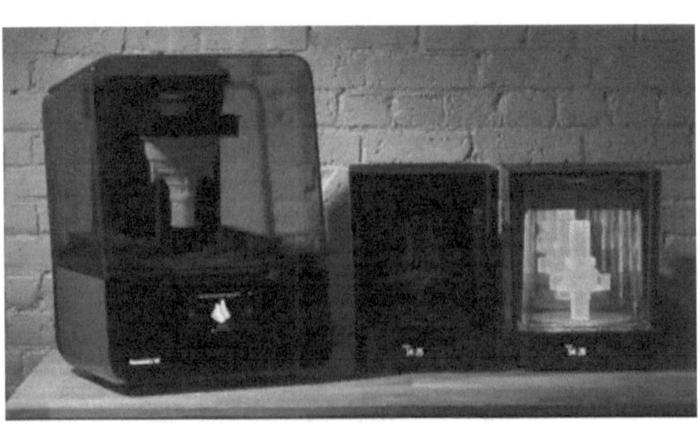

Figure 12.5 Postcuring unit.

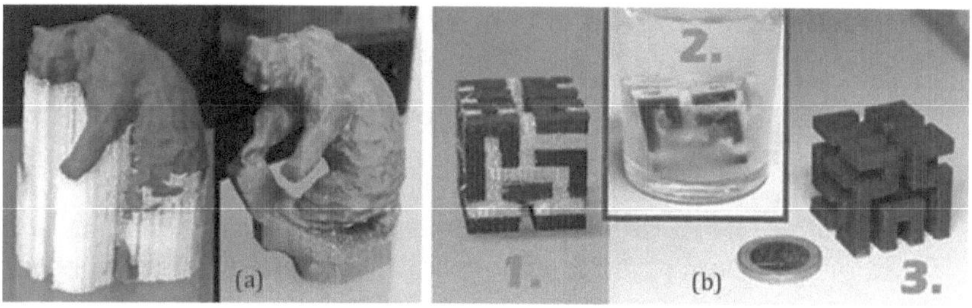

Figure 12.6 (a-b) Support removal.

melts away in limonene solution based on citrus, or PVA (polyvinyl alcohol), which dissolves in water, as shown in Figure 12.6(b). This greatly simplifies the process of removing support structure, especially in confined spaces.

c. **Surface Treatment:** Surface finish in 3D printing can significantly impact the appearance and functionality of the final product. Post-processing is often necessary to achieve a smooth and refined surface; some common methods for improving surface finish after 3D printing are sanding, filling and priming, chemical smoothing, heat treatment, coating, casting, and molding. The robotic soft end effector's glossy surface texture is seen in Figure 12.7. are as follows

12.4.5 Integration and testing

a. **Integration:** The printed actuator is integrated with its control systems, sensors, and other components. This step ensures that the actuator functions as intended within the larger system.
b. **Testing:** The actuator is tested for its performance characteristics such as flexibility, range of motion, response to stimuli, and load-bearing capacity. Adjustments may be needed based on the results.

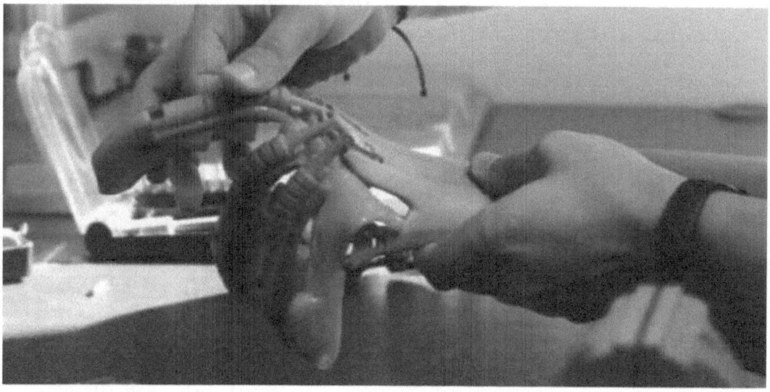

Figure 12.7 Surface-finished robotic soft end effector.

12.4.6 Applications and customization

a. **Customization:** With 3D printing, wearables, prostheses, and soft robots can all be customized and prototyped quickly to fit the needs of their particular applications.
b. **Integration with Electronics:** Soft actuators can be combined with electronics for more advanced functionality, such as adding sensors or control systems to enhance their performance in real-world applications.

By combining these fabrication processes, researchers and engineers can develop highly specialized soft actuators that meet a wide range of needs, from intricate robotic movements to adaptable prosthetic limbs.

12.4.7 Fundamentals of bio-inspired soft robotics design

Bio-inspired soft robots draw inspiration from various biological systems, such as the locomotion of octopuses, the gripping ability of geckos, and the resilience of plants.

12.4.8 Material selection

Typically, elastomers, silicone, and hydrogels are used to build soft robots because they offer the required compliance and flexibility. These materials can be engineered to exhibit specific mechanical properties, enabling robots to adapt to diverse tasks.

12.4.9 Actuation mechanisms

Actuation is the fundamental component of soft robots, converting energy into mechanical motion. In soft robotics, the actuation system influences many points. From the tasks that soft robots can complete in their workspace to the necessary manufacturing procedure.

a. **Pneumatic Actuation:** Pneumatic actuation plays a pivotal role in soft robotics, leveraging the use of air or other gases to control the movement of flexible structures made from elastomeric materials, as shown in Figure 12.8. This approach allows for versatile and biomimetic motion, enabling soft robots to perform tasks with compliance and adaptability. This strategy has multiple benefits in terms of energy efficiency, versatility, compliance, and safety.
b. **Flexible Fluidic Actuation:** Flexible fluidic actuation refers to a method of actuating or controlling movement using flexible structures that can deform in response to fluid pressure. In the flexible fluidic actuation, each actuator is typically inflated and deflated independently and

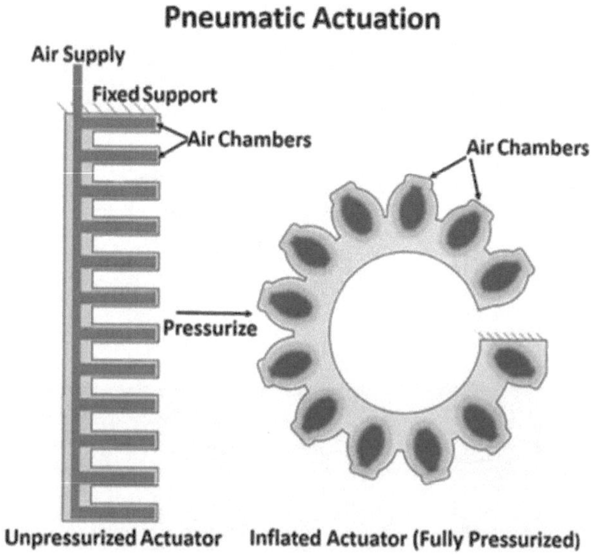

Figure 12.8 Pneumatic actuation.

(source: [16]).

individually, as shown in Figure 12.9(a), and inflated with a single pressure input, as shown in Figure 12.9(b). This approach leverages the flexibility of materials, often elastomers or soft polymers, to achieve a variety of mechanical motions or tasks. This method has various benefits, including low weight, quiet operation, flexibility, and adaptability.

c. **Cable-Driven Actuation:** Cable-driven actuation is a method of actuating mechanical systems using flexible cables instead of rigid mechanical linkages or direct drives, as shown in Figure 12.10. This method has multiple benefits that can be used to a range of situations, including cost-effectiveness, weight reduction, smooth operation, remote actuator, flexibility, and maneuverability.

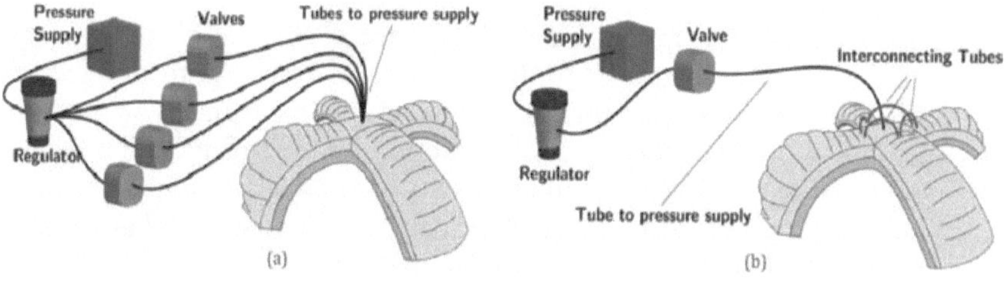

Figure 12.9 Flexible fluidic actuation. (a) Each actuator is typically inflated and deflated independently and individually. (b) Inflated with a single pressure input.

(source: ref. [17]).

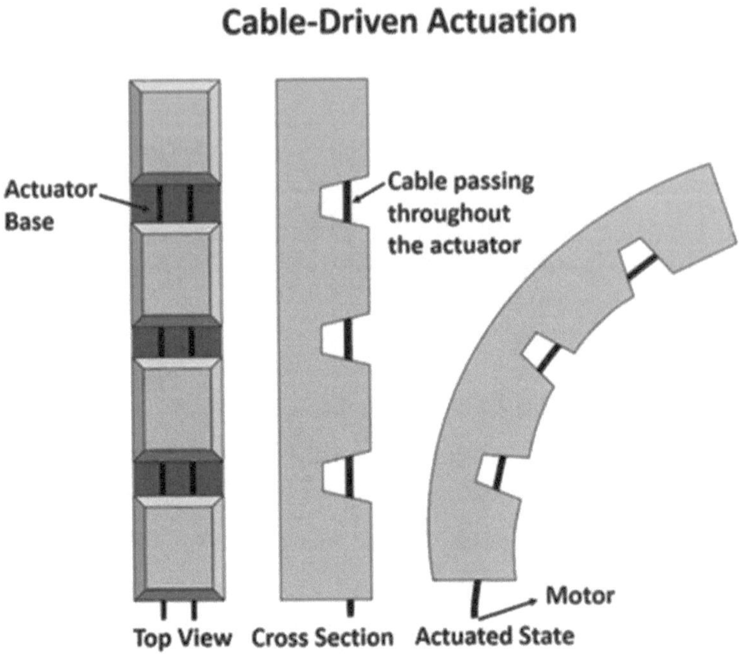

Figure 12.10 Cable-driven actuation.

(source: ref. [16]).

d. **Shape-Memory Materials:** A class of materials known as shape-memory materials (SMMs) is renowned for its extraordinary capacity to recall and regain its original shape following deformation. This unique property is due to a solid-state phase transformation, typically involving a change between martensitic and austenitic crystal structures, which is reversible under certain conditions such as stress or temperature changes. Numerous benefits are provided by this method in terms of energy efficiency, durability, and versatility. Figure 12.11 shows the shape-memory alloy–based actuation.

a. **Electro-active Polymers (EAPs):** EAPs are a class of materials that exhibit significant size or profile changes in response to an electric field. Unlike traditional materials that rely on mechanical or thermal actuation, EAPs undergo electrostriction or electrodynamics when subjected to an electrical stimulus. This method has multiple benefits, including biocompatibility, quick response, lightweight, and flexibility. Figure 12.12 shows the EPA-based actuation.

b. **Magneto- and Electro-rheological Materials (M/E-RMs):** Smart materials that display reversible changes in their rheological properties (viscosity, stiffness, etc.) in reaction to external magnetic or electric fields are known as magneto-rheological (MR) and electro-rheological (ER) materials, respectively. This method has multiple benefits, including

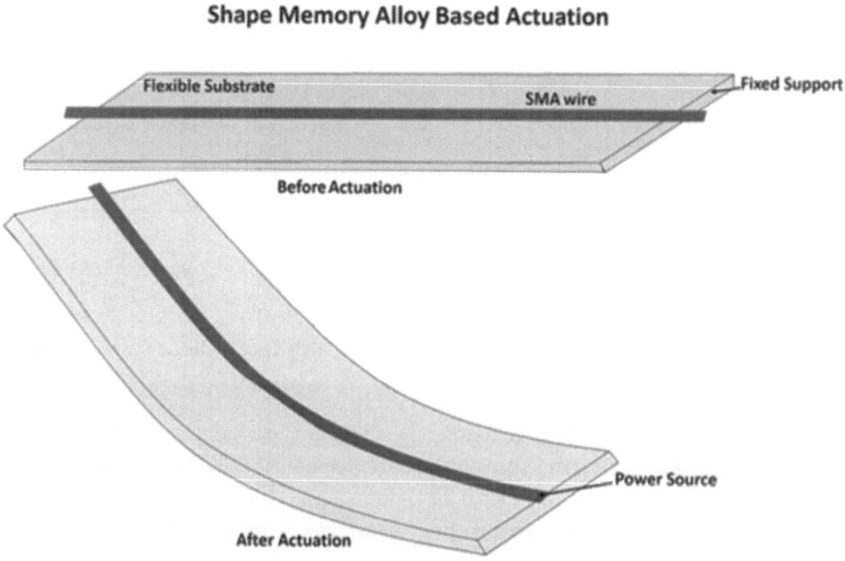

Figure 12.11 Shape-memory alloy–based actuation.
(source: ref. [16]).

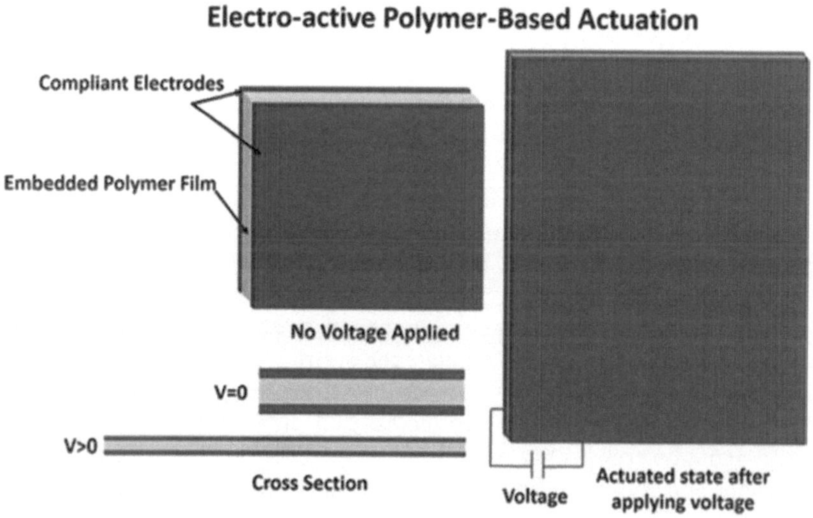

Figure 12.12 Electro-active polymer–based actuation.
(source: ref. [16]).

biocompatibility, quick response, lightweight, and flexibility [18]. Materials in a related family that react to magnetic fields are called MR fluids. Usually, these fluids are made up of ferrous particles, the size of which are measured in microns, suspended in a carrier fluid like water or oil. These particles align in the presence of a magnetic field, causing

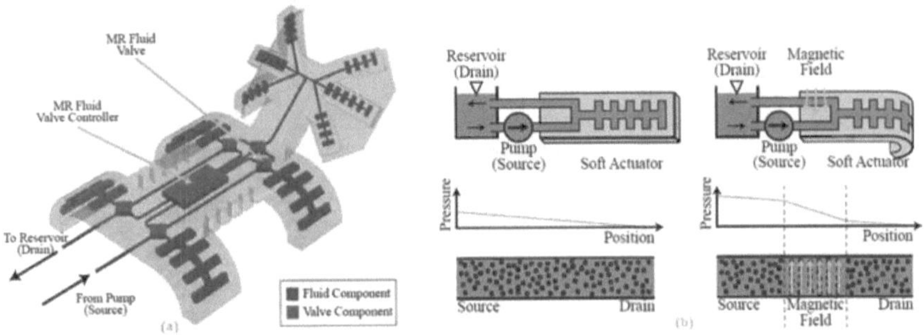

Figure 12.13 (a) MR fluid valves. (b) Soft actuator with and without magnetic field.

the fluid to show an increasing yield stress with field strength [19]. A platform for operating soft robotic devices with MR fluid as the working fluid is depicted in Figure 12.13(a). Thus, the pressure drop across a specific flow zone can be directly affected by the application of a magnetic field, enabling the integration of flow control elements like on-board valves. The soft actuator in Figure 12.13(b) on the left displays pressure and MR fluid behavior when there is no magnetic field, whereas the soft actuator on the right displays pressure and MR fluid behavior when there is a magnetic field [19].

Smart materials known as electro-rheological fluids (ERFs) have applications in soft robotics. By applying an electric field that alters their rheological properties, these fluids can undergo reversible and repeatable transitions from liquid to solid phases, usually within a matter of milliseconds. Because ER fluids phase shift quickly, ER valves offer a straightforward drawing and speedy execution. With the recommended basic valves, it is likely to build robots by numerous single-valve control of fluidic actuators. This concept may have a number of uses in continuum arms and soft robotics. More precisely, a group of these tiny valves might create a soft continuum arm, with several fluidic actuators installed on each valve to regulate the position and value of the bending. A portion of the fluid in the actuator on the other side should be released as the volume of the actuator increases. A different hose is required for evacuation (reverse) flow in the interim. Therefore, to control the forward and backward flow of the ER fluid, each actuator on a continuum arm would need two different ER valves (Figure 12.14(a)). ER valves can also be utilized to regulate how flexible a robot's body structure is. ER valves and a fluidic system can be used to connect several cells embedded in a structure as an initial idea. The suggested schematic in Figure 12.14(b) depicts a continuum arm driven by a tendon [20].

c. **Sensing and Control:** Integrating sensors into soft robots enhances their ability to interact with their environment. Tactile sensors, proprioceptive sensors, and bio-inspired control algorithms are crucial for precise manipulation and navigation in medical contexts.

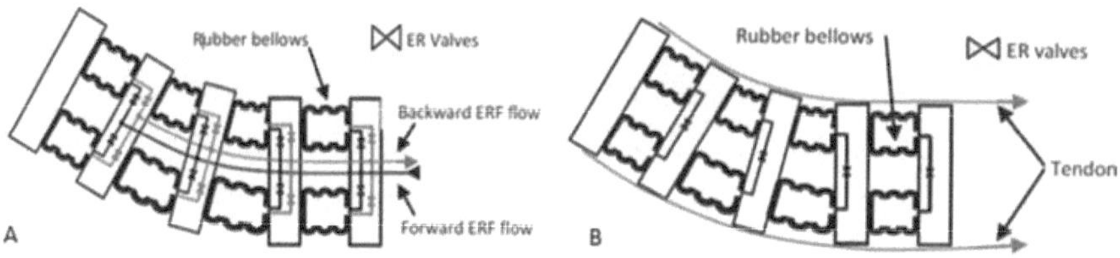

Figure 12.14 (a) Soft fluidic continuum arm and (b) soft tendon–driven continuum arm.

(source: ref. [20]).

12.5 MAJOR APPLICATIONS OF SOFT ROBOTICS

12.5.1 Medical applications

Soft robots offer significant advantages in minimally invasive surgery (MIS). Their flexibility and adaptability allow for better maneuverability within the human body, reducing trauma and improving patient outcomes.

- **Surgical Assistance:** Soft robots can be used in minimally invasive procedures, such as laparoscopic surgery, to access confined spaces and perform delicate manipulations with greater dexterity and precision.
- **Soft Endoscopes:** Equipped with flexible, steerable tips, these devices can navigate complex anatomical pathways, providing high-resolution imaging and enabling precise surgical interventions.
- **Cardiac and Vascular Interventions:** Soft robotic catheters equipped with flexible actuators can navigate through blood vessels with reduced risk of damage or discomfort to patients, aiding in diagnostic imaging or delivering therapeutic agents.
- **Heart Assist Devices:** Soft robots can assist in pumping blood or providing mechanical support to the heart, improving cardiac function in patients with heart failure or during cardiac surgeries.
- **Robot-Assisted Catheters:** These catheters can navigate through blood vessels with minimal risk of injury, enhancing the precision and safety of procedures such as angioplasty and cardiac ablations.
- **Assistive Robotics in Elderly Care:** These robots can assist elderly individuals with activities of daily living, such as dressing, feeding, and mobility support, while ensuring safe interaction and comfort.
- **Pain Management and Therapy:** Devices incorporating soft actuators and sensors can provide targeted pain relief through controlled pressure or heat application, aiding in chronic pain management.

12.5.2 Drug delivery systems

Bio-inspired soft robots have the capacity to transform targeted drug delivery by emulating the locomotion of microorganisms. This enables them to navigate through bodily fluids with precision, delivering drugs to specific sites and thereby Increasing the effectiveness of treatment while minimizing adverse consequences.

- **Microswimmers:** Tiny, soft robots that swim through bodily fluids, directed by external magnetic fields or chemical gradients, to deliver drugs precisely where needed.
- **Hydrogel-Based Carriers:** These carriers ensure controlled and sustained delivery by encasing medications and releasing them in response to particular physiological stimuli.

12.5.3 Types of soft robotic drug delivery systems

- **Capsule Robots:** Soft capsule robots are ingestible devices that can navigate through the gastrointestinal tract to deliver drugs or perform diagnostic procedures. They can be controlled externally or autonomously to navigate through the digestive system.
- **Soft Grippers and Manipulators:** These are used for handling and positioning drug-loaded microcarriers or nanoscale drug delivery vehicles within targeted tissues or organs.
- **Microfluidic Devices:** Soft microfluidic systems can mimic physiological fluid dynamics and be used to transport and release drugs in a controlled manner.

12.5.4 Rehabilitation and assistive devices

Soft robotics can significantly enhance rehabilitation and assistive technologies. Their adaptability and compliance make them ideal for interacting with the human body, providing support and facilitating recovery.

- **Exoskeletons:** Soft, wearable exoskeletons can assist patients with mobility impairments, providing support and augmenting muscle strength during rehabilitation exercises.
- **Soft Orthotic Devices:** Customizable and flexible orthotic devices can provide support to joints and muscles, aiding in the recovery of patients with musculoskeletal injuries.

12.5.5 Tissue engineering

Tissue engineering is another field in which soft robotics has promise for creating dynamic, biomimetic environments for tissue creation and cell growth.

- **Bioprinting:** In bioprinting technology, soft robotic actuators can be utilized to accurately deposit cells and biomaterials to create intricate tissue structures that resemble genuine tissues.
- **Dynamic Scaffolds:** These scaffolds can change shape and stiffness in response to environmental cues, promoting cell differentiation and tissue maturation.

- **Bioreactors with Soft Robotic Components:** Soft robotic actuators are integrated into bioreactor systems to provide mechanical stimulation (e.g., stretching, compression) to cultured cells. This mechanical conditioning promotes tissue maturation and enhances tissue functionality.
- **Soft Robotic Surgical Tools:** By delicately interacting with sensitive tissues, these instruments lessen trauma during surgical procedures and increase surgical precision.

12.6 CHALLENGES AND FUTURE DIRECTIONS

12.6.1 Bioinspired soft robotics: Challenges

Despite promising advancements, bio-inspired soft robotics encounters several challenges

- **Material Limitations:** One significant hurdle is the development of materials that can replicate the complexity and functionality of biological tissues. It is difficult to design materials with the strength, flexibility, and resilience of biological tissues. Soft robotics often relies on polymers and elastomers, which need to balance flexibility with durability. Finding or engineering materials that can perform well under various conditions without degrading is a key challenge.
- **Control Systems:** Creating control systems that can manage the complex, adaptive movements of soft robots is difficult. Traditional control methods might not be directly applicable, requiring innovative approaches such as artificial intelligence (AI), machine learning, or bio-inspired algorithms.
- **Sensing and Feedback:** Soft robots often lack rigid structures, which makes it harder to incorporate sensors and feedback systems. Developing sensors that can conform to flexible surfaces and provide accurate, real-time data is a significant challenge.
- **Manufacturing Techniques:** Fabricating soft robots involves advanced manufacturing techniques like 3D printing or molding, which need to be precise and scalable. Achieving high fidelity and consistency in these processes can be technically demanding and costly.
- **Durability and Reliability:** Soft robots often face issues with wear and tear due to their flexible materials. Ensuring long-term reliability and maintaining performance over time requires innovative approaches to material science and design.
- **Energy Efficiency:** Because they require constant deformation and movement, soft robots may require more energy than rigid robots. Developing energy-efficient actuators and power sources is crucial for practical applications.
- **Integration with Existing Systems:** Integrating soft robots into existing systems or environments, particularly those designed for traditional

rigid robots, can be complex. Soft robots may require new interfaces or modifications to existing infrastructure.

- **Biomechanical Modeling:** Accurately modeling the biomechanics of soft robots to predict their behavior and interactions with the environment can be difficult. This involves complex simulations and an understanding of how soft materials deform and respond to forces.
- **Ethical and Safety Considerations:** As with any advanced technology, ethical and safety concerns must be addressed. Ensuring that soft robots are used responsibly and do not pose unforeseen risks to humans or the environment is important.
- **Regulatory Hurdles:** Ensuring that soft robotic devices meet stringent medical regulatory standards is essential for their clinical adoption.

12.6.2 Future directions of bio-inspired soft robotics

The field of bio-inspired soft robotics is advancing rapidly, and several promising directions are emerging for its future development

- **Advanced Materials:** Future research will likely focus on developing new materials with enhanced properties. This includes materials with greater flexibility, strength, self-healing capabilities, and responsiveness to environmental stimuli. Smart materials that can adapt their characteristics to the environment will be especially useful.
- **Integration with AI and Machine Learning:** Soft robots' functionality and flexibility could be revolutionized by using AI and machine learning to control them. AI algorithms can help soft robots learn from their environment and optimize their behavior in real time, making them more autonomous and efficient.
- **Improved Actuation Techniques:** Exploring new actuation methods, such as those inspired by natural muscle movements or hydraulic systems, could lead to more precise and efficient control of soft robots. Developments in soft actuators and hybrid actuators combining soft and rigid components are areas of active research.
- **Biohybrid Systems:** Combining biological tissues with synthetic materials to create biohybrid robots is an exciting area of research. These systems could harness the advantages of both biological and artificial components, leading to more efficient, adaptable, and responsive robots.
- **Enhanced Sensory Systems:** Developing more sophisticated sensory systems that can provide comprehensive feedback in real-time will be crucial. Future soft robots may integrate advanced sensors for touch, pressure, temperature, and chemical detection, allowing them to interact more naturally and effectively with their environment.

- **Modular and Reconfigurable Designs:** Creating soft robots with modular and reconfigurable designs could enhance their versatility and adaptability. Modular robots have a wide range of applications since they may adapt their design or functioning to the work at hand and the surrounding conditions.
- **Wearable Robotics:** Soft robotics has potential applications in wearable technology, including exoskeletons and prosthetics. Future developments may focus on creating more comfortable, adaptable, and efficient wearable robots that can enhance human capabilities or assist those with disabilities.
- **Biomedical Applications:** The development of soft robotics applications for surgery that is minimally invasive, rehabilitation, and drug delivery systems is one possible direction for medical technology. Compared to conventional rigid robots, soft robots might negotiate complicated biological settings more precisely and with greater ease.
- **Environmental and Disaster Response:** When it comes to responding to environmental emergencies and disasters, soft robots may be quite important. They could be especially helpful in situations requiring flexibility and adaptability, including search and rescue operations in dangerous or cramped areas.
- **Energy Efficiency and Sustainability:** Soft robotics must address sustainability and energy consumption if they are to be widely used. To lessen the environmental impact of soft robotics, future research may concentrate on creating actuators, power sources, and recyclable materials that are more energy efficient.
- **Interdisciplinary Collaboration:** In the future, more cooperation between the fields of biology, materials science, robotics, computer science, and engineering will be beneficial for bio-inspired soft robotics. Such multidisciplinary methods will stimulate creativity and result in more sophisticated and useful solutions. are shown as follows

12.7 FUTURE STUDIES OUGHT TO CONCENTRATE ON

- **Multifunctional Materials:** developing materials that can simultaneously offer mechanical flexibility, biocompatibility, and functional responsiveness.
- **Advanced Sensing:** utilizing cutting-edge sensor technologies to enhance soft robot control and feedback in medical applications.
- **Clinical Trials:** carrying out comprehensive clinical experiments to confirm the security and effectiveness of bio-inspired soft robotic devices in actual healthcare environments.

12.8 OUTLOOK

The development of sophisticated controls, precise modeling, and streamlined production techniques are essential for the advancement of soft robotics. The progress of sensor and actuator technologies is also critical to the development of soft robots. Alternatives with high performance and mass production capabilities will come from further advancements in soft materials [21]. In soft robotics, pneumatic energy systems are currently used. Pneumatic technologies may eventually take the lead in all fields. Consequently, the systems' capacity would rise [22]. Because soft robots have so many DoF, modeling soft robotic systems has proven to be challenging. Large deformation of the materials and the nonlinear kinematics of the system's actuation must be examined in order to model a soft robotic system. To date, a number of methods have been employed to approximate the system's behavior. Nonetheless, the models continue to be intricate, and the approximations provide room for significant analytical errors. To enable in-depth research on soft robots and expand design capabilities, new models must be created [23]. The need for biocompatible systems and materials in the medical profession is only growing. It will take more investigation into possible soft materials to find materials that can sustain live tissues and cells. With the development of novel materials, approaches for rapid prototyping are needed. Bio-inspired soft robotics signifies a revolutionary approach to tackling diverse medical challenges. Their intrinsic flexibility, adaptability, and biocompatibility position them as ideal candidates for applications spanning from MIS to drug delivery and rehabilitation. Despite existing challenges, ongoing interdisciplinary research and technological progress hold the promise of unlocking the complete potential of these innovative systems, heralding a new era in medical care.

REFERENCES

[1] Iida, F., Laschi, C., "Soft robotics: Challenges and perspectives." *Procedia Computer Science* 7 (2011): 99–102. https://doi.org/10.1016/j.procs.2011.12.030

[2] Trivedi, D., Rahn, C.D., Kier, W.M., Walker, I.D., Soft robotics: Biological inspiration, state of the art, and future research, *Applied Bionics and Biomechanics* 5 (3) (2008) 99–117. https://doi.org/10.1080/11762320802557865

[3] Ilievski, F., Mazzeo, A.D., Shepherd, R.F., Chen, X., Whitesides, G.M., Soft robotics for chemists, *Angewandte Chemie, International Edition* 50 (2011) 1890–1895. https://doi.org/10.1002/anie.201006464

[4] Floreano, D., Zufferey, J.C., Srinivasan, M.V., Ellington, C. (Eds.), *Flying insects and robots*, Springer, 2009. DOI: https://doi.org/10.1007/978-3-540-89393-6

[5] Yim, M., Shen, W. M., Salemi, B., Rus, D., Moll, M., Lipson, H., Klavins, E., Chirikjian, G.S., Modular self-reconfigurable robot systems: Challenges and opportunities for the future, *IEEE Robotics and Automation Magazine* (2007) 43–52. https://doi.org/10.1109/MRA.2007.339623

[6] Ansari, Y., Hassan, T., Manti, M., Falotico, E., Cianchetti, M., Laschi, C., Soft Robotic Technologies for Industrial Applications, 2019. https://doi.org/10.5220/0007900900350064
[7] Alici, G., Softer is harder: What differentiates soft robotics from hard robotics? *MRS Advance* 3 (28) (2018) 1557–1568. https://doi.org/10.1557/adv.2018.159
[8] Rus, D., Tolley, M. Design, fabrication and control of soft robots. *Nature* 521 (2015) 467–475. https://doi.org/10.1038/nature14543
[9] Schmitt, F., Piccin, O., Barbé, L. and Bayle, B., Soft robots manufacturing: A review. *Frontiers in Robotics and AI* 5 (2018) 84. https://doi.org/10.3389/frobt.2018.00084
[10] Majidi, Carmel. "Soft-matter engineering for soft robotics." *Advanced Materials Technologies* 4 (2) (2019) 1800477. https://doi.org/10.1002/admt.201800477
[11] Wallin, T.J., Pikul, J. & Shepherd, R.F. 3D printing of soft robotic systems. *Nature Reviews Materials* 3 (2018) 84–100. https://doi.org/10.1038/s41578-018-0002-2
[12] Hawkes, Elliot W., et al. "A soft robot that navigates its environment through growth." *Science robotics* 2(8) (2017) eaan3028. http://robotics.sciencemag.org/
[13] Zhao, Wenchuan, Zhang, Yu, and Wang, Ning. "Soft robotics: Research, challenges, and prospects." *Journal of Robotics and Mechatronics* 33 (1) (2021) 45–68. https://doi.org/10.20965/jrm.2021.p0045
[14] Razavykia, A., Brusa, E., Delprete, C., Yavari, R., An overview of additive manufacturing in numerical study of selective laser melting (September, 2020). https://doi.org/10.3390/ma13173895
[15] Elkaseer, Ahmed, et al. "Effect of process parameters on the performance of drop-on-demand 3D inkjet printing: Geometrical-based modeling and experimental validation." *Polymers* 14 (13) (2022): 2557. https://doi.org/10.3390/polym14132557
[16] Zaidi, Shadab, et al. "Actuation technologies for soft robot grippers and manipulators: A review." *Current Robotics Reports* 2 (3) (2021) 355–369. https://doi.org/10.1007/s43154-021-00054-5
[17] Vasios, Nikolaos, et al. "Harnessing viscous flow to simplify the actuation of fluidic soft robots." *Soft Robotics* 7 (1) (2020) 1–9. https://doi.org/10.1089/soro.2018.0149
[18] Youn, J.H., et al., Dielectric elastomer actuator for soft robotics applications and challenges, *Applied Sciences* 10 (2) (2020). https://doi.org/10.3390/app10020640
[19] McDonald, Kevin, et al. "Magnetorheological fluid-based flow control for soft robots." *Advanced Intelligent Systems* 2 (11) (2020) 2000139. https://doi.org/10.1002/aisy.202000139
[20] Sadeghi, Alì, Beccai, Lucia, and Mazzolai, Barbara. "Innovative soft robots based on electro-rheological fluids." *2012 IEEE/RSJ International Conference on Intelligent Robots and Systems*. IEEE, 2012. https://doi.org/10.1109/IROS.2012.6385846
[21] Trivedi, D., Rahn, C.D., Kier, W.M., Walker, I.D. Soft robotics: Biological inspiration, state of the art, and future research. *Applied Bionics and Biomechanics* 2008;5 (3) 99–117. https://doi.org/10.1080/11762320802557865

[22] Wehner, M. et al. Pneumatic energy sources for autonomous and wearable soft robotics. *Soft Robotics* 2014;1 (4) 263–274. https://doi.org/10.1089/soro.2014.0018

[23] Ashuri, T. et al. "Biomedical soft robots: current status and perspective." *Biomedical Engineering Letters* 10 (2020) 369–385. https://doi.org/10.1007/s13534-020-00157-6

Chapter 13

Advances in design and manufacturing of soft robotic applications

Shaik Himam Saheb and Tharakeshwar Appala

13.1 INTRODUCTION

The field of soft robotics has remarkable advancements in recent years, driven by the increasing demand for flexible, adaptable, and safe robotic systems that can seamlessly integrate with human environments and perform a wide range of tasks. The key principle underlying soft robotics is the incorporation of compliance, which enables these systems to interact with their surroundings with greater adaptability and robustness, much like natural organisms.

One of the primary areas of focus in soft robotics research has been the development of novel materials and actuation mechanisms that can provide the necessary flexibility and deformability. Soft materials, such as elastomers, hydrogels, and shape-memory alloys, have been extensively explored for their ability to undergo large deformations without compromising structural integrity [1, 2]. These materials have enabled the creation of soft robotic actuators that can mimic the movements and functionalities of biological systems, opening up new possibilities for applications in areas like biomedical robotics, adaptive manufacturing, and assistive technologies [3, 4].

The field of soft robotics has also benefited from advancements in computational modeling and simulation tools. These tools have helped researchers and engineers understand the complex dynamics and control challenges associated with soft systems, allowing for the design and optimization of soft robotic components and systems.

13.2 IMPORTANCE OF SOFT ROBOTICS DESIGN

For any product or mechanism or machine, the need and design are most crucial elements. The diabetic and blood pressure cases are increasing in the world because of which the importance of minimally vascular surgery is increased. The medical industries need precise and accurate tools to cover these issues. Soft robotics covers all the major problems of medical diagnosis including minimally vascular surgery and rehabilitation. The soft robotics

DOI: 10.1201/9781003539612-13

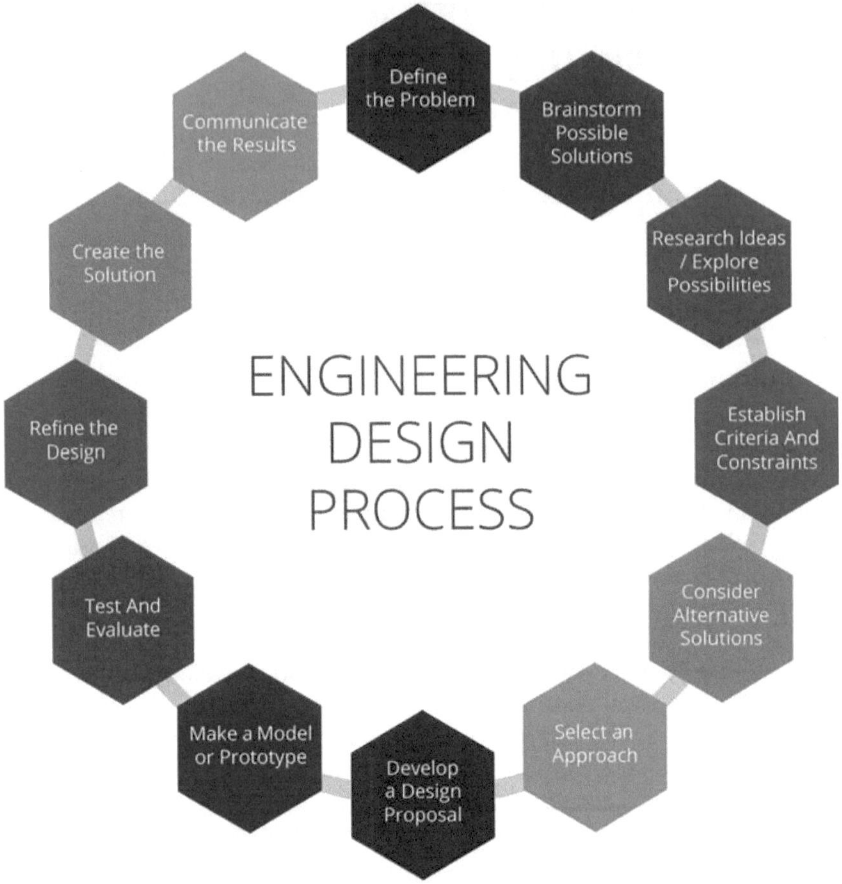

Figure 13.1 The design process.

represents a significant advancement in robotic technology, focusing on creating robots made from flexible materials that can safely interact with humans and delicate environments. The design of these soft robotic systems is crucial for their effectiveness and applicability, particularly in fields like healthcare, rehabilitation, and assistive technologies [5]. The design always starts from need or defining of the problem. The detailed design process is shown in Figure 13.1. The integration of various mechanical and electrical design software plays a vital role in this process, enhancing both the design and the functionality of soft robots [6].

13.2.1 Enhanced design accuracy

The advent of computer-aided design (CAD) software, including tools like SolidWorks and AutoCAD, has significantly transformed the engineering landscape, particularly in the design of soft robotic systems. These software platforms enable engineers to create intricate and precise three-dimensional (3D) models, which are essential for visualizing the complex geometries often found in soft robotics. By providing a detailed representation of the robotic components, CAD software allows engineers to explore design possibilities and refine their concepts before any physical prototypes are built.

One of the advantages of CAD software is its capability to calculate geometric tolerances with a high degree of accuracy. In soft robotics, where flexibility and adaptability are key, ensuring that all parts meet specified dimensional tolerances is critical. CAD tools allow engineers to simulate and analyze how variations in dimensions might affect the performance of the system. This attention to detail not only ensures a proper fit among the components but also contributes to the overall reliability and functionality of the robot [7]. By identifying and addressing tolerance issues early in the design process, engineers can mitigate potential complications during assembly and operation. CAD software plays a crucial role in assessing weight distribution and space availability for various components. Soft robotic systems often require careful consideration of how weight is distributed across the design to maintain balance and efficiency during movement [8]. CAD programs provide engineers with tools to analyze and optimize this distribution, ensuring that the robotic system performs as intended. Furthermore, these software tools help determine the spatial constraints for miscellaneous parts, such as sensors, actuators, and control systems, allowing engineers to design compact, efficient solutions without sacrificing performance.

The precision achieved through CAD modeling is vital for ensuring that all components of the robotic system fit together seamlessly. In soft robotics, even minor misalignments can lead to significant performance issues or operational failures. By enabling engineers to simulate the interactions between various parts within the virtual environment, CAD software helps identify potential conflicts or design flaws before they manifest in physical prototypes. This foresight is crucial for creating robots that can operate effectively in real-world conditions, where flexibility and adaptability are essential [9].

The accuracy of CAD modeling directly contributes to cost and time savings throughout the development process. By allowing for comprehensive design validation and modification in the virtual space, engineers can significantly reduce the likelihood of costly errors that might arise during the prototyping and manufacturing phases. The ability to troubleshoot and refine designs before moving to production not only prevents expensive reworks but also accelerates project timelines. This efficiency is particularly important in industries where rapid innovation is a competitive advantage, as it allows teams to bring their soft robotic solutions to market more swiftly and effectively [10].

The use of CAD software such as SolidWorks and AutoCAD is indispensable in the design and development of soft robotic systems. These tools facilitate precise 3D modeling, enable accurate calculations of geometric tolerances, and assist in evaluating weight distribution and spatial constraints. The resulting precision ensures seamless integration of components, crucial for the functionality of the robotic system. Furthermore, the accurate modeling capabilities of CAD software help prevent costly errors during prototyping and manufacturing, ultimately leading to significant time and resource savings. As the field of soft robotics continues to advance, the importance of such sophisticated design tools will only become more pronounced, underpinning the creation of increasingly capable and innovative robotic solutions [11].

13.2.2 Complex geometries and topologies

Soft robotics represents a captivating intersection of engineering and biology, where the aim is to create robotic systems that mimic the flexibility and movement of natural organisms. This pursuit often demands intricate designs that traditional rigid robots simply cannot achieve. Advanced modeling software such as Rhino and Blender have emerged as essential tools in this field, empowering designers to craft complex geometries and innovative topologies that enhance the functionality of soft robots [12].

One of the features of software like Rhino and Blender is their ability to manipulate curves and surfaces with a level of precision and flexibility that is vital for soft robotic design. Unlike traditional CAD programs, which may be more suited to linear and rigid shapes, these advanced modeling tools allow designers to explore organic forms and fluid structures. This capability is particularly important in soft robotics, where the goal is often to replicate the nuanced movements and adaptable shapes found in nature. For instance, the design of a soft robotic gripper might require intricate curves and folds that can conform to various objects, providing a secure grip without damaging delicate items.

These software applications facilitate the optimization of designs for performance. By enabling designers to simulate and analyze how different geometries respond to forces and motions, Rhino and Blender support the development of soft robots that are not only aesthetically pleasing but also functionally superior. This optimization process is critical when designing robots intended for delicate manipulation tasks, such as surgical applications or handling fragile objects. The ability to fine-tune designs based on simulated performance ensures that the resulting soft robots can achieve the necessary dexterity and responsiveness required for these specialized tasks.

Designers can quickly create and modify their models, testing various configurations without the need for extensive physical trials. This iterative approach not only accelerates the development timeline but also fosters innovation, as designers can experiment with unconventional shapes and mechanisms that might not have been considered feasible with traditional design methods. The ability to visualize and manipulate designs in real time enhances collaboration among interdisciplinary teams, bringing together engineers, biologists, and artists to create more effective soft robotic solutions [13].

13.2.3 Simulation and testing

Simulation tools such as ANSYS or COMSOL Multiphysics allow engineers to test their designs virtually under various conditions. By simulating the physical behaviors of soft robotic components such as deformation and movement, designers can assess performance metrics and identify potential failure points before creating physical prototypes. This ability to conduct virtual testing enhances the reliability of the final product and accelerates the development process. The operation of soft robots relies heavily on sophisticated control systems. Software like MATLAB/Simulink provides tools for modeling and simulating control algorithms, enabling engineers to develop systems that manage the interactions between soft actuators and sensors. This capability is crucial for achieving precise movements and adapting to varying environmental conditions [14].

13.2.4 Material optimization

The choice of materials is critical in soft robotic design. Software that incorporates material properties helps engineers select appropriate elastomers, hydrogels, or other flexible materials tailored for specific applications. This optimization ensures that the soft robot not only performs well but also meets safety and durability standards. Soft robots often incorporate sensors and actuators for enhanced functionality. Electrical design software, such as Altium Designer or Eagle, enables engineers to create efficient circuit designs and PCB layouts that can be integrated into soft robotic systems. This integration is essential for ensuring that the robotic system operates smoothly and responds accurately to user inputs.

13.2.5 Collaboration and prototyping

Collaboration is key in multidisciplinary teams working on soft robotics projects. Platforms like Fusion 360 facilitate real-time collaboration, allowing mechanical, electrical, and software engineers to work together seamlessly. This collaborative environment fosters innovation and leads to more comprehensive design solutions. The integration of design software with 3D printing technology allows for rapid prototyping of soft robotic systems. This capability accelerates the iteration process, enabling designers to quickly test and refine their concepts based on real-world performance. Rapid prototyping not only speeds up development but also encourages experimentation and creativity. The importance of soft robotic design cannot be overstated, particularly when enhanced by mechanical and electrical design software. These tools enable accurate modeling, complex simulations, and effective integration of materials and components, ultimately leading to more effective and innovative soft robotic solutions. As technology continues to advance, leveraging these software tools will be essential in unlocking the full potential of soft robotics across various applications, especially in healthcare and rehabilitation, where the need for safe and adaptable robotic systems is growing rapidly [15].

13.3 MANUFACTURING OF SOFT ROBOTS

Soft robotics is an innovative field that focuses on the design and creation of robots from flexible, compliant materials. These robots are particularly beneficial in applications that require gentle interactions, such as in healthcare and rehabilitation. The manufacturing of soft robots involves various techniques, each suited to specific materials and applications. This chapter details the most prominent methods for fabricating soft robotic systems.

- **Additive Manufacturing Process:** 3D printing, or additive manufacturing, is one of the most versatile methods for creating soft robotic components. It allows for the production of complex geometries that are difficult to achieve with traditional manufacturing methods. The additive manufacturing process is shown in Figure 13.2. Materials include flexible thermoplastics (like TPU) and specialized silicones that provide the necessary compliance. Fused deposition modeling (FDM) and stereolithography (SLA) are widely used. FDM is particularly effective for producing soft structures with varying stiffness, while SLA can achieve high-resolution details. Rapid prototyping, customization, and reduced material waste make 3D printing an attractive option for soft robotics.

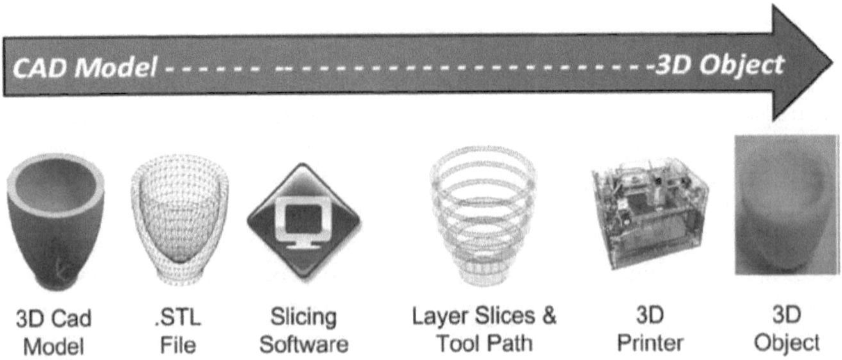

Figure 13.2 Stages in additive manufacturing [16].

3D printing and soft robotics are at the forefront of technological innovation, merging to create flexible, adaptive systems that can revolutionize various fields. The ability to 3D print complex, customized geometries is particularly advantageous for soft robotics, which relies on materials that can deform and mimic natural movements. This technology allows for rapid prototyping, enabling engineers to quickly iterate on designs tailored for specific applications. Soft robots have numerous applications, particularly in medicine, where they are being developed for minimally invasive surgeries, reducing damage to surrounding tissues due to their flexible structures. Wearable soft exosuits are being designed to assist individuals with mobility impairments, combining support with comfort. In industrial settings, soft robots excel at delicate tasks like gripping fragile objects, making them ideal for agriculture and electronics assembly. The field faces challenges, including the need for effective actuation methods, such as pneumatic or hydraulic systems, to replicate natural movements, as well as ensuring the durability of soft materials for long-term use. Moreover, advanced control systems are required to manage the intricate dynamics of soft robots, which adds complexity to their design and functionality. Looking ahead, integrating artificial intelligence (AI) into soft robotics can enhance their adaptability and autonomy, while bio-inspired designs and the use of sustainable materials in 3D printing promise to push the boundaries of innovation. Together, 3D printing and soft robotics offer exciting opportunities to develop more efficient, versatile, and environmentally friendly solutions across a wide range of industries, paving the way for future advancements in technology.

- **Soft Lithography** [17]: Soft lithography is a microfabrication technique that utilizes elastomeric materials to create detailed structures. It involves creating a mold from a hard substrate (often using photolithography), which is then filled with a liquid silicone elastomer. After curing, the mold is removed to reveal the soft robotic component. Typically, polydimethylsiloxane (PDMS) is employed due to its excellent mechanical properties and biocompatibility. This method is particularly effective for creating soft actuators and sensors with intricate designs, such as those used in soft grippers.

These techniques allow researchers to design compliant materials that can deform and adapt to their environments, which is vital for soft robots that mimic biological systems. Soft lithography is particularly effective for fabricating microfluidic systems, enabling precise control over pneumatic or hydraulic actuation in soft robots. This capability supports rapid prototyping, allowing for quick iterations and testing of innovative designs. Additionally, the technique facilitates the integration of sensors within soft structures, enhancing their ability to perceive and respond to environmental changes. Applications of soft robots developed through soft lithography span various fields, including medical devices for minimally invasive surgeries, delicate grippers for fragile objects, and wearable technology for rehabilitation. As soft lithography continues to evolve, it holds great promise for advancing soft robotics, paving the way for more sophisticated, adaptable, and efficient robotic systems.

Inflation techniques are used to create soft actuators that can expand and contract, mimicking biological movement. This method involves creating a sealed, flexible structure that is inflated with air or liquid to produce motion. The design often includes valves or chambers that control the inflation process. Soft polymers or elastomers are used to ensure compliance and flexibility. Inflation-based soft robots are widely used in applications requiring soft gripping or delicate interactions, such as in medical devices [18].

- **Knitting and Weaving:** Textile techniques like knitting and weaving are gaining traction in soft robotics for creating soft actuators and structures. These techniques involve crafting soft robotic components from fibers, which can then be infused with materials like silicone for added functionality. Fabrics made from elastic fibers or yarns are common, often combined with silicone coatings to enhance performance. This method allows for lightweight and highly flexible designs, making it suitable for wearable robotics and soft exoskeletons.
- **Electrospinning [19]:** Electrospinning is a versatile technique used to create nanofibers from various materials, and it plays a significant role in advancing soft robotics. This process involves applying a high-voltage electric field to a polymer solution, which stretches the solution into fine fibers that can be collected on a surface. These nanofibers can be arranged in various architectures, leading to lightweight, flexible materials that mimic biological tissues. In soft robotics, electrospun materials are crucial for developing soft actuators, sensors, and other components. The unique properties of electrospun fibers, such as high surface area and tunable mechanical properties, enable the creation of highly responsive soft robotic structures. For example, electrospun mats can be used to fabricate actuators that respond to stimuli like heat or electricity, allowing for smooth and adaptive movements. This technique facilitates the incorporation of functional elements, such as conductive fibers for sensing or actuation. Applications range from medical devices that adapt to the human body to robots designed for delicate handling tasks. As electrospinning technology advances, it promises to enhance the capabilities and performance of soft robotics, opening new avenues for innovation in various fields.
- **Bio-inspired Manufacturing:** Bio-inspired manufacturing draws inspiration from natural processes and organisms to create soft robots. This approach often involves mimicking biological structures and mechanisms, such as the way muscles contract or how certain animals move. Techniques like self-assembly, where components spontaneously

organize into functional structures, can be used to create soft actuators that mimic muscle movement. This method allows for the creation of highly adaptive and efficient robotic systems that can perform complex tasks similar to their biological counterparts.

- **Origami and Kirigami Techniques:** Origami and kirigami techniques involve folding and cutting materials to create complex 3D structures. By strategically folding or cutting flat sheets of material, designers can produce soft robots that change shape and functionality when manipulated. These techniques can be applied to various materials, including polymers and textiles. Soft robots designed using origami principles can be deployed in confined spaces and expand when needed, such as in minimally invasive surgical applications. This method allows for lightweight structures that can transition between multiple configurations, enhancing versatility [20].
- **Self-Healing Materials:** The use of self-healing materials in soft robotics introduces an innovative approach to maintaining robotic functionality. Self-healing materials can automatically repair damage after being cut or punctured. This involves incorporating microcapsules containing healing agents that react upon rupture. Soft robots made with self-healing materials can maintain operational integrity in dynamic environments, such as underwater exploration or surgical applications where wear and tear are common. This capability extends the lifespan of soft robotic systems and reduces maintenance needs, enhancing reliability.
- **Shape Memory Alloys (SMAs):** SMAs are materials that can return to a predetermined shape when exposed to a specific stimulus, such as temperature changes. SMAs can be integrated into soft robotic designs to create actuators that respond dynamically to environmental conditions. These materials can be used in soft grippers that adapt their shape based on the objects they handle, providing a gentle touch in applications like prosthetics or rehabilitation devices. The ability to change shape allows for high adaptability and responsiveness, essential for interacting with variable environments [21].
- **Electroactive Polymers (EAPs):** EPAs change shape or size when an electric field is applied, providing a mechanism for actuation in soft robots. EAPs can be designed into soft actuators that contract or expand in response to electrical stimuli, enabling controlled movement. These materials are particularly useful in soft robotics applications requiring precision movements, such as in surgical tools or soft exoskeletons. EAPs offer lightweight, low-power solutions for actuation, making them ideal for mobile and wearable robots [22].
- **Liquid-Based Manufacturing:** Liquid-based manufacturing methods involve the use of liquid materials that can solidify into soft structures. Techniques such as liquid deposition modeling (LDM) or using hydrogels allow for the creation of soft robots that can change shape

and functionality based on fluid dynamics. Soft robots that utilize liquid-based materials can perform tasks that require flexibility and compliance, such as in robotic surgeries or drug delivery systems. This method can lead to the development of robots that are highly adaptable to their environments, with the ability to reconfigure based on task requirements.

13.3.1 Manufacturing intelligence

Manufacturing intelligence and soft robotics are converging to revolutionize production processes, enhancing efficiency, adaptability, and precision in various industries. Manufacturing intelligence encompasses advanced data analytics, AI, and machine learning, enabling smarter decision-making and optimized operations. When integrated with soft robotics, which employs flexible, adaptive structures, this synergy creates a powerful framework for modern manufacturing. The key capabilities of this integration are shown in Figure 13.3. Manufacturing intelligence systems can analyze data from sensors embedded in soft robots to monitor performance, detect anomalies, and predict maintenance needs.

This capability minimizes downtime and ensures continuous operation, which is critical for maintaining production schedules. Soft robotics, known for their gentle handling and versatility, can adapt to a variety of tasks, making them ideal for assembly lines that require the manipulation of fragile or irregularly shaped objects. Their inherent flexibility allows for seamless

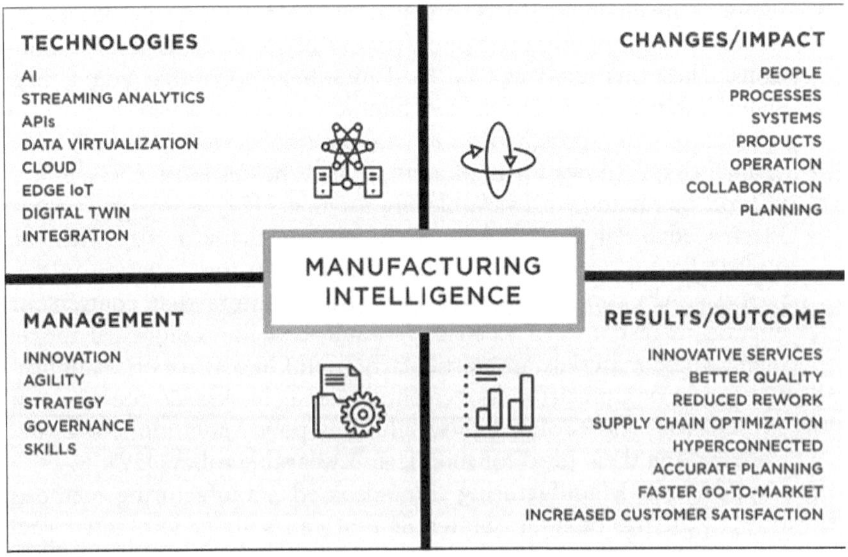

Figure 13.3 Capabilities of manufacturing intelligence.

collaboration with human workers, enhancing safety and productivity in shared workspaces. Additionally, the ability to quickly reprogram soft robots for different tasks offers manufacturers the agility needed to respond to changing demands. This combination of manufacturing intelligence and soft robotics facilitates advanced automation. Intelligent algorithms can optimize the movements and actions of soft robots, leading to improved efficiency and reduced energy consumption. This optimization can be particularly beneficial in sectors like food processing, electronics, and healthcare, where precision and care are paramount.

The integration of manufacturing intelligence with soft robotics is poised to drive innovation, enabling smarter factories that are more responsive to market needs. This synergy not only enhances productivity but also contributes to sustainable manufacturing practices by minimizing waste and optimizing resource usage. Together, they represent a significant leap forward in the future of manufacturing.

13.4 MECHANISMS USED IN SOFT ROBOTICS

The mechanism of any robot plays a major role for desirable motions. The researchers [23–26] studied various soft robotic motions. The field of soft robotics has gained significant attention due to its potential to create flexible, adaptable systems that can safely interact with humans and navigate complex environments. Central to the effectiveness of these robots is the mechanism by which they operate, influencing their design, functionality, and manufacturing processes. Understanding the importance of mechanisms in soft robots is crucial for developing systems that can perform tasks efficiently while ensuring safety and adaptability.

The mechanism of a soft robot dictates its ability to perform specific tasks. Unlike traditional rigid robots, soft robots rely on flexible materials and novel mechanisms to achieve motion and interaction. Various actuation methods, such as pneumatic, hydraulic, and SMAs, enable soft robots to achieve movements that mimic biological organisms. For instance, pneumatic actuators allow for smooth, gentle movements that are essential in applications like surgical assistance or rehabilitation. The choice of mechanism directly impacts the robot's motion capabilities. Mechanisms that allow for multi-directional movement, such as those inspired by octopus limbs or insect legs, enhance the robot's versatility. By integrating compliant mechanisms, designers can create robots that not only perform complex tasks but also adapt to unpredictable environments.

Soft robots are designed to operate in close proximity to humans, making safety a paramount consideration. The mechanisms employed in these robots play a crucial role in ensuring that they can operate safely without causing harm. Mechanisms that allow for compliance—such as soft actuators—enable robots to absorb impacts and adapt their shapes during interactions.

This characteristic is particularly important in healthcare settings, where soft robots can assist patients without risking injury. Implementing feedback mechanisms that provide real-time data about the robot's interaction with its environment enhances safety. For example, incorporating sensors that detect pressure or proximity allows soft robots to adjust their movements dynamically, preventing accidents.

13.5 CONCLUSIONS

The rapid evolution of soft robotics presents transformative potential, particularly in the medical and healthcare sectors. By focusing on the design and manufacturing processes of soft robotic systems, this chapter underscores their distinct advantages over traditional rigid robots, such as adaptability, safety, and user-friendly interaction. The exploration of advanced materials, including silicones and hydrogels, alongside innovative actuation strategies like pneumatic systems and SMAs, highlights the technical progress driving the field forward.

The integration of sophisticated sensors is pivotal in enhancing the functionality and responsiveness of soft robots, enabling them to interact more effectively with users in various applications. However, the chapter also addresses critical challenges in scaling production and ensuring the reliability of these systems, which are essential for their widespread adoption in medical environments. Design aspects and software used in design of robots and analysis also covered in this chapter. The advancements discussed promise significant implications for future medical applications, particularly in minimally invasive surgeries, rehabilitation therapies, and improved patient care. The advancements in the mechanical, mechatronics, and metallurgical processes enhance the application range of soft robots due to their added flexibilities in the healthcare industries.

REFERENCES

[1] Korde, J. M., & Kandasubramanian, B. (2020). Naturally biomimicked smart shape memory hydrogels for biomedical functions. *Chemical Engineering Journal*, 379, 122430.

[2] Huang, X., Ford, M., Patterson, Z. J., Zarepoor, M., Pan, C., & Majidi, C. (2020). Shape memory materials for electrically-powered soft machines. *Journal of Materials Chemistry B*, 8(21), 4539–4551.

[3] Cianchetti, M., Laschi, C., Menciassi, A., & Dario, P. (2018). Biomedical applications of soft robotics. *Nature Reviews Materials*, 3(6), 143–153.

[4] https://www.twi-global.com/technical-knowledge/faqs/engineering-design-process

[5] Cianchetti, M., Laschi, C., Menciassi, A., & Dario, P. (2018). Biomedical applications of soft robotics. *Nature Reviews Materials*, 3(6), 143–153.

[6] Schegg, P., & Duriez, C. (2022). Review on generic methods for mechanical modeling, simulation and control of soft robots. *PLoS One*, 17(1), e0251059.
[7] Bock, T., & Linner, T. (2015). *Robot oriented design.* Cambridge university press.
[8] Polygerinos, P., Correll, N., Morin, S. A., Mosadegh, B., Onal, C. D., Petersen, K., ... & Shepherd, R. F. (2017). Soft robotics: Review of fluid-driven intrinsically soft devices; manufacturing, sensing, control, and applications in human-robot interaction. *Advanced Engineering Materials*, 19(12), 1700016.
[9] Ostrowski, A. K. (2023). *How Do We Design Robots Equitably? Engaging Design Justice, Design Fictions, and Co-Design in Human-Robot Interaction Design and Policymaking Processes* (Doctoral dissertation, Massachusetts Institute of Technology).
[10] Jin, B. E., Cedrola, E., & Kim, N. (2019). Innovation: Hidden Secret to Success and Efficiency. In: Jin, B., Cedrola, E. (eds) *Process Innovation in the Global Fashion Industry. Palgrave Studies in Practice: Global Fashion Brand Management.* Palgrave Pivot, New York. https://doi.org/10.1057/978-1-137-52352-5_1
[11] Rajagopalan, P., Muthu, M., Liu, Y., Luo, J., Wang, X., & Wan, C. (2022). Advancement of electroadhesion technology for intelligent and self-reliant robotic applications. *Advanced Intelligent Systems*, 4(7), 2200064.
[12] Kim, J. (2019). *Modular Systems for Fabrication: Toward a Collaborative Partnership between Humans and Machines* (Doctoral dissertation, University of Colorado at Boulder).
[13] Kim, Y. E., Morton, B. G., Gregorio, J., Rosen, D. S., Edouard, K., & Vallett, R. (2019). Enabling creative collaboration for all levels of learning. *Proceedings of the National Academy of Sciences*, 116(6), 1878–1885.
[14] Hines, L., Petersen, K., Lum, G. Z., & Sitti, M. (2017). Soft actuators for small-scale robotics. *Advanced Materials*, 29(13), 1603483.
[15] Chandrashekhar, A. S., Pavan Kishore, M. L. (2021). Investigation of the static and dynamic path planning of mobile and aerial robots. *Computer Networks and Inventive Communication Technologies: Proceedings of Third ICCNCT 2020*, 1033–1044.
[16] Saheb, S. H. (2024). Applications of 3D printing in medical, engineering, agricultural, and other sectors. In *Additive Manufacturing of Bio-implants: Design and Synthesis* (pp. 159–176). Singapore: Springer Nature Singapore.
[17] Xia, Y., & Whitesides, G. M. (1998). Soft lithography. *Angewandte Chemie International Edition*, 37(5), 550–575.
[18] Babu, S. H., & Raju, N. S. (2018, December). Relative kinematic analysis of serial and parallel manipulators. In *IOP Conference Series: Materials Science and Engineering* (Vol. 455, No. 1, p. 012040). IOP Publishing.
[19] Sarkar, K., Gomez, C., Zambrano, S., Ramirez, M., De Hoyos, E., Vasquez, H., & Lozano, K. (2010). Electrospinning to forcespinning™. *Materials Today*, 13(11), 12–14..
[20] Plocher, J., & Panesar, A. (2019). Review on design and structural optimisation in additive manufacturing: Towards next-generation lightweight structures. *Materials & Design*, 183, 108164.
[21] Mazzolai, B., Mondini, A., Del Dottore, E., Margheri, L., Carpi, F., Suzumori, K., ... & Lendlein, A. (2022). Roadmap on soft robotics: multifunctionality, adaptability and growth without borders. *Multifunctional Materials*, 5(3), 032001.

[22] Bar-Cohen, Y. (2002, July). Electroactive polymers: current capabilities and challenges. In *Smart Structures and Materials 2002: Electroactive Polymer Actuators and Devices (EAPAD)* (Vol. 4695, pp. 1–7). SPIE.
[23] Fei, Y., & Xu, H. (2016). Modeling and motion control of a soft robot. *IEEE Transactions on Industrial Electronics*, 64(2), 1737–1742.
[24] Yao, D. R., Kim, I., Yin, S., & Gao, W. (2024). Multimodal soft robotic actuation and locomotion. *Advanced Materials*, 36(19), 2308829.
[25] Garriga-Casanovas, A., Shakib, F., Ferrandy, V., & Franco, E. (2024, June). Hybrid Control of Soft Robotic Manipulator. In *Actuators* (Vol. 13, No. 7, p. 242). MDPI.
[26] Qin, L., Peng, H., Huang, X., Liu, M., & Huang, W. (2024). Modeling and simulation of dynamics in soft robotics: A review of numerical approaches. *Current Robotics Reports*, 5(1), 1–13.

Chapter 14

Soft robotics

Current opportunities and challenges

Prateek Mishra and Harpal Singh Kalra

14.1 INTRODUCTION

Robots are typically manufactured using rigid materials such as composites, various metals and nonmetals. Natural systems are composed of flexible components. These natural components are full of elasticity and flexibility, which help ensure survival in diverse environments. The bodies of living organisms are made up of soft components, such as skin and hair, which are formed from flexible fibers. Conventional robots operate based on pre-programmed instructions, while natural systems continuously learn and provide input to their neural circuitry, allowing for surprising modifications in body structures. Traditional robots, built with hard materials, often lack accessibility, adaptability, freedom of movement, and effective communication. (Ahmed et al., 2022).

Soft robots are more flexible and more capable compared to hard robots. Soft robots dynamically change its shape and tolerate elastic pressures. Optimum flexibility in soft robots makes such robots more dynamic and smarter and conforms to bending and twisting around obstacles in divergent fields such as extremely narrow medical surgery where access of human is impossible.

Soft robots are better updated versions of hard robots. Hard-bodied robots are usually programmed to perform specific tasks but these robots have generally limited capability due to the hardness of the substances used to manufacture these robots that is why these robots encounter difficulties in the sudden changing conditions. Since delicate robots are manufactured using highly elastic materials, they perform quick and secure interaction even in changing conditions with optimum degree of freedom. Smooth robots have a greater impact in day-to-day human life. For example, noninvasive smooth robots are being used in the healthcare field such as in endoscopy, in Neuro and Cardiac surgery, and in the transportation of drugs in sensitive and delicate places in the human and animal body.

DOI: 10.1201/9781003539612-14

Soft robotics is an emerging field and is in its nascent state. The domain of soft robotics usually deals machines that are optimally gentle (Collins et al., 2005). Gentle characteristics in robots offer benefits such as reduced injury risk, noninvasive interaction, enhanced adaptability, etc. (Pfeifer et al., 2007). Soft robots can also have capability to prevent accidents and are natural enough of being biocompatible and compliant resistant. This field is basically under experiment and under test and not much literature is available about this field till date. According to Trivedi et al. (2008) & Ilievski (2011), novel developed smart materials, sensing components, and actuating parts are combined into microrobots of divergent kinds. The replica design of animal bending and movement (Floreano et al., 2009) has been developed for re-configurable robots (Hara and Pfeifer, 2003; Yim et al., 2007).

Requirements of soft robotic functions (Albu-Schaffer et al., 2008) demand more biocompatibility with the further requirements of the development of trustworthy novel technologies in multiple sectors such as social sector, medical sector, and industrial sector. The main purpose of designing soft robots is the efforts to create the exact copy of natural creatures (Laschi et al., 2009) but it is still a herculean task. Arithmetic developed over the past centuries for the design of rigid bodies commonly fails to extend to smooth robots. Smooth robots are still not performing as per expectations. Hence more research and development is needed to be focused (Brown et al., 2010): (i) In re-engineering novel materials for better interfacing between gentle and hard robotic components that must allow multifunctional delicate robots for autohealing, autosensing, and autogrowth. (ii) In the development of optimum algorithms for optimum performance. (iii) In the development of adaptive architectures for situation-based performance. The ongoing phase of robotics is the transition phase from hard robots to soft robots as shown in Figure 14.1. During this transition phase, limitations (Cons) of hard robots such as complexity and rigidity (limited flexibility) are being removed with the development of technology, and concepts and softness (Pros) such as adaptability and flexibility are being increased.

14.2 LITERATURE REVIEW

- According to Iida & Laschi (2011), implementing delicate raw materials to create robots presents new technological issues and challenges. Among these challenges are the development of novel technologies for soft materials actuation to implant sensors into delicate parts of soft robots and to gently control soft robots.
- Lipson (2014) elaborated that unlike hard robotics the soft robotics presents new opportunities and new challenges and demands out-of-the-box research and development of novel technology.

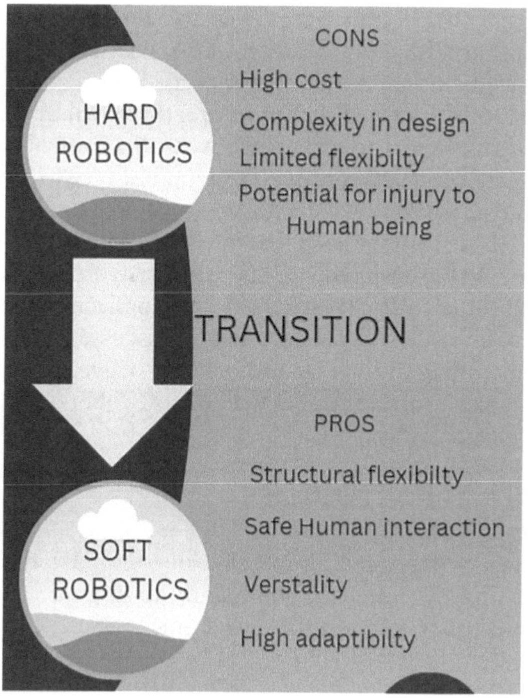

Figure 14.1 Transition from hard robotics to soft robotics (original figure).

- Feinberg (2015) presented a study on complexity and functionality of natural systems so as to encourage the creation of replica of these features in biological soft robots.
- Laschi et al. (2009) stated that soft robotics is in its nascent research and development stage. Research and development in soft robotics presents new challenges and demands for new technological development.
- Polygerinos et al. (2017) put their focus on intrinsically soft robots due to its compliant independent nature, reduced control complexity, and low manufacturing cost.
- Wang et al. (2018) mentioned that there is a gap between availability of numerous soft sensing technologies and its effective utilization in practical scenarios.
- Appiah et al. (2019) proposed that a new version of soft robots "bio-hybrid soft robots" can address the recent challenges of self-healing, enabling soft touch, or showing situational adaptability.
- Yang et al. (2020) explain that soft robots are the better version of hard robots as diverse features are added in the harder version of robots to build the robots more and more softer.

- Tawk & Alici (2021) expect that in establishing functional soft robotic systems, soft and functional materials can be used that meet the applications and functional requirements of the robotic systems.
- Zhu et al. (2022) asserted that in future, there will be opportunities to develop wearable soft robots. These wearable soft robots such as tiny healthcare robots may improve the troubles faced in the day-to-day human life.
- Chen et al. (2023) emphasized that intelligent microrobots can be developed by adding bio-inspired intelligence with hydrogel soft microrobots.
- López-Díaz et al. (2024) analyzed the applications of hydrogel in incurring softness in soft robots and also discussed the limitations that prevent edits utilization. The authors also suggested future improvements to achieve softness in the field of soft robotics.

14.3 CURRENT OPPORTUNITIES

Based on the review presented above, the following are the opportunities for the research and development community to upgrade and enhance the capability of hard robots toward the development of complete soft robots.

14.3.1 Soft robotics compatible technology development

The development of soft robots requires the advancement in the current technologies especially that contributes toward the softness of hard robots. For being softer, the substances to be applied in delicate robots reduce stress and internal pressure and increase reformation (Majidi, 2019). Soft matter engineering can play a vital role in the development of soft robots as soft matter engineering reproduces stretchable materials (Majidi, 2019).

14.3.2 Complete conversion from hard robots to soft robots

For researchers, it is an opportunity to build a completely soft robot without any hardness such as a living being without bone, Octopus Robot. But in the development of these types of robots, there will also be the opportunities to solve the issues such as no locomotion (Majidi, 2019). The requirements of fully flexible and independent soft robots provide an opportunity to integrate flexible electronic devices (El-Atab et al., 2020).

14.3.3 Soft actuator development

Soft actuators (El-Atab et al., 2020) enable soft robots to deform, stretch, and compress, consequently allowing gentle interaction with the environment, for example, Pneumatic Actuators and Soft Textile Actuators. Various active, delicate, and elastic substances, for example, polymers and gels, have capacity to perform soft actuation.

14.3.4 Soft robots' control

Soft robots rely on autonomous control. To fully implement autonomous control, there is an opportunity to establish the highest level of coordination among actuator, model, sensor, and controller (Wang & Chortos, 2022). The highest level of coordination is now possible to maintain using rapidly emerging technology stretchable electronics.

14.3.5 μ-Organism-like soft robots' development

Microorganism-like robots generally have hard actuators (Ahmed et al., 2022) which provide an opportunity to replace it with soft actuators so as to increase the flexibility, adaptability, and autonomy and also to decrease the probability of damage. High power consumption in autonomous flight in μ-robots provides an opportunity either to develop contactless continuous energy resource for continuous energy consumption or to modify the architecture for optimum energy consumption.

14.3.6 Wearable soft robots' development

Bendable and delicate robots, such as RoboGlove and Rewalk, worn on the body of living beings are commonly called as wearable soft robots. There are opportunities to solve issues (Cianchetti et al., 2018) such as unexpected high temperature, exceptionally strong electric fields, and dangerous high electric currents so as to increase the usability of wearable soft robots. Technologies can be developed to solve these issues such as natural energy sources utilization to avoid electric socks so as to increase the usability of such wearable devices.

14.3.7 Untethered soft robots' development

These robots are battery dependent and its functionality is based on the Internet of Things (IoT). These robots perform contactless navigation without any hurdle and perform tasks such as search, rescue, etc. (Majid, 2019). But hurdle-free navigation needs an infinite energy source of battery. No such battery exists having infinite power. The lightweight low resource μ-soft robots have low-power battery that discharges rapidly. There are opportunities either to develop the technology of inbuilt recharge facility within the soft robot or a contactless recharge facility must be developed as the battery discharges. Using nanotechnology it is possible to develop a battery which will never discharge.

14.4 ENCOUNTERED CHALLENGES

14.4.1 Wearable soft robots' challenges

Wearable contactless soft robots are resource deficient as they have limited capacity components such as low-power battery. Battery power decay is the biggest hurdle in the active life cycle and in the autonomy of wearable devices. On the other hand, connected energy resources are again hurdle in autonomy of wearable soft robots. Connected energy resources present issues of unexpected high temperature, exceptionally strong electric fields, and dangerous high electric currents that not only damage wearable devices but also cause damages to the living being who wears these devices.

14.4.2 M-Organism-like soft robots' development challenges

According to Ahmed et al. (2022), generally μ-Organism-like soft robots such as aerial robots face the challenge of being hard actuators. Reduction in flexibility, adaptability thus increases in the probability of damage and denial of locomotion. Another challenge is a power autonomous flight in μ-soft robots that consumes high power which reduces time of flight (Ahmed et al., 2022).

14.4.3 Soft actuator development challenges

The portability (Cianchetti et al., 2018) of soft robots is confined and most of the actuation technologies are not compatible with soft robotics applications. There is no standard protocol that exists to standardize the characteristics of soft actuators. Hurdles in meeting the challenges of soft actuators are their mechanical properties such as strain & stress, actuator's response time, its noise sensitivity, actuator's size, its reliability, and its life cycle. Robots performance depends on stimuli parameters such as frequency, amplitude of the driving signals (El-Atab et al., 2020).

14.4.4 Soft materials development challenges

It is one of the challenging tasks to develop a completely soft robot because it requires completely soft material having no hardness at all. But completely soft materials present another challenge of denial of locomotion as experienced in the soft octopus robot (Majidi, 2019). Smart soft materials should be designed to achieve medical requirements in the soft robots used in health medical field (Cianchetti et al., 2018).

14.4.5 Untethered soft robots' challenges

Contactless navigation without any hurdle becomes a challenge since the soft materials used in soft robots do not support self-controlled functionality (Majid, 2019). Because soft materials need interfacing with hard microelectronics to perform signal processing and to allow communication. Hard microelectronics is a hurdle for flexibility. Battery power decay is another challenge in the freedom of action and autonomy of soft robots. Infinite contactless battery source and inbuilt battery recharging facility are still a challenge.

14.4.6 Soft robots control challenges

Control of soft robots is an ever-challenging issue due to elasticity, bending, twisting, stretching, compressing, buckling, wrinkling, etc. These motions need freedom of infinite degrees. Various new and advance methods have been proposed by Research & Development community to control soft robots' modeling, control, and dynamics. An ideal model considered for mobile soft robot is caterpillar (Rus & Tolley, 2015). But the control system is particularly affected by actuator, model, sensor, and controller (Wang & Chortos, 2022) which requires high coordination among these to attain autonomy in soft robots which is a challenging task; hence, fully controlled soft robots have not been built till date.

14.5 SOFTNESS CHARACTERISTICS

Unique characteristics that contribute to the softness of the soft robots are: (i) flexibility, (ii) adaptability, and (iii) autonomy in the components of soft robots in particular. Better the flexibility, adaptability, and autonomy, better will be the softness in the whole soft robotics system. Thus, mathematically these three characteristics are directly proportional to the softness of the soft robotics system as shown in Figure 14.2.

Thus, to maximize the softness in the soft robotics system, flexibility, adaptability, and autonomy of the soft robotics system need to maximized.

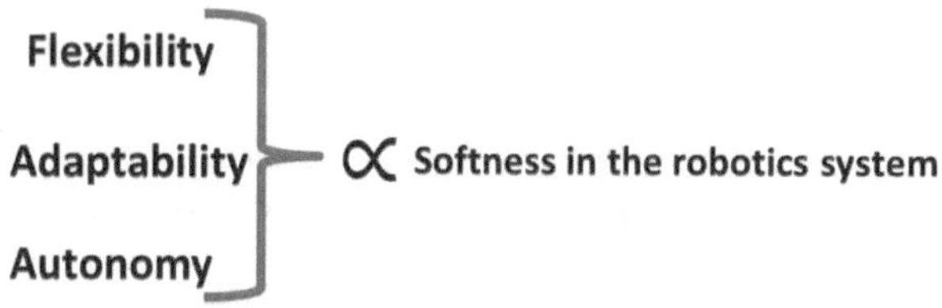

Figure 14.2 Relation between flexibility, adaptability, autonomy, and softness (original figure).

14.6 CONCLUSION

Soft robotics represents a promising frontier in robotics, with the potential to revolutionize a range of applications, particularly in fields such as medicine. The primary goal is to develop soft robots that exhibit complete softness, which entails achieving optimal flexibility, self-repairing capabilities, and self-healing properties. However, significant challenges remain in realizing these attributes. Key areas requiring further research include exploring innovative materials that enhance flexibility and studying the morphing structures that enable self-controlled systems. Currently, self-control remains a critical unresolved issue, necessitating new methodologies and concepts that facilitate the development of fully autonomous soft microrobots (μ-robots).

These μ-robots could have transformative effects in medical applications, particularly in prosthetics and rehabilitation devices, provided they achieve the requisite levels of flexibility, strain resistance, and safety under varying conditions. The challenge of modeling soft robots and expanding their degrees of freedom further complicates the landscape of soft robotics. To address these challenges, a dual focus on comprehensive training alongside research and development is essential. As the field of soft robotics is still in its infancy, sustained efforts will be crucial to unlock its full potential and achieve the goal of complete softness in soft robots. This journey will pave the way for groundbreaking advancements that could significantly enhance the quality of life in numerous sectors.

REFERENCES

Ahmed, F., Waqas, M., Jawed, B., Soomro, A. M., Kumar, S., Hina, A., ... & Choi, K. H. (2022). Decade of bio-inspired soft robots: A review. *Smart Materials and Structures*, 31(7), 073002.

Albu-Schaffer, A., Eiberger, O., Grebenstein, M., Haddadin, S., Ott, C., Wimbock, T., ...& Hirzinger, G. (2008). Soft robotics. *IEEE Robotics & Automation Magazine*, 15(3), 20–30.

Appiah, C., Arndt, C., Siemsen, K., Heitmann, A., Staubitz, A., & Selhuber-Unkel, C. (2019). Living materials herald a new era in soft robotics. *Advanced Materials*, 31(36), 1807747.

Brown, E., Rodenberg, N., Amend, J., Mozeika, A., Steltz, E., Zakin, M. R., ...& Jaeger, H. M. (2010). Universal robotic gripper based on the jamming of granular material. *Proceedings of the National Academy of Sciences*, 107(44), 18809–18814.

Chen, Y., Zhang, Y., Li, H., Shen, J., Zhang, F., He, J., ...& Guo, Z. (2023). Bioinspired hydrogel actuator for soft robotics: Opportunity and challenges. *Nano Today*, 49, 101764.

Cianchetti, M., Laschi, C., Menciassi, A., & Dario, P. (2018). Biomedical applications of soft robotics. *Nature Reviews Materials*, 3(6), 143–153.

Collins, S., Ruina, A., Tedrake, R., & Wisse, M. (2005). Efficient bipedal robots based on passive-dynamic walkers. *Science*, 307(5712), 1082–1085.

El-Atab, N., Mishra, R. B., Al-Modaf, F., Joharji, L., Alsharif, A. A., Alamoudi, H., ... & Hussain, M. M. (2020). Soft actuators for soft robotic applications: A review. *Advanced Intelligent Systems*, 2(10), 2000128.

Feinberg, A. W. (2015). Biological soft robotics. *Annual Review of Biomedical Engineering*, 17(1), 243–265.

Floreano, D., Zufferey, J. C., Srinivasan, M. V., & Ellington, C. (Eds.). (2009). *Flying insects and robots* (pp. 127–142). Berlin: Springer.

Hara, F., & Pfeifer, R. (Eds.). (2003). *Morpho-functional machines: The new species: Designing embodied intelligence*. Tokyo: Springer Science & Business Media.

Iida, F., & Laschi, C. (2011). Soft robotics: Challenges and perspectives. *Procedia Computer Science*, 7, 99–102.

Ilievski F., Mazzeo A.D., Shepherd R.F., Chen X., Whitesides G.M. Soft robotics for chemists, *Angewandte Chemie International Edition*, 50 (2011), pp. 1890–1895.

Laschi, C., Mazzolai, B., Mattoli, V., Cianchetti, M., & Dario, P. (2009). Design of a biomimetic robotic octopus arm. *Bioinspiration & Biomimetics*, 4(1), 015006.

Lipson, H. (2014). Challenges and opportunities for design, simulation, and fabrication of soft robots. *Soft Robotics*, 1(1), 21–27.

López-Díaz, A., Vázquez, A. S., & Vázquez, E. (2024). Hydrogels in Soft Robotics: Past, Present, and Future. *ACS Nano*, 18(32), 20817–20826.

Majidi, C. (2019). Soft-matter engineering for soft robotics. *Advanced Materials Technologies*, 4(2), 1800477.

Pfeifer, R., Lungarella, M., & Iida, F. (2007). Self-organization, embodiment, and biologically inspired robotics. *Science*, 318(5853), 1088–1093.

Polygerinos, P., Correll, N., Morin, S. A., Mosadegh, B., Onal, C. D., Petersen, K., ...& Shepherd, R. F. (2017). Soft robotics: Review of fluid-driven intrinsically soft devices; manufacturing, sensing, control, and applications in human-robot interaction. *Advanced Engineering Materials*, 19(12), 1700016.

Rus, D., & Tolley, M. T. (2015). Design, fabrication and control of soft robots. *Nature*, 521(7553), 467–475.

Tawk, C., & Alici, G. (2021). A review of 3D-printable soft pneumatic actuators and sensors: research challenges and opportunities. *Advanced Intelligent Systems*, 3(6), 2000223.

Trivedi, D., Rahn, C. D., Kier, W. M., & Walker, I. D. (2008). Soft robotics: Biological inspiration, state of the art, and future research. *Applied Bionics and Biomechanics*, 5(3), 99–117.

Wang, H., Totaro, M., & Beccai, L. (2018). Toward perceptive soft robots: Progress and challenges. *Advanced Science*, 5(9), 1800541.

Wang, J., & Chortos, A. (2022). Control strategies for soft robot systems. *Advanced Intelligent Systems*, 4(5), 2100165.

Yang, Y., Wu, Y., Li, C., Yang, X., & Chen, W. (2020). Flexible actuators for soft robotics. *Advanced Intelligent Systems*, 2(1), 1900077.

Yim, M., Shen, W. M., Salemi, B., Rus, D., Moll, M., Lipson, H., ... & Chirikjian, G. S. (2007). Modular self-reconfigurable robot systems [grand challenges of robotics]. *IEEE Robotics & Automation Magazine*, 14(1), 43–52.

Zhu, M., Biswas, S., Dinulescu, S. I., Kastor, N., Hawkes, E. W., & Visell, Y. (2022). Soft, wearable robotics and haptics: Technologies, trends, and emerging applications. *Proceedings of the IEEE*, 110(2), 246–272.

Chapter 15

Current and future market trends in soft robotics

A management perspective

Suresh Chandra Ch, Shaik Mahaboob Syed, and Shaik Himam Saheb

15.1 INTRODUCTION

The field of soft robotics has witnessed a remarkable surge in recent years, with its flexible and adaptive nature transforming various industries, from healthcare to manufacturing and beyond. As organizations increasingly recognize the value of soft robotics in enhancing operational efficiency and safety, understanding the present and future market trends is crucial for managers and decision-makers navigating this rapidly evolving landscape.

This chapter begins by outlining the current state of the soft robotics market, highlighting the key players, applications, and technological advancements that are driving growth [1]. The flexibility and adaptability of soft robots have made them valuable assets in diverse sectors, catering to a wide range of tasks that traditional rigid robots struggle to tackle [2]. As the industry continues to evolve, the economic implications of soft robotics, including cost structures and return on investment, are explored.

The adoption of soft robotics is not without its challenges. Technological limitations, market perceptions, and regulatory considerations must be addressed to unlock the full potential of these transformative technologies. Recognizing these barriers, this chapter examines strategies for overcoming them, emphasizing the need for collaborative approaches and sustainable business models [3]. The field of soft robotics has experienced significant growth and innovation in recent years, driven by advancements in materials science, control systems, and artificial intelligence. Soft robots, characterized by their flexible and adaptive structures, are uniquely suited to perform tasks in environments where traditional rigid robots may falter. This versatility has led to their adoption across a diverse array of industries, including healthcare, manufacturing, agriculture, and logistics [4].

As organizations increasingly recognize the potential of soft robotics to enhance operational efficiency, improve safety, and reduce costs, understanding the present and future market trends becomes essential for managers and decision-makers. The unique capabilities of soft robots such as gentle handling of delicate objects and adaptability to complex environments position them as valuable assets in sectors facing rapid change and

DOI: 10.1201/9781003539612-15

increasing demands. This chapter provides a comprehensive overview of the current state of the soft robotics market, highlighting key players, technological advancements, and application areas that are driving growth. It also examines the economic implications of adopting soft robotics, including considerations of cost structures and return on investment.

The path to widespread adoption is not without challenges. Technological limitations, market perceptions, and regulatory hurdles must be addressed to fully unlock the transformative potential of soft robotics. This chapter will explore these barriers and discuss strategies for overcoming them, emphasizing the need for collaborative approaches and sustainable business models [5].

15.2 CURRENT MARKET OVERVIEW

The soft robotics market is projected to grow from approximately USD 1.49 billion in 2024 to around USD 6.53 billion by 2029, representing a remarkable compound annual growth rate (CAGR) of 34.45% during this period. The adoption of soft robots is anticipated to rise significantly due to their numerous advantages over traditional robotic systems [6, 7].

Several key factors are propelling the growth of the soft robotics market. There is an increasing demand for enhanced safety measures across various industries, coupled with a rising need for automation in sectors such as food processing and e-commerce [8]. Substantial investments in research and development (R&D) from multiple countries are driving innovation and expansion in this field. Exoskeleton technology is emerging as a promising solution aimed at protecting warehouse and manufacturing workers from common injuries associated with heavy lifting and repetitive tasks. Researchers are actively developing soft, wearable robots that mimic human muscle movements. For instance, a team from Queen's University in Canada designed an exoskeleton in May 2021 that effectively reduces the metabolic cost of walking by compensating for the energy lost during movement. Figure 15.1 shows the world's expected growth region wise [9].

Both medical and nonmedical exoskeletons must adhere to international safety standards set by organizations like ISO and IEC. Compliance with these regulations is essential for successful commercialization, but the process can be lengthy and subjective, delaying market growth due to the absence of a centralized regulatory authority. In the food sector, many companies are focusing on developing soft, pneumatic-powered grippers that are ideal for handling delicate items that rigid robots might damage. The COVID-19 pandemic has heightened interest in automation within the food industry, driven by labor shortages and concerns over disease transmission. June 2021, soft robotics secured USD 10 million in funding to advance their soft grasping, 3D perception, and AI technologies, citing increased demand stemming from pandemic-related challenges [10, 11].

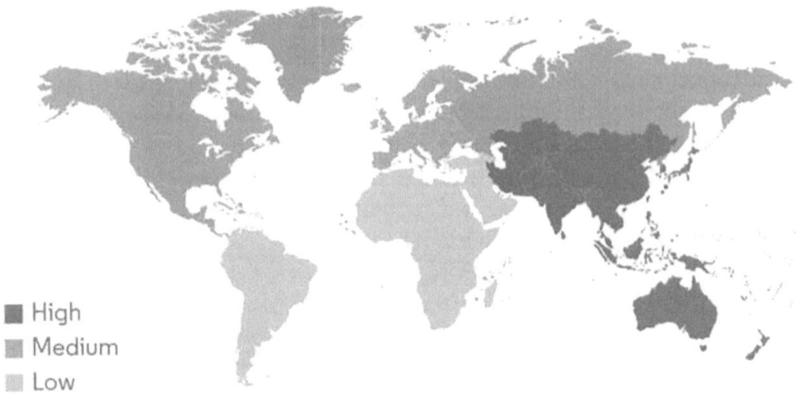

Figure 15.1 Expected growth of robotics market separated country region [12].

15.3 ECONOMIC IMPLICATIONS AND VALUE CREATION

The adoption of soft robots in healthcare brings transformative economic implications, primarily through cost savings and enhanced operational efficiency. By automating routine tasks such as patient handling and medication delivery, soft robots significantly reduce labor costs. This automation not only alleviates the burden on healthcare staff but also minimizes the risk of injuries associated with manual handling, thus lowering liability expenses. Soft robots improve precision in delicate procedures, particularly in minimally invasive surgeries and rehabilitation. This increased accuracy leads to better patient outcomes, resulting in quicker recoveries and fewer complications. Enhanced patient care reduces long-term healthcare costs associated with chronic conditions, creating substantial value for healthcare providers [13, 14].

The integration of soft robotics also encourages innovation through investment in R&D. As healthcare organizations explore new applications for these technologies, they drive advancements that can lead to improved solutions and more personalized patient care. Collaborations between healthcare providers and technology firms can facilitate knowledge sharing and amplify the impact of investments in soft robotics. The initial costs of acquiring and implementing soft robotic systems can be a barrier for some facilities. Understanding the return on investment is crucial to justifying these expenses. Regulatory compliance adds another layer of complexity, requiring careful navigation to ensure successful deployment. The long-term benefits of adopting soft robots in healthcare are significant, paving the way for improved efficiency and enhanced patient care in a rapidly evolving industry [15, 16].

15.3.1 Case studies of economic impact

- **Surgical Assistance at Johns Hopkins University:** At Johns Hopkins University, researchers integrated soft robotic systems in surgical settings to assist surgeons during minimally invasive procedures. The economic impact was significant: operating times were reduced by an average of 20%, resulting in lower surgical costs and faster patient recovery. Additionally, fewer complications led to shorter hospital stays, decreasing overall healthcare costs. The initial investment in the robotic system was offset by the savings generated from improved operational efficiency and enhanced patient outcomes.
- **Rehabilitation with Soft Exoskeletons:** A study conducted at the University of California, Berkeley, examined the use of soft exoskeletons in rehabilitation for stroke patients. By implementing these wearable devices, facilities reported a 30% increase in patient adherence to rehabilitation protocols. This improvement translated into shorter recovery times and reduced long-term therapy costs. The economic analysis indicated that the investment in soft robotics paid off within two years due to lower rehabilitation expenses and higher throughput of patients.
- **Soft Robotic Grippers in Food Service within Hospitals:** In a pilot program at a large metropolitan hospital, soft robotic grippers were introduced to automate meal delivery to patients. This innovation reduced labor costs by 25% and minimized food waste by ensuring precise handling. The hospital reported savings of over $100,000 annually from reduced staffing needs and improved meal accuracy. The success of this program not only demonstrated the financial benefits of adopting soft robotics but also enhanced patient satisfaction through timely and accurate meal service.
- **Telehealth and Remote Monitoring Solutions:** A healthcare provider in Europe implemented soft robotic systems for remote patient monitoring, especially for elderly patients. By enabling continuous monitoring without requiring frequent in-person visits, the provider reduced hospitalization rates by 15%. The economic impact was substantial, with estimated savings of over €500,000 per year due to decreased emergency room visits and hospital admissions. This case highlights how soft robotics can lead to cost-effective care while improving patient outcomes and satisfaction.

15.4 COMPETITIVE LANDSCAPE AND MARKET ENTRY CHALLENGES

The soft robotics market in healthcare is characterized by a diverse array of players, ranging from established medical device manufacturers to innovative startups. Major firms such as Intuitive Surgical and Medtronic are investing in soft robotics to enhance their surgical offerings. Their strong market presence and extensive distribution networks provide them with a competitive advantage. Emerging companies like Soft Robotics [17] and Re Walk Robotics [18] focus on niche applications, such as automated food handling and rehabilitation exoskeletons. These startups often drive innovation through specialized solutions, attracting attention for their cutting-edge technologies [19].

Academic institutions play a vital role in the competitive landscape by developing groundbreaking soft robotic technologies. Collaborations between universities and commercial entities are increasingly common, leading to the commercialization of advanced prototypes. Partnerships between tech companies and healthcare providers are fostering innovation. For instance, collaborations with AI firms are enhancing the functionality of soft robots, improving their adaptability and operational efficiency. The costs associated with developing and implementing soft robotic systems can be significant. Many healthcare facilities face budget constraints, making it challenging to justify the initial expenditure despite potential long-term savings. Soft robots used in healthcare must comply with stringent regulatory standards set by bodies like the FDA and ISO. The complex and often lengthy approval processes can delay market entry and increase development costs. Navigating these regulations requires expertise, which may not be readily available in smaller firms. Integrating soft robotics into existing healthcare workflows can be complex. Staff may require training to work effectively with new technologies, and compatibility with current systems must be ensured. This can lead to resistance to change from healthcare professionals who are accustomed to traditional methods [20, 21].

Market Awareness and Acceptance soft robotics offer significant advantages; there is still a lack of awareness among healthcare providers regarding their benefits. Educating stakeholders about the capabilities and economic advantages of soft robots is essential to facilitate adoption. Established methods and technologies in healthcare can be difficult to displace. Soft robotics must demonstrate clear advantages over traditional robotic systems and manual processes to gain traction in a competitive market [22]. The competitive landscape for soft robotics in healthcare is dynamic and diverse, featuring a mix of established players, innovative startups, and research institutions. However, the path to market entry is fraught with challenges, including high costs, regulatory complexities, and the need for technological integration. Addressing these challenges through strategic partnerships, effective marketing, and robust training programs will be crucial for stakeholders looking to capitalize on the opportunities presented by soft robotics in the healthcare industry [23].

15.5 ANTICIPATED MARKET GROWTH AND OPPORTUNITIES

The soft robotics market is expected to experience significant growth in the coming years, driven by technological advancements and increasing demand across various sectors. Below are key insights into market growth projections and opportunities, supported by industry reports and references.

According to a report by Mordor Intelligence, the global soft robotics market is anticipated to grow from approximately USD 1.49 billion in 2024 to about USD 6.53 billion by 2029, reflecting a CAGR of 39% during this period [12]. This growth is attributed to the increasing adoption of soft robots across industries such as healthcare, manufacturing, and logistics. The year-wise growth prediction is depicted in Figure 15.2. The healthcare industry is a primary driver of soft robotics adoption. A report by Markets and Markets highlights that the healthcare robotics market is expected to grow significantly.

Soft robots facilitate minimally invasive surgeries, improving precision and reducing recovery times [25]. Wearable soft exoskeletons are emerging as effective tools for rehabilitation, enhancing patient adherence to recovery protocols (ReWalk Robotics) [18]. Continuous innovations in materials and AI are expanding the capabilities of soft robots. Research published in the journal *Nature* discusses advancements in soft actuators and sensing technologies, which are crucial for developing more sophisticated robotic systems. The demand for automation across sectors is accelerating the adoption of soft robotics. According to a report by ABI Research, the food processing industry is increasingly leveraging soft robotic solutions for gentle handling and packaging, particularly following disruptions caused by the COVID-19 pandemic. As industries focus on sustainable practices, soft robotics offers eco-friendly solutions. A study in the journal *Advanced Robotics* emphasizes the potential for soft robots to be made from biodegradable materials, positioning them as sustainable alternatives in manufacturing and other sectors (Grand View Research) [26].

Emerging markets are increasingly investing in automation technologies, creating significant growth opportunities for soft robotics. A report by Grand View Research forecasts a substantial increase in demand for automation

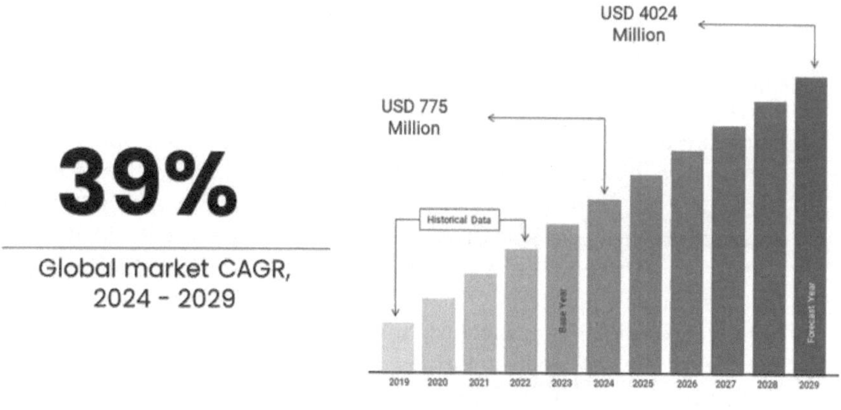

Figure 15.2 Global soft robotics market size prediction [24].

solutions in Asia-Pacific, which will benefit the soft robotics sector (O'Brien et al.) [27]. Increased investments in R&D are vital for innovation in soft robotics. The National Science Foundation (NSF) has been funding research initiatives focused on soft robotics, highlighting the importance of collaborative efforts between academia and industry to drive advancements. The anticipated growth of the soft robotics market offers substantial opportunities across various sectors, particularly in healthcare and manufacturing. As technological advancements continue and demand for automation rises, soft robotics is set to play a pivotal role in shaping the future of industries. Stakeholders who capitalize on these opportunities can position themselves advantageously in this rapidly expanding market.

15.6 STRATEGIC MANAGEMENT APPROACHES

With the integration and efficacy of soft robotics in healthcare, organizations can adopt several strategic management approaches. These strategies focus on fostering innovation, optimizing operations, and ensuring effective stakeholder engagement.

- **Encouraging R&D Investment:** Establishing a culture that prioritizes R&D can lead to breakthroughs in soft robotics technology. Healthcare organizations should allocate funds and resources to innovative projects that explore new applications of soft robotics. To encourage R&D investment in soft robotics, strategic management should focus on fostering innovation through partnerships with academic institutions and industry leaders. Implementing agile project management can enhance responsiveness to market needs, ensuring research remains relevant. Securing diverse funding sources, including government grants and venture capital, is essential to support long-term initiatives. Additionally, cultivating a culture of innovation within the organization—where employees are empowered to explore new ideas—can drive internal R&D efforts. By showcasing the potential for efficiency gains and cost savings, companies can attract investment and strengthen their competitive position in the soft robotics market.
- **Cross-disciplinary Collaboration:** Partnering with academic institutions and tech companies can foster knowledge exchange and accelerate the development of cutting-edge solutions. Collaborative research initiatives can lead to more effective soft robotic systems tailored to specific healthcare needs. Cross-disciplinary collaboration is vital for advancing soft robotics, as it brings together diverse expertise from fields such as engineering, materials science, biology, and artificial intelligence. By integrating insights from different disciplines, teams can develop innovative solutions that enhance robot functionality and adaptability. This collaboration fosters creativity and accelerates

problem-solving, enabling the design of soft robots that can perform complex tasks in real-world environments. Additionally, engaging stakeholders from various sectors, including healthcare, manufacturing, and academia, can ensure that research aligns with practical applications and market needs, ultimately driving the successful development and adoption of soft robotic technologies. Implementing comprehensive training programs for healthcare staff is essential for successful integration. Educating staff on the capabilities and operation of soft robots will enhance their comfort and effectiveness in using these technologies.

- **Patient Involvement:** Engaging patients in the design and testing of soft robotic solutions ensures that the products meet real-world needs. Collecting feedback from patients can inform further improvements and enhance user acceptance. Conducting thorough analyses of existing workflows to identify areas where soft robotics can add value is crucial. Streamlining operations can enhance productivity and reduce costs, allowing healthcare providers to serve more patients effectively.
- **Interoperability with Existing Systems:** Ensuring that soft robotics systems can seamlessly integrate with current healthcare technologies (e.g., electronic health records, imaging systems) is vital for maximizing their utility and minimizing disruption. Understanding and anticipating regulatory requirements is essential for the successful commercialization of soft robotics in healthcare. Organizations should engage with regulatory bodies early in the development process to ensure compliance and expedite approvals.
- **Robust Quality Management Systems:** Implementing quality assurance protocols can help maintain high standards for soft robotic systems. Continuous monitoring and improvement of these systems will ensure their reliability and effectiveness in clinical settings. Conducting thorough market research to identify trends, customer needs, and competitive landscapes will help healthcare organizations position their soft robotics offerings effectively. Understanding market dynamics allows for informed strategic decisions.
- **Differentiation and Value Proposition:** Developing a clear value proposition that highlights the unique benefits of soft robotics can differentiate products in a competitive market. Focusing on patient outcomes, operational efficiency, and cost savings will resonate with healthcare stakeholders. Adopting environmentally friendly practices in the development and operation of soft robotics will appeal to a growing segment of socially conscious consumers and organizations. This includes using biodegradable materials and energy-efficient designs.
- **Ethical Considerations:** Addressing ethical concerns related to the use of robotics in healthcare, such as patient privacy and autonomy, is essential. Developing policies that ensure ethical practices will build trust and acceptance among patients and healthcare professionals.

Implementing strategic management approaches to improve soft robotics in healthcare involves fostering innovation, enhancing stakeholder engagement, and ensuring operational efficiency. By focusing on these areas, healthcare organizations can effectively integrate soft robotics into their operations, leading to improved patient outcomes, enhanced efficiency, and overall advancements in healthcare delivery.

15.7 CONCLUSIONS

The market for soft robots is experiencing robust growth, projected to reach approximately $3.9 billion by 2026, with a CAGR of 32.6% from 2021 to 2026. This expansion is driven by the increasing demand for automation across various sectors, including healthcare, manufacturing, and agriculture, where the need for adaptable and safe robotic solutions is paramount. Soft robots' unique capabilities to navigate complex environments and interact gently with humans make them an attractive option for industries aiming to enhance efficiency and reduce operational risks.

Technological innovations in materials and design are significantly enhancing the functionality of soft robots. For instance, advancements in soft actuators and sensors have led to improved dexterity and responsiveness, allowing robots to perform tasks previously thought impossible. A recent study indicated that 70% of businesses in the automation sector are actively investing in soft robotics technology, highlighting the sector's momentum and the strategic importance of adopting these innovative solutions to remain competitive. As the soft robotics market grows, organizations must navigate regulatory and ethical challenges. Safety standards and guidelines for human–robot interaction will be crucial to ensuring public trust and widespread adoption. Furthermore, companies must be prepared to address potential job displacement concerns, as automation continues to evolve. Research indicates that over 50% of employees in industries susceptible to automation express concerns about job security, underscoring the importance of transparent communication and workforce retraining initiatives.

Strategic collaborations between technology developers and end-users will be essential for fostering innovation and ensuring that soft robotics solutions meet real-world needs. By leveraging partnerships, companies can combine expertise and resources, driving the development of tailored solutions that address specific industry challenges. Additionally, the focus on sustainability is becoming increasingly important, with a growing emphasis on eco-friendly materials and processes. A survey revealed that 62% of consumers are more likely to support brands that prioritize sustainable practices, indicating a clear market trend toward environmentally conscious innovations.

The future of soft robotics is promising, with potential applications expanding into areas such as elderly care, search and rescue, and consumer products. Organizations that prioritize R&D, adapt to evolving market demands, and implement sustainable practices will be well-positioned to capitalize on the significant opportunities that this burgeoning sector offers. As the landscape of automation continues to shift, the management of soft robotics will play a crucial role in shaping the future of work and enhancing human–robot collaboration.

REFERENCES

[1] Hartmann, F., Baumgartner, M., & Kaltenbrunner, M. (2021). Becoming sustainable, the new frontier in soft robotics. *Advanced Materials*, 33(19), 2004413.

[2] Xiloyannis, M., Alicea, R., Georgarakis, A. M., Haufe, F. L., Wolf, P., Masia, L., & Riener, R. (2021). Soft robotic suits: State of the art, core technologies, and open challenges. *IEEE Transactions on Robotics*, 38(3), 1343–1362.

[3] Lin, Z., Wang, Z., Zhao, W., Xu, Y., Wang, X., Zhang, T., ... & Peng, Z. (2023). Recent advances in perceptive intelligence for soft robotics. *Advanced Intelligent Systems*, 5(5), 2200329.

[4] Sharma, S., Malik, A., Sharma, C., Batra, I., Kaswan, M. S., & Garza-Reyes, J. A. (2023). Adoption of industry 4.0 in different sectors: a structural review using natural language processing. *International Journal on Interactive Design and Manufacturing* (IJIDeM), Volume 18, 6069–6091.

[5] Chataut, R., Phoummalayvane, A., & Akl, R. (2023). Unleashing the power of IoT: A comprehensive review of IoT applications and future prospects in healthcare, agriculture, smart homes, smart cities, and industry 4.0. *Sensors*, 23(16), 7194.

[6] Bakhshalipour, M. (2024). *Bridging Real-Time Robotics and Computer Architecture* (Doctoral dissertation, Carnegie Mellon University).

[7] Bakhshalipour, M. (2024). *Bridging Real-Time Robotics and Computer Architecture* (Doctoral dissertation, Carnegie Mellon University).

[8] Majidi, C. (2014). Soft robotics: a perspective—current trends and prospects for the future. *Soft robotics*, 1(1), 5–11.

[9] Chow, S. W. C. (2022). Design and development of a non-powered exoskeleton device to cater to the physical needs of puppeteers, IOP Conf. Ser.: Mater. Sci. Eng. Vol.612 DOI: 10.1088/1757-899X/612/3/032114

[10] Barfoot, T., Burgner-Kahrs, J., Diller, E., Garg, A., Goldenberg, A., Kelly, J., ... & Waslander, S. L. (2020). Making sense of the robotized pandemic response: a comparison of global and canadian robot deployments and success factors. arXiv preprint arXiv:2009.08577.

[11] Lopez Solano, J., Martin, A., Ohai, F., de Souza, S., & Taylor, L. (2022). Digital disruption or crisis capitalism? Technology, power and the pandemic. https://doi.org/10.26116/gdj-euaifund

[12] https://www.mordorintelligence.com/industry-reports/robotics-market

[13] https://www.marketsandmarkets.com/

[14] de Groot, J. A., Bossuyt, P. M., Reitsma, J. B., Rutjes, A. W., Dendukuri, N., Janssen, K. J., & Moons, K. G. (2011). Verification problems in diagnostic accuracy studies: consequences and solutions. BMJ, 343.

[15] Majidi, C. (2014). Soft robotics: a perspective—current trends and prospects for the future. *Soft robotics*, 1(1), 5–11.
[16] Chen, S., Fan, S., Chan, H., Qiao, Z., Qi, J., Wu, Z., ... & Lim, C. T. (2024). Liquid metal functionalization innovations in wearables and soft robotics for smart healthcare applications. *Advanced Functional Materials*, 34(31), 2309989.
[17] https://www.startus-insights.com/innovators-guide/5-top-soft-robotics-startups/
[18] https://www.rewalkrobotic.com/
[19] Valavanidis, A. (2020). Universities as innovation drivers for major disruptive technological transformations and economic development. *Scientific Reviews*, 2, 1–48.
[20] Schweyer, A. (2010). *Talent management systems: Best practices in technology solutions for recruitment, retention and workforce planning*. John Wiley & Sons.
[21] Lee, D. M., Trauth, E. M., & Farwell, D. (1995). Critical skills and knowledge requirements of IS professionals: A joint academic/industry investigation. *MIS Quarterly*, Vol. 19, No. 3, Special Issue on IS Curricula and Pedagogy (Sep., 1995), pp. 313–340.
[22] Gorissen, B., Reynaerts, D., Konishi, S., Yoshida, K., Kim, J. W., & De Volder, M. (2017). Elastic inflatable actuators for soft robotic applications. *Advanced Materials*, 29(43), 1604977.
[23] Ochuba, N. A., Okafor, E. S., Akinrinola, O., Usman, F. O., & Amoo, O. O. (2024). Strategic partnerships in the satellite and telecommunications sectors: a conceptual review of data analytics-enabled identification and capitalization of synergies. *Engineering Science & Technology Journal*, 5(3), 716–727.
[24] https://www.zionmarketresearch.com/report/soft-robotics-market
[25] Qiu, Y., Ashok, A., Nguyen, C. C., Yamauchi, Y., Do, T. N., & Phan, H. P. (2024). Integrated sensors for soft medical robotics. *Small*, 20, 22.
[26] https://www.grandviewresearch.com/
[27] O'Brien, A., & Arnold, S. (2024). *Combining motherhood and work in the creative industries: Mothers have the problem*. Media, Culture & Society, 01634437241229327.

Index

Pages in *italics* refer to figures.

actuators
embedded, 179
hydrogel-based, 173
adaptive grippers, 175
adaptive structures, 212
additive manufacturing, 170, 172
Advanced Robotics, 231
ATARO, 111
Augmented Reality, 24

bibliometric analysis, 25
biocompatibility, 174
biodegradable materials, 178
bio inspired design, 179
bio printing, 179, 197
biomimetic research, 179

cancer treatment, 53
closed-loop 4D printing, 179
clubfoot, 29
collaborative robotics, 175
control systems, 179
control strategies, 73
customized Implants, 174

Digital Light Processing (DLP), 172
digital twin, 3
Direct-Ink Writing, 133–134, 172, 187
disaster response applications, 175
dressing assistance, 88
drug delivery, 174

electroactive polymers (EAP), 14, 73, *193*
Electron Beam Melting, 22
electrospinning, 210
Endogenous Laser Therapy, 5
endoscopic soft robots, 50
environmental applications, 179
environmental exploration, 175
exoskeletons, 175

fabrication techniques, 178–179
finite-element analysis, 136
FNPN controller, *65*
fused deposition modeling (FDM), 171–172
fuzzy neural network, 63

gait training, 86
genetic syndromes, 34
grippers, 175

hand rehabilitation, 1, 18
healthcare applications, 174–175
high-resolution printing, 179
Hull, Charles, 171
human-robot interaction, 85, 179
hydrogels, 39, 120, 173

idiopathic clubfoot, 33
implants, 174
industrial applications, 175

knitting and weaving, 210

Laser Therapy, 5
liquid deposition modelling, 211
liquid printing, rapid, 179

machine learning, 179
magnetic responsiveness, 173
material optimization, 207
materials
  biodegradable, 178
  multifunctional, 178
  self-healing, 178
  stimuli-responsive, 178
minimally invasive surgery, 4, 174
micromolding, 133
microscale soft robots, 52
microstepping, 73
microstructures, 174
mild cognitive impairment (MCI), 87
multi-material printing, 134, 174
musculoskeletal factors, 32

neurological factors, 32
neuromuscular, 34
non idiopathic clubfoot, 34–35

ocean exploration, 146
Octobot, 162
omnidirectional printing, 173
origami and kirigami techniques, 211

PARO, 91
Petri net, 64
photosensitive actuators, 19
PneuNets, 18, *18*, 164
post stroke rehabilitation, 87
potentiometer, 71
precision agriculture, 6, 159

rapid liquid printing, 179
regenerative medicine, 174
rehabilitation, 229
rehabilitation and therapy, 85
reinforcement learning, 139
RIBA, 108, *108*
Robo-Mate Project, 106
Robust Quality Management Systems, 233

silicone rubber, 16, 31, 37, 132
selective laser melting, 22
selective laser sintering (SLS), 171–172
self-healing materials, 178
sensors, soft, 179
servo motors, 70
shape-memory
  alloys (SMAs), 173
  effect, 173
SMPs, 171, 173
Snake-like Locomotors, 13
socially assistive robotics (SAR), 80–90
soft lithography, 129, 209
soft robotic exoskeletons, 82
soft wearable devices, 83
space exploration, 180
stereolithography (SLA), 171–172
stretch sensors, 136
stimuli-responsive materials, 173, 178
swarm robotics, 179
swelling and de swelling, 173

talipes equinovarus, 30, *30*
tenotomy, 34
therapeutic efficacy, 47
therapeutic robotics, 87
thermal expansion, anisotropic, 173
thermally responsive actuators, 122
Tibbits, Skylar, 170–171
two-photon polymerization, 179

UltiCast method, 173
underwater exploration, 175
untethered soft robots, 221

Wearable Assistants, 101